TOX-SICK

TOX-SICK

From Toxic to Not Sick

SUZANNE SOMERS

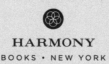

HARMONY
BOOKS • NEW YORK

The information presented in this work is in no way intended as medical advice or as a substitute for medical counseling. The information should be used in conjunction with the guidance and care of your physician. Your physician should be aware of all medical conditions that you may have, as well as the medications and supplements you are taking.

Library of Congress Cataloging-in-Publication Data

Somers, Suzanne, 1946–
Tox-sick: from toxic to not sick / Suzanne Somers.
        pages   cm
1. Detoxification (Health) 2. Environmental toxicology.
3. Environmentally induced diseases. 4. Environmental health. 5. Toxins.
I. Title.
RA784.5.S72 2015
613'.1—dc23   2014047109

ISBN 978-0-385-34772-3
Ebook ISBN 978-0-385-34773-0

Printed in the United States of America

Jacket design by Caroline Somers and Danielle Shapero-Rudolph
Jacket photograph by Cindy Gold

10 9 8 7 6 5 4 3 2 1

First Edition

For the last several years I have sat by helplessly, watching members of my family battle debilitating environmental diseases. I wrote this book for them.

To Alan, my husband, the healthiest guy on the planet who was hit hard by black mold. To my granddaughters, Camelia and Violet, both suffering with environmentally induced brain conditions. To their parents, Caroline and Bruce, who had their serene and tranquil family life torn apart by worry and hopelessness. And to Leslie, my daughter, who has also been blindsided by toxicity.

Watching all of them regain their health from the depths of today's "mystery diseases" brings joy to my life and gives hope to all who read this book. You can win and you can get well again.

ACKNOWLEDGMENTS

SO MANY PEOPLE MAKE A BOOK: THE PUBLISHER, THE EDITOR, THE doctors, the scientists, my staff, my family, and more.

My editor, Heather Jackson, is the best in the business. We have done seven books together and each time our rapport gets smoother and our methods faster. She sees what I don't; she has the gift of structure and organization, moving the puzzle around, creating and making order so readers' queries all get answered. She does this by questioning me. She is tough yet easy. She is sweet yet strong. She is above all extremely talented and I am grateful once again to have her on my team, and she came up with this amazing title.

Can't expect people to read a book if they don't know it's out there. That's where Sandi Mendelson comes in, my publicist extraordinaire. We have done eighteen books together, and with so many bestsellers under my belt I have to thank Sandi for corralling the media, cherry-picking the best, and booking those with the most coverage, never wasting my time, and allowing me to present my hard work in a way that gives each book the widest exposure not just nationally but globally. As a result my books are in print all over the world. There is no one better than Sandi and she's a cool chick too, which makes touring so much fun with her.

My literary lawyer, Marc Chamilin, is always on scene, protecting, negotiating, making sure all the legalities are perfectly lined up. We have done ten books together and I'm sure there will be ten more.

Thanks to Dave Henson, my IT computer troubleshooter.

Bill Faloon and the scientific advisory board are of invaluable assistance in the writing of all my books, this one being no exception. They make sure I can never be stupid. I'm not a doctor, so I rely on interviews and research for my information. The scientific advisory board at Life Extension goes over each page with a fine-tooth comb, finding any inaccuracies. At times we have differences of opinion and it is at those times we hash it out until we all feel comfortable. They also provided their own chapter of supplements for survival that will prove invaluable to the reader. Thanks to:

Bill Faloon, editor of *Life Extension* magazine and founder of Life Extension Foundation; Blake Gossard; Kira Schmid, ND; Lori Feldman, RD, CCRC; Richard Stein, MD, PhD; Daniel Heller, ND; Emily Gonzalez, ND; Luke Huber, ND, MBA.

Thank you to Jim England, president of my company, The Somers Companies, and Caroline Somers, executive vice president of The Somers Companies, who is also head of branding and marketing. She works closely with our in-house graphics designer, Danielle Shapero, to create my beautiful book jackets as well as all branding design. Together Danielle and Caroline came up with the brilliant jacket design. Between the two of them and a lot of back-and-forth with me, they were able to design a jacket that subliminally conveys my message: Toxins kill! Brilliant!

President and publisher, Maya Mavjee; Aaron Wehner, senior vice president and publisher; Diana Baroni, editorial director and vice president; Christine Tanigawa, production editor of my last six books; Debbie Glasserman, interior designer; Jessica Morphew, Harmony art director; Candace Chaplin and Christine Edwards in sales; and Tammy Blake in publicity—my deepest appreciation to all of my team at Crown.

Thank you to Mooney for my hairstyles and to the girls in the office: Julie Turkel, my fabulous assistant, and Jordyn Goodman—we will miss you.

And now, my family, an integral part of this book; their stories, heartbreaking though they may be, were told to me with total candor and honesty. All of them have been tenacious and focused on getting well from an environment that is trying to do them in.

My husband, Alan Hamel, is my everything. He runs the businesses and directs all the departments. He's always got my back. We are partners in the truest sense of the word. To say I love and appreciate him does not seem to cover it. But in this book, he vulnerably tells his story of black mold and the years it took to clear. He has faithfully practiced his protocols under the guidance of Dr. Nick Gonzalez, a feat that is daunting to most doctors.

My granddaughters Camelia and Violet have both fought this invisible enemy and did what they had to do to get well. It hasn't been easy but, as you will read, they did it. Violet was so hard hit that she missed crucial months of school because mold, Lyme, and toxins grabbed her health. I get teary-eyed when I see her functioning, catching up, and upbeat about having fought her internal enemy and knowing that she is winning.

Caroline Somers, their mother, and Bruce Somers, my son and their father, both have a story to tell from the perspective of what these mystery diseases do to the family unit, including worry, and a loss of safety because the planet has betrayed them. Theirs is a story of hard work, tenacity, lots of anxiety, and winning. And Leslie, my daughter by marriage, who seemingly overnight lost control of her body, not knowing the culprit but knowing that nothing about her life and health was the same. Many are going to see what is wrong with them through her saga.

And finally, the doctors, the courageous ones featured in this book, all of whom have embarked on a new and important path. These are the new doctors in the trenches, each with their own specialties that combine their areas of expertise to combat the environment. These are the doctors who understand the changed planet and how it has affected our bodies: Dr. Stephen Sinatra, Dr. Nick Gonzalez, Dr. Sherry Rogers, Dr. Garry Gordon, Dr. Ritchie Shoemaker, and Dr. Walter Crinnion. I thank them all for the time they gave to me and the back-and-forth they all so graciously endured so I could get it right for my readers. The other doctors who allowed me to pick their brains: Dr. Russell Blaylock, Dr. Michael Galitzer, and Dr. Jonathan Wright.

These are all important cutting-edge doctors who understand the limitations of orthodox medicine and at the risk of ridicule by their peers move forward anyway, knowing they are actually getting their patients well. Bravo.

The other doctors quoted throughout who gave me expertise can all be found at the Foreverhealth.com website.

I profoundly and deeply appreciate everyone involved in helping me to put out this book, which for me was life changing.

CONTENTS

A PEEK AT WHAT'S INSIDE

LIFE IS A BLESSING IF YOU ARE HEALTHY. IF YOU ARE OF AN AGE TO have some wisdom, and most of the challenges of your life have been worked out, it's a glorious experience. But sadly, in today's world, people look to their future with their fingers crossed.

We are younger at midlife today than ever before thanks to modern technology and advanced science. With midlife our children have for the most part left home and we have our lives to ourselves again. If you are lucky, a level of enjoyment follows that is unlike anything those who preceded us were ever able to entertain.

Aging is great if you know how to do it. I feel very satisfied with the work I've been privileged to do in delivering the message of making people's lives better.

But things have begun changing at lightning speed, and some of that change is not good. Suddenly, replacing hormones isn't enough to keep up with the demand of the environmental insults bombarding us on a daily basis. Women have begun to complain that even though they are on hormone replacement, they aren't feeling as well as they used to, they can't lose weight, and their moods are not as stable.

What is happening? It's become clear that due to the toxic assault of today's world, it's going to take more work to feel the "sweet spot" of great health again, that place of bliss where you used to wake up feeling energized and upbeat, healthy and primed for the day. Why would we settle for anything less? If you want to regain optimal health for you and your entire family, then you will find the answers in this book.

Maybe you are noticing that your hair has lost its luster, or your nails are brittle, yet you are eating right (you think). You are exercising but you keep gaining weight, and, worst of all, you are forgetting things. Brain fog!

These symptoms are just some of what I call being *tox*-sick. And this tox-sickness is the result of a massive environmental chemical assault that is permeating every cell and orifice in everyone, including your children.

For years I have been on a mission to educate women and men about the joys of replacing declining hormones with bioidentical (natural) hormones. Millions of people all around the globe listened, and a movement started. People threw away their dangerous pharmaceutical hormones and went natural. They lost weight, their bellies went flat, they got their sex drives back, their moods improved, and they learned that aging could be something to look forward to. Now true health is more challenging. We aren't feeling well, and our doctors are stymied. The environment has caught up with us and we are feeling the effects. Sadly, we've become *tox*-sick!

We've been told chemicals are safe yet we know something is not right.

Why are so many people bloated and constipated and experiencing flatulence, unexplained weight gain, headaches, rashes, brain fog, brain diseases, ADD, ADHD, OCD, asthma, autism, bipolar disorder, schizophrenia, hormone imbalances, and autoimmune diseases? And why the *epidemic of cancer*?

Why?

Although it's a dirty little secret, the one no one wants to acknowledge, courageous cutting-edge doctors and scientists know the truth about why we're not feeling well and will tell you the answers in this book.

The research is very clear: We are sick as a result of being under the greatest environmental assault in the history of humanity and our bodies have reached their tipping point. Our livers are groaning and exhausted. Like a glass that cannot hold another drop, the next smallest chemical exposure causes overflow, and then the symptoms, big and small, start plaguing us. We go to the doctor and are given pills, then more pills. Soon we are sluggish, toxic, and feeling worse. The illnesses take many forms, but they all go back to the original cause. Toxins.

Professionals—scientists, drug manufacturers, doctors, and so on—told us these toxic chemicals were safe.

This book will unravel the confusion and give the solution to a *whole life detox*. You can get back balance, plus great health, if you know what to do. It's all here.

INTRODUCTION

How We Got So *Tox*-Sick

One year, in a tournament near Miami, I had to withdraw after thirty-six holes. The course had been heavily sprayed, and there was weed killer in the lake. When I got to the course for the third round, I couldn't hit a wedge shot thirty yards—I didn't have enough strength. My eyes were bloodshot, my complexion was very ruddy, and my right hand was swollen from taking balls from the caddie. My doctor said it was acute pesticide poisoning.

—BILLY CASPER, TOP U.S. PROFESSIONAL GOLFER
(HE WON FIFTY-ONE MAJOR TOURNAMENTS DURING HIS CAREER
AND IS IN THE WORLD GOLF HALL OF FAME.)

HOW HAVE YOU BEEN FEELING? MOST PEOPLE ARE COMPLAINING these days that they just don't feel right. Some aren't sleeping. Some have stomach problems. Some have headaches . . . or fatigue, rashes, bloating, cramping, or constipation. People also complain of allergies, hay fever, sinusitis, unexplained weight gain, puffy faces and bodies, dark circles under the eyes, acid reflux and heartburn, restless sleep, itchy skin, stiff joints and muscles, depression, foggy brain, and the list goes on! And then the sickness amps up all the more: heart disease, cancer, Alzheimer's. What has happened? Why is our collective health so challenged? **We're not sick. But we're not well, either.** When did this become the new "normal"?

These everyday symptoms are now considered such a part of everyone's day, followed by "I'm allergic to something" kinds of excuses, that we don't even think about it. The sum total of this *dysfunction* all adds up, however, until one day you find yourself in real trouble.

Don't despair. The answers are in this book.

How do you know if toxicity is affecting *you*? The symptoms vary from person to person. My daughter was puffy, bloated, and lethargic; my granddaughter had an inability to think and unbelievable fatigue. My other granddaughter was unable to sleep and had hyper episodes that took away her quality of life. I had bloating, cramping, and unexplained weight gain, what I call "chemical belly." My husband had fatigue and facial tics. If you experience any of these signs and symptoms, pay attention; these are indicators of a body in distress. The symptoms are the "language," your body's *wisdom*; it's trying to talk to you.

All these signs and symptoms could have a disease label attached to them if you go to visit an unevolved doctor. So many people are walking around on severe pharmaceutical drugs for conditions they don't even have, given to them by clueless doctors who are just guessing. They are doing their best, but today's orthodox medicine in relation to toxicity is fifty years old. When faced with patients not "feeling well," today's doctors reach in their allopathic arsenal for the only tools they have, drugs. How many people are on Parkinson's medications (which are debilitating) when in reality they are suffering from toxic overload? The symptoms of accumulated toxicity mimic Parkinson's; how many know this?

Toxins tend to bioaccumulate, meaning they build up in our tissues and cells more quickly than they are eliminated. Since they bioaccumulate over time, lingering and gathering in the fat cells, people have no idea why they can't lose weight or why they feel so lousy. What people often think of as their culprit is usually just the one that tipped the toxic scales, the one more agent that, when added to the total toxic burden, puts it over the top and throws your health out the window.

Today's scientists admit that we are fundamentally ignorant of the ways the thousands of chemicals we are exposed to interact once inside our tissues or cells. As humans we have multiple toxins constantly combining in our bodies, altering and shifting our inner environments in ways that new environmental doctors are just starting to figure out. We don't realize that chemical reactions are happening throughout our bodies in thousands of small ways at the same time, and that is why everyone is so mystified about our ill health. It's hard to pinpoint. Everybody reacts differently; there is no "textbook" case.

It's not simple anymore, but it's not hopeless. Remember that.

A THREAT YOU CAN'T SEE

Toxins are the invisible enemy. You can't see them, but they are there wreaking havoc on your health and your environment. We are exposed to more than six thousand common everyday chemicals, and each alone can lead to a laundry list of possible symptoms. Toxins have many ways of interfering with the normal physiology of life. Maybe they block the usage of oxygen needed for the full metabolism of glucose. Or maybe they block an enzyme needed for an important body function, or stimulate a specific bodily function in such persistent ways that it begins to cause damage.

Tragically, we are all overloaded with toxins, and the chickens have finally come home to roost. We've reached the tipping point. Yet big business and many in the government do not want to acknowledge that the planet—just like our bodies—has become *tox*-sick!

One of the most extensive studies of Americans' toxic burden was funded by the Environmental Working Group (EWG) and conducted at the Mount Sinai School of Medicine. Researchers tested nine adults, none of whom worked in industries that would expose them to high levels of environmental poisons; well-known journalist Bill Moyers was one of them. All were tested for the presence of 210 contaminants that have been globally recognized as persistent pollutants (like DDT). The results of the participants' blood and urine showed the presence of 167 of the 210 contaminants, with an average of 91 in any given person. Each person tested had an average of

- 53 chemicals that have been linked to cancer.
- 63 compounds toxic to the central nervous system, including the brain.
- 58 compounds toxic to the endocrine (hormonal) system.
- 55 compounds that are toxic to the immune system and frequently lead to autoimmunity (fibromyalgia, lupus, multiple sclerosis) and an impaired ability to fight infections.

The whole story of the public deception is brilliantly explained in *Trade Secrets*, the documentary film produced by Bill Moyers on this experiment.

Our parents and grandparents did not experience this bombardment. Sadly, there is not a single space left on the planet today that has not been contaminated with pollution by humans. I've said it before, but it's worth repeating: we are under the greatest environmental assault in the history of humanity.

I'll say it again, don't despair. The purpose of this book is to unravel the mystery illnesses in your body and give you the recipes for health.

Sadly, chemicals are in the water and the air. Our food is contaminated from pesticides and/or the plastic wraps covering it; the fruits, vegetables, and meats in our grocery carts are encased in plastic wrap like sleeping bags. These chemicals outgas and leach into our food. Then there are the Styrofoam trays that hold these foods; they look harmless because we are so used to them, as do the plastic bottles for baby formula. But these products are outgassing dangerous phthalates (pronounced: thal-ates).

To make matters worse, the water supply is polluted, as is most every liquid we consume: sodas, milk, ketchup, fruit juices. Glass bottles, which *are* safe, are few and far between. Everything is bottled in plastic. No longer can kids collect empty glass bottles for return and a deposit. We have become a "disposable" society, polluting the planet with packaging that does not biodegrade while also making our bodies sick. Food and beverage packaging is so ubiquitous that we forget to factor in that these chemical products can turn even beautiful fresh organic foods into toxic substances never meant for human consumption. Because of general ignorance and big business interests we find ourselves with genetically modified foods (GMO stands for genetically modified organism), or those loaded with plastics, chemicals, and bleaching agents (the same chemicals used to make yoga mats).

I feel ripped off, don't you?

But it doesn't stop there. Toxins have invaded our homes, from our household cleaners to our carpets; even the paint on our walls is toxic. Then add in our so-called smart meters from the gas companies that are putting dangerous electromagnetic fields over our homes like a toxic grid. Cell phones are not safe . . . research now clearly shows the connection of cell phones' electromagnetic rads to brain tumors. Later in this book I will tell you how to protect yourself with Matrix 2, a simple, inexpensive product you put in your cell phone case to protect you from dangerous radiation.

At the office, dioxins and PCBs outgas in our daily lives from carbonless copy paper, plastics, inks, paints, furnishings, and construction glues as well as common contaminants in the food chain. Dichlorobenzene can be breathed in from that noxious odor of "air freshener" in public bathrooms, and xylene outgases from plastics, carpeting, furnishings, construction materials, industrial and traffic exhaust, and much more.

My husband was exposed to black mold for four years (unbeknownst to him), which created his tipping point. The black mold was the final trigger that tipped the scale of toxins accumulated over years in his body. From that moment on he, like so many others with toxic accumulation, could be thrown into an "episode" from seemingly benign things like car exhaust, industrial solvents, plasticizers, paint, a new-car smell here, fresh laundry detergent smell there, new carpeting that outgases for years, rush-hour exhaust fumes, a microwaved leftover wrapped in plastic, pesticide-laden berries. You never know; any of these chemicals can set off an "episode" in those with allergies. For chemically sensitive people or people with MCS (multiple chemical sensitivities), these fumes, outgassing, and toxins make them very sick. My family has been hard hit by toxicity; but they are not alone. The list of people with MCS is growing exponentially not just in the United States but around the globe. But you don't have to have MCS to be sensitive or susceptible to these toxins. We are *tox*-sick from the bombardment of chemicals never meant to be processed by the human body. What did we expect?

If you are like me, for so long you figured that all these substances must be safe; otherwise, the agencies in control would not allow them to be used or sold. Now I know better. It's time for us to grow up and realize that nobody's going to save us; we've got to save ourselves. It's up to each of us to control the amount of our individual toxic exposures. To live and thrive, we need to truly think about every product we use and every bite of food we take.

Let me tell you a little story before we really get going. You will probably relate:

I had front-row seats for one of my favorite female entertainers! The room was sold out and you could feel the anticipation. Everybody loves her. Excitement was in the air. The musicians appeared onstage; one by one, magically sheltered by smoke, caught in a cloud, all moving to their designated places. Then the singers walked onstage: cute, darling girls, in tight, sexy, black sequin dresses. They walked in unison, moving perfectly, dancing to the intense rhythm. You could feel the build—it was almost time for the star to make her entrance to what would be thunderous response—but something caught my eye. I was transfixed by the singers!

Each girl was a different size, each girl unique and darling, and all of them in great shape, but I couldn't help but notice they all had huge, protruding chemical bellies!

Bloated bellies, sticking out visibly. How could this be after all the exercise they did night after night? Here were these trim, young darling girls with big bloated stomachs that clearly looked uncomfortable.

But then I thought, why wouldn't these girls have bloated bellies? They lived on the road. I know what "road food" is: I spent thirty-five weeks a year on the road for twenty years doing my musical act. The food from room service is never organic, and after a performance when you've just exercised for an hour and a half onstage, usually preceded by a rigorous rehearsal in the afternoon, you feel you "deserve" that chocolate bomb cake or the french fries. Or maybe all the road manager could find was some Frankenfood from a fast-food joint. So you gobble it down because you are ravenous and now you are in trouble, except you don't know it: trans fats, chemicals, pink slime in the meat. All these substances are designed so that bad food will taste scrumptious. Once you get a "taste" for them, you start to crave them.

When you are young, like these singers, your body doesn't hang on to the weight. Unlike what we've heard, it's not the calories that are the problem: it's the chemicals. The chemicals load up your liver and then get shunted to the GI tract (gut), where they play havoc with the balance in your ecosystem. The result of this buildup of chemicals in the GI tract is a leaky gut and bloating, along with constipation, chronic discomfort, and eventually disease. The process is slow but insidious. . . . That's how the chemical belly is created.

On the night of that concert, my journey to this book began. I wanted to find the answer to the medical mystery plaguing not only my family members, but people all over; why were everyone's bellies exploding? I heard it from all the people I interviewed: "It doesn't matter what I do, how little I eat, or how much I exercise, I just can't get my belly to go flat."

But a chemical belly isn't the only thing we've got to worry about in this toxic soup. And this really got me digging.

Scarily, there are even newer dangers: disease, mold toxicity, and more!

We are finally beginning to realize the harmful effects of mold. It is common in so many of today's homes and is highly underrated as a dangerous toxin to the brain and body. Left unchecked, mold toxins can silently eat through the intestines, causing massive stomach and brain damage. You must get mold toxins out of your body.

Then there's Lyme disease. When did that become an epidemic? Why can't our immune systems fight this horrible invader and why can't anyone cure it? I suspect it's because we are so toxic. Taken together, you start to see how pervasive this problem has become.

> It's as if we are all on a big, chemical drunk, and the hangover
> is a killer!

That's what the scientists and researchers are saying. Pretty frightening. I wrote this book because *tox*-sickness is hurting adults and our children, compromising our health and quality of life, and I wanted to find answers for you and for my family.

Why are younger and younger people contracting cancer? The childhood cancer rate has risen 67.1 percent since 1950 (the United States has the fourth-highest rate in the world). Now kids are even born with a toxic burden! Toxins are passed from mother to child in utero, just as an imbalanced microflora system in the mother is passed to the newborn. The rise of C-sections is also depriving children of their very first microbial protection, gotten only from the natural journey through their moms' birth canals.

Toxic chemicals may be triggering recent increases in
neurodevelopmental disabilities among children—such as
autism, attention deficit hyperactivity disorder, and dyslexia. . . .
The researchers say a new global prevention strategy to control
the use of these substances is urgently needed. "The greatest
concern is the large numbers of children who are affected by
toxic damage to brain development in the absence of a formal
diagnosis," said Philippe Grandjean, adjunct professor of
environmental health at HSPH. "They suffer reduced attention
span, delayed development, and poor school performance.
Industrial chemicals are now emerging as likely causes." . . . The
authors say it's crucial to control the use of these chemicals to
protect children's brain development worldwide.
                    —Harvard School of Public Health, February 14, 2014

In one study, the EWG (Environmental Working Group) examined the cord blood, which circulates between a baby and its mother's
placenta, of infants born in U.S. hospitals to study how many toxins
are passed on. The results were startling: EWG researchers found that
newborns begin their lives with exposure to as many as 287 of the 413
toxic chemicals being studied. An average of 200 toxins were found
per baby, and 101 toxins were found in all of the babies. The 287 toxins included 180 chemical compounds that have been shown to cause
cancer in either animals or humans. (Incidentally, all chemicals that
cause cancer in humans were initially found to cause it in animals.)
The babies also had 217 compounds that have been found to damage the central nervous system and 208 compounds that lead to developmental problems. No one has studied the effects of these toxic
combinations yet. Obesity rates have more than doubled in the past
thirty years among children aged two to five, and twelve to nineteen;
they've more than tripled among those aged six to eleven. And "they"
say there's no connection to toxins? I think we've been duped!

Today's young mothers are at their wits' ends trying to figure out
the puzzle of their children's health. We now have an epidemic of
environmentally poisoned people. Food allergies abound, and brain
fog makes the normal course of going to school virtually impossible
for some. Our children have been exposed to chemicals and toxins

from birth and the negative effects are coming to their logical conclusion.

Don't despair. My grandchildren and children have fought these environmentally induced conditions and won. But we have to pay attention because children's brains are not fully formed until around age twenty-five. Every choice you make on their behalf has a consequence. We are talking about their brains! Taking this precious unformed resource and making it tox-sick with dangerous chemicals is not only stealing their brains, but disturbing the delicate balance of the GI tract and the overall health of everybody. The youngest among us are taking the hardest hit.

> **Clearly our children deserve optimum health! So do you!**

The baby boomers aren't escaping this: If you're a boomer, beware; your brain is also under attack and has been for some time! Toxins and the low-fat craze have accelerated brain damage, and 50 percent of boomers are expected to get Alzheimer's in the upcoming years. If individuals already have diabetes, they are at an additional increased risk of 50 percent!

Do you still wonder why you aren't feeling well?

Take heart, there are solutions coming.

We did not know that this massive chemical assault was permeating every cell and orifice of our bodies. Most people don't realize that even their weight gain is a result of their toxic burden, and even more alarming is that it is a sign of distress of the GI tract (gut). This distress comes from the toxins that eventually are making their way to the brain and are helping cause brain diseases and conditions, even cancers. Yes, it is now a fact validated by the Columbia University School of Public Health that

> **95% of cancer is caused by diet and the environment!**

That's the bad news. But there is good news. Really good news. So don't get discouraged.

The good news is you do not have to fall victim to the chemical diseases and the obesity crisis that are taking away our quality of life, including the loss of our precious brains. Nondrug solutions exist. If toxins in the diet and the environment are the culprits, then it makes sense that a change of diet, proper supplementation, and whole-life detoxification to undo this damage are now essential. The human body was never meant to process the volume of dangerous toxins, chemicals, and overabundance of pharmaceuticals permeating our lives. But learning to detox your body—and your life—effectively will allow you to fight and reverse the effects of this phenomenon.

You do not have to expect Alzheimer's as the end point of your life. You do not have to accept the present negative paradigm of aging and illness. We deserve good health and quality for our entire lives.

Leading scientists, professionals, and doctors will validate the information put forth here in these pages. I have sourced for you the brightest and most cutting-edge minds on environmental sickness. Fortunately, these new specialty doctors are responding to the needs of these unique conditions and diseases. These environmental doctors understand the effects of toxicity in the human body and have found new ways of detoxing to regain balance and optimal health.

If you want to get better, you must accept that toxic chemicals are not safe for the human body. You must know that the center of all immunity is your gut, and that it has to function optimally for the rest of you to do so. Diet is crucial to success in clearing the body of toxins. In this book, you will learn about nutrition and balancing the ecosystem in your GI tract.

Each interview will read as though you have a private appointment with the world's greatest specialist in his or her medical arena. The new-thinking doctors already know what we're up against. They know toxins are killing us. But these doctors and professionals also know something else: You can fight these toxins and you can win.

Keep reading.

Your health is in your hands. It's your life. It's your choice. You can get your good health back. I did it, my husband did it, my daughter did it, my granddaughters did it . . . and you can, too!

You can detox your way to health. But the time to make a change is now. There is no time to lose.

WHAT YOU CAN DO RIGHT *NOW*

The goal of this book is to identify the toxic threats one by one and dismantle them. You'll also learn how to heal the damage toxicity has done to your body, stop new toxins from coming into your body, get the accumulated toxins out, and clean up your personal sphere to protect you from future toxicity. You can live, thrive, and survive in this toxic soup that man has created. You can come out on the other side healthier than ever and remain so permanently, if you adopt the changes you will learn from this reading. In this book, we are not going to focus on what we can't have or do, but rather on what we *can* achieve together.

What you *can* have is exciting: enjoyable, sustainable, vibrant health. Individually, none of us has the power to turn around the damage done to our precious planet; that would be overwhelming and cause hopelessness, but on a positive note, each of us has the power to change our own and our family's health. You'll lead by example, and others will want what you have. That's how things change: through people at the grassroots level, providing inspirational and aspirational personal examples. One step at a time, one person at a time, good health will return, as opposed to the present poor health of so many. To heal your brain, your digestive tract, your immune system, your hormonal system, your autoimmune "conditions," and to take the steps to help "manage" cancer, will require a major detoxification, **with the end goal being to thrive in optimal health!**

I have promised solutions in this book, so here is my list of what we can do together:

CAN'S

1. You *CAN* heal and restore your gut and thus your immune system through dietary changes and eliminating toxins.
2. You *CAN* repair memory loss, brain fog, and "senior moments."

3. You *CAN* get your energy back.

4. You *CAN* help reverse ADD, ADHD, OCD, and even asthma.

5. You *CAN* heal your ailing and leaky digestive tract and protect your stomach from the toxins that are causing your discomfort, as well as your bloating, flatulence, and abdominal pain.

6. You *CAN* live without taking a pill for every ailment. Let's dispel the myth that has had us all brainwashed that allopathic (drug) medicine is the only way to go.

7. You *CAN* protect yourself from dangerous cell-phone radiation.

8. You *CAN* protect yourself from EMFs (electromagnetic fields).

9. You *CAN* eat delicious healthy fats again. (Think steak and butter!)

10. You CAN detoxify your home and make it a safe, toxic-free zone.

11. You *CAN* help reverse autoimmune diseases.

12. You *CAN* get your sex drive back.

13. You *CAN* help manage cancer through detoxification.

And you *can* get back optimum health!

To accomplish the preceding requires a commitment to make some major changes in the way you are living. But if you do commit and do the work, you *can* get the life you want and the joys of optimal health.

Oh, and you *can* and will LOSE WEIGHT! Yes, the weight. Unexplained weight gain will disappear when you reduce your chemical load. When you clean up your diet, clean out your body, and clean out your home of chemicals and toxins, that unexplained weight you've been carrying around will melt away. Yes, your toxic burden is likely the culprit; the bigger your exposure, the bigger the effect on your health and your weight.

> The secret to survival in today's world is to get your body so chemically unloaded and primed with nutrients that it heals itself.
> —Dr. Sherry Rogers

Consider this book your crash course in curing whatever ails you as you heal your insides by ridding your body of the toxins.

PART I

TOTALLY
TOX-SICK

CHAPTER 1

THE NEW TOXIC THREATS

The time has come when we are waking up to an alarming truth. We are killing ourselves with the same chemicals we invented to make our lives easier.

—DR. ALEJANDRO JUNGER, *CLEAN*

THERE ARE SIX MAJOR TOXIC THREATS:

1. Plastics and Other Chemicals
2. The Low-Fat Food Movement and Processed, Sugar-Filled Foods
3. Toxic Mold
4. The Overuse of Pills
5. GMOs (Genetically Modified Organisms)
6. EMFs (Electric and Magnetic Fields) and Cell Phones

These toxic threats are seemingly benign because we use and interact with all of them on a daily basis. How could these everyday things pose danger?

We were told chemicals were safe. We have been encouraged to consume low-fat products and low-fat diets. Sugar isn't that bad (we think), so why should we be deprived of it? And GMOs are how we are going to "feed the world"; isn't that great? Drugs and pills? Well, they are prescribed by our doctors; surely they are okay. Same for over-the-counter drugs—they wouldn't be for sale if they weren't safe, would they? Electromagnetic fields? But the gas company installs these grids in our homes; surely they are safe. And our cell phones, we can't leave home without them. We are so addicted we can't leave a room without them. But no one told us that talking on a cell phone is like putting a microwave oven next to your ear every time you use it. Or how about putting a microwave in your pocket next to your breast? Does that seem safe? And mold, who has even heard of it? So how harmful can it be?

You are already thinking . . . I can feel it as I write. Keep reading: there's a lot we've been misinformed about. But I'm going to dismantle, one by one, each of these threats so you can see the damage they have caused and then learn how you can clean out your body.

Let's start with toxic threat number one.

TOXIC THREAT #1: PLASTICS AND OTHER CHEMICALS

Our bodies were not meant to metabolize chemicals that were invented yesterday. Disbelievers in the harm of toxins say these chemicals we absorb and ingest daily are in such tiny amounts that the body hardly even notices them. "They" say the body can easily detoxify and get rid of these chemicals, but studies prove otherwise. The EPA (Environmental Protection Agency) has done biopsy studies of chemicals stored in the fat of human beings; these have shown that 100 percent of people studied had dioxins, PCBs, dichlorobenzene, and xylene in their bodies. To translate: dioxins and PCBs are among the most potent causes of cancers known to man.

Shocking! We know in our "gut" that this has to be true, but when you see it in print the facts are sobering.

When "they" say the body can handle the small amounts, they are not considering the stockpiling of chemicals day after day, month after month, that all adds up to why you are not feeling well on a daily basis. You may not be sick . . . *yet*, but you aren't *well*, either. Sadly, this accumulation takes decades in some cases to produce disease. At that point no one points the finger at the toxic buildup that began years ago. We have blindly accepted chemicals into our world, wrongly thinking that if the FDA said these substances were safe, then, in fact, they were.

Think about our lawns. With chemicals, our grass grows greener, thicker, fuller. It's beautiful and you don't have to water as much. But what is it doing to the environment? What is it doing to us? Nature intended that grass needs only water and sunlight. Why have we interfered so as to have it be greener than green? Our pets and children walk and play on these grasses. Then we bring it into our homes, the chemicals invisibly sticking to our feet and our skin. We never connect the dots to the rashes and dry skin and itchiness, and we NEVER connect the dots as to the migration of these seemingly benign chemicals that make their way to our fragile and already compromised GI tract systems and how these toxins eat through our gut lining and make their way up to our brains.

Our food has been hijacked by pesticides, herbicides, and the "miracle" of Roundup weed killer (according to my friend renowned neuroscientist Dr. Russell Blaylock, "The only miracle with Roundup is the statistic of an 800 percent increased risk of multiple myeloma").

The pesticides on vegetables and fruit are often sprayed with organophosphate. Studies have shown that children who live in homes where organophosphate pesticides, the most common class, are used have a higher rate of brain tumors. The higher the pesticide levels in your blood, the slower you burn calories while you are sleeping. They mess with your insulin. That's why you can't lose weight.

Remember "an apple a day keeps the doctor away"? Well, not so fast. Organic apples still pack their punch, but nonorganic apples aren't so healthy anymore. They are typically grown in soil that's been degraded by pesticides and toxic fertilizers. The USDA reports the nutritional content of American produce has declined significantly since the 1950s when these chemicals came on the scene. Insufficiencies of vitamins and minerals can damage DNA according to Dr. Bruce Ames at the University of California at Berkeley, who also states that these insufficiencies prompt people to overeat because their bodies desperately try to gain the nutrients they are not getting.

Other EPA studies show that human fat samples contain styrene, a substance that can cause any number of perplexing symptoms, as well as cancer. Styrene outgases from our computers (I'm getting hit right now as I write). Then factor in all the everyday plastics, including the plastic bottles that are such a part of our daily lives. The very water we go out of our way to drink as a healthier choice is contaminated from the plastic bottles it's contained in!

People with symptoms think it's because they are getting older, but it's often not the years that are the problem, it's the addition of significant amounts of toxic exposure with more being added every year. In the last two decades, the percentages of toxin-caused ailments have skyrocketed, including things such as allergies, asthma, infertility, Parkinson's, Parkinson's-like symptoms, even bone marrow cancers, lymphomas, leukemias, and multiple myeloma. There's more; autoimmune diseases like Hashimoto's thyroiditis and rheumatoid arthritis are linked to this chemical assault. In fact, studies have found that the levels of pesticides in people's blood prior to diet and stomach stapling correlate with age, not weight, with the most pesticides accumulated in the oldest people—not the heaviest.

As mentioned, toxins bioaccumulate over time, lingering and gathering in the fat cells, and people have no idea why they can't lose weight or why they feel so lousy. Most of us now learning about toxins worry that it's only a matter of time before we ingest or inhale the chemical that creates the "tipping point." This book is going to teach you how to detox regularly so you never have to reach your tipping point.

TOXIC THREAT #2: THE LOW-FAT FOOD MOVEMENT AND PROCESSED, SUGAR-FILLED FOODS

> The diet-heart (low-fat) hypothesis is the greatest scientific deception of this century, perhaps of any century.
> —George Mann, eminent American physician and scientist

I've found in life that when the time comes to say "I told you so," it's too late. The problem has been created. In all of my nine Somersize books, I stressed the value of healthy dietary fats. Now the facts are out. In order to "thrive" in today's world, you need to understand the effects of foods on your health. You also need to know that since the low-fat movement started we have gotten sicker and fatter. We've been brainwashed into believing that fat is the enemy. Let's look at what the science *really* says:

- In 2013, a prominent London cardiologist by the name of Aseem Malhotra argued in the *British Medical Journal* that you should ignore advice to *reduce* your saturated fat intake, because it's actually increasing your risk for obesity and heart disease.
- March 2014, a new meta-analysis published in the *Annals of Internal Medicine,* using data from nearly eighty studies and more than a half-million people, found that those who consume higher amounts of saturated fat have *no more heart disease* than those who consume less.

About 800,000 Americans die from cardiovascular disease annually. A quarter of these deaths could be prevented through simple lifestyle changes such as maintaining a healthy weight, exercising, and managing insulin and leptin levels.

Your body needs saturated fats for proper function. Consider what foods humans consumed during their evolution. We evolved as hunter-gatherers, eating animal products for most of our existence on earth. That's why the low-fat movement makes no sense, especially from an evolutionary perspective. We're designed to eat these foods! As recently as 2010, the U.S. Department of Agriculture (USDA) suggested reducing saturated fat intake to a mere 10 percent of total calories or less. The USDA bought into this myth! Research shows that this is the opposite of what most people require for optimal health! Fats provide a number of important health benefits, including the following:

- Provide building blocks for cell membranes, hormones, and hormonelike substances
- Help mineral absorption such as calcium
- Carry important fat-soluble vitamins, A, D, E, and K
- Act as an antiviral agent
- Modulate genetic regulation and help prevent cancer

We need fats for our brains, too! Without the vital protective barrier they provide to our GI tract, toxins can make their way up to our brains and start causing damage. Fats are protective? Yes! And to think we've been talked out of enjoying them all these years and instead have been given harmful drugs to keep the myth alive!

Healthy, delicious organic fats that are *not* altered and chemical-
ized, fats that come pure from nature, are the answer to health. The
complete lack of understanding about healthy fats as essential for sealing the barrier wall in the GI tract and the necessity for the brain to be
satiated with fat to operate at optimum is how we have been misled to
believe low-fat, no-fat, is the way to go.

The Cholesterol Myth

Dispelling the myth about cholesterol as the culprit in heart disease is
the latest effort in a long line of science proving saturated fat is not the
enemy. Dr. Stephen Sinatra, author of the book *The Great Cholesterol
Myth,* explains in a later chapter why the cholesterol myth has been
propagated, and dispels the information. In 2012, researchers at the
Norwegian University of Science and Technology examined the health
and lifestyle habits of more than 52,000 adults ages 20 to 74, concluding that women with "high cholesterol" (greater than 270 mg/dl) had
a *28 percent lower mortality risk* than women with "low cholesterol"
(less than 183 mg/dl). Researchers also found that, if you're a woman,
your risk for heart disease, cardiac arrest, and stroke are *higher* with
lower cholesterol levels.

Cholesterol is beneficial and mandatory for your body. Every cell
in our body requires fat as an essential component. Our bodies also
require cholesterol for health. The low-fat myth is so ingrained that
people have died as a result of stringent low-fat diets, and the FDA has
been bamboozled into believing the culprit in poor health is cholesterol and our high-fat diets!

By consuming a diet of healthy fats and grass-fed protein, you are
feeding your body what it needs to perform a number of critical functions. We need a balance of healthy dietary fats and vegetables to be
healthy and to provide sufficient nutrition to make our bodies run
efficiently. But fats that we've been told are healthy in the past are
instead problematic; trans fats, hydrogenated oils, or those found in
processed foods or fast foods are *not* healthy fats.

Healthy fats are organic and wild caught, such as fresh salmon or
grass-fed proteins like beef, pork, lamb, and the by-products of these
animals: butter, cream, sour cream, full-fat cream cheese, full-fat yogurts. We need a sufficient daily intake of omega-3 fatty acids from

extra-virgin cold-pressed olive oil, cold-pressed flaxseed oil, and virgin, organic coconut oil.

> Fats will heal and seal the protective barrier in your GI tract, essential for keeping toxins from entering your bloodstream and causing damage.

There is also strong evidence that people have a higher risk for heart attacks by having their cholesterol levels driven too *low*, as is being done with drugs like statins. Cholesterol plays important roles such as building your cell membranes, interacting with proteins inside your cells, and helping regulate protein pathways required for cell signaling. Having too little cholesterol may negatively impact your brain health, hormone levels, heart disease risk, and more. Therefore, placing an upper limit on dietary cholesterol, especially such a *low* upper limit as is now recommended, is likely causing far more harm than good.

It's all been a big fat lie!

We don't want to wait until the proponents of the low-fat movement die off to make a change, so let's settle the "fat is bad" myth once and for all. First, let me remind you of what you have been missing that I am going to urge you to reincorporate into your diet forever. Remember steak? Succulent, tender, grass-fed, delicious steak drowning in its pan juices with a melting pat of butter on top? Remember how it literally melted in your mouth, each bite a sensory experience, as though your body recognized that this is what it was designed to consume? Have you longed to return to those glorious days when steak was considered "healthy"? Well, now you can.

> A new scientific truth does not triumph by convincing its opponents but rather because its opponents eventually die, and a new generation grows up that is familiar with it.
> —Max Plank, German physicist, 1949 Nobel Prize winner

It's never too late to reverse the damage of the low-fat movement. You have to start now, today, with a shift in your thinking. Lucky for all of us, there is now an "army" of cutting-edge Western doctors, naturopaths, cardiologists, neuroscientists, oncologists, and others who all understand the health benefits of a diet rich in healthy fats. If your current doctor is not on board, it's probably time to find a new one who is better informed about the effects of toxins on the planet and our bodies. (To find a new thinking, qualified doctor, go to ForeverHealth.com.)

You can bring back butter, and enjoy lightly steamed fresh vegetables tossed in it. Or use those yummy pan juices deglazed with a wine reduction and a pat of butter—yummm! Remember baby lamb chops, panfried in their own fat, pink and juicy inside with the fat on the sides cooked till crispy? Remember how with just one bite, your eyes would roll back into your head in ecstasy? What about chicken piccata in lemon butter sauce, or pork chops marinated in garlic and olive oil then quickly grilled until the fat gets crispy and delicious? Well, bring them back to your plate. Your body will thank you.

We've been duped, and it boggles the mind to understand how trusting we were to let ourselves be so indoctrinated.

Why did we stop eating these yummy foods? We grew up with them, right? Your parents and grandparents ate this way and none of them had the diseases of today. The kids in our classes weren't fat. Or maybe there was one kid, but the rest ate these delicious healthy fats and good-quality proteins, and we were well and full of energy when we exercised daily by going outside to play.

When we were kids, it wasn't common for any of our elders to end up with Alzheimer's and/or in nursing homes. It was rare for our grandparents to die of heart attacks or cancer. It was rare to even know of someone who *had* cancer. People used to die peacefully in their sleep, with lives that had run a natural course, not experiencing long, drawn-out expensive deaths, lost in a haze of pills, tubes, and torture, not knowing who they were or are.

What happened???

The answer is simple. . . . The low-fat campaign and the deception regarding the dangers of cholesterol, along with toxins that have shredded our digestive tracts like a tire that has blown on a freeway. The new so-called healthy guidelines have been a recipe for disaster for humanity and now the chickens are coming home to roost.

We bought into the low-fat advice. We wanted to be healthy. So we switched from butter to chemicals called margarine because we were told it was healthier. We believed experts when they said meat was dangerous, that fats were the enemy. Dutifully we bought low-fat treats, low-fat yogurts, low-fat milk, "better than butter" chemical substitutes, diet sodas, processed foods. We stopped eating real food, or real animal fats, and switched to high-carb diets loaded with hydrogenated dangerous oils.

Look at what has happened. . . . We got sicker . . . and fatter.

Diabetes has skyrocketed.

Cancer is now the number two killer in the world.

Heart disease is the number one killer.

Alzheimer's is an epidemic and it is predicted that 50 percent of the baby boomers can expect to lose their precious minds to Alzheimer's.

The "experts" were wrong—and it wasn't just about low-fat. It's what resulted from trying to eat this way. The low-fat craze in turn promoted excessive consumption of refined carbohydrates and sugars, resulting in increased inflammation and disease.

The Real Problem: Sugar and Processed Foods

The problem is sugar, not fats. A high-sugar diet raises your risk for heart disease by promoting metabolic syndrome—a cluster of health conditions that includes high blood pressure, insulin and leptin resistance, high triglycerides, liver dysfunction, and visceral fat accumulation. Insulin and leptin resistance is caused by factors inherent in our modern lifestyle, including diets heavy in processed carbohydrates, sugars or fructose, refined flours, and industrial seed oils.

Making matters worse, the average American gets inadequate exercise to offset consumption of sugar and processed foods, suffers from chronic stress and sleep deprivation, is exposed to environmental toxins, and has poor gut health (dysbiosis). This is the perfect storm for chronic disease.

Again, we believed what we were told. Low-fat food products, which are highly processed and filled with sugar, are good for business, profits, and selling fear, but sadly, have nothing to do with what is good for us.

Let me ask you: Have you felt well since chemicals have bombarded your life?

Do you feel better since you gave up things like butter and real healthy fats and instead began eating more processed, sugary products?

Have you felt better on cholesterol-lowering drugs?

We gave up healthy fats and we got fat. We started eating more processed, sugar-laden foods and we got sick. "They" told us fats were harmful and detrimental to our health; how wrong they have been. Let's be clear; the "fat is bad" myth is exactly that . . . a myth. As you are learning, toxins destroy the GI tract and are leading to a multitude of illnesses and conditions; the elimination of healthy fats in our diets has exacerbated the problem.

We started life on a high-fat diet from our mother's breast, yet science has tried to outthink the perfection of nature and told us for the last fifty years that nature was wrong, that low-fat was the way to go. Butter was replaced by margarine, and healthy grass-fed protein was replaced by high-carb pastas.

> Much of our food system depends on our not knowing much about it, beyond the price disclosed by the checkout scanner; cheapness and ignorance are mutually reinforcing. And it's a short way from not knowing who's at the other end of your food chain to not caring—to the carelessness of both producers and consumers that characterizes our economy today.
> —Michael Pollan, *The Omnivore's Dilemma: A Natural History of Four Meals*

TOXIC THREAT #3: TOXIC MOLD

Before I dive into this newest of the toxic threats, I wanted you to read about how mold affected my husband's health. Alan is a healthy guy who has eaten correctly all his life, exercises, and lives a happy life. When you read his story, it might help you to piece together the puzzle of your own degraded health. Mold is insidious and can cause immeasurable damage. His is a story of triumph, so take heart. If you're not sure what's making you ill, this may hold the answer.

After our home burned down five years ago, we moved into this spectacular hillside property with views for miles. I was very happy sharing this great new adventure with my fabulous Suzanne. We loved our life there. Wonderful light. Fresh ocean breezes. Fun family times on weekends. We enjoyed a few romantic dates a week at our bar with a little tequila and a martini. It was perfect.

Soon I noticed that every time I walked into certain rooms in the house, my eyes would water, my nose would run, and my tongue swelled up. I thought this was some allergy from all our plants that I would get over, but it got worse. Then I started blinking. Watery eyes, runny nose, and now blinking. . . . What's next? I wondered. "Next" arrived in the form of grimacing. Whenever I drove more than twenty minutes, it would begin, and because my eyes were closed for seconds at a time, Suzanne freaked. I did too. She then took the wheel and I sat in what I jokingly call "the death seat." It's not that Suzanne is a bad driver, it's that she rarely drives. She's also a little dyslexic, so she changes lanes first and then looks behind her.

Then the odyssey began.

I was diagnosed with black mold (from an unfinished section below the house that had standing water) that had invaded my body and brain. We spent two weeks in Dallas, a week at a time, with the father of environmental medicine, Dr. Bill Rae, getting detoxed and injected and spec scanned. It seemed to help. Then we did daily far infrared saunas to detox all the heavy metals. Then daily oxygenations with tubes up my nose.

Then I added all the detox foods and smoothies I could think of. Then I patched myself with LifeWave glutathione patches to detox. They helped a lot and I still wear them every day. But it was only when my dear friend Dr. Nicholas Gonzalez, an oncologist who manages cancer with a nutritional program, told me that half his patients have mold that I went on his program and, eureka, it has calmed down my grimacing by 90 percent and I am now driving most of the time.

This morning I drove the winding mountain roads of Malibu in my "midlife crisis car" and since Suzanne was not with me, I powered around the curves and straightaways and no blinking and no grimacing. I was smiling and laughing all by myself, realizing that we may be able to take our long 3,000-mile drives through the southwestern part of this great country after all.

Mold . . . the new mystery disease. It can lead to devastating conditions. Mold, as well as Lyme disease, are two conditions my family knows about firsthand. My granddaughter Violet, whose story you'll hear a little later, had both and they destroyed the eco balance in her GI tract, as well as my husband Alan's. I am addressing the two conditions together because the treatment for both diseases is essentially the same, and they are treatments that require diligence and patience. Chronic illnesses such as these are caused by biotoxins manufactured by invisible microorganisms in our environment. You can be exposed in so many ways, from your school as happened to Violet, or your home as happened to Alan (and to me to a lesser extent), or even local recreational areas. Below is an anonymous letter that is just one of the many we have received about the horrors of mold:

> We bought a house three years ago. Did a stupid thing, trusted our real estate agent. Coming from a different state, not knowing anything about where we were moving, we trusted the agent's inspector. End result, yesterday we had to walk away from our home because of black mold. We had a baby two months ago, born two months early and after a very difficult pregnancy. I now wonder if breathing the mold was partly responsible. No one knows. The mold won when I became too sick from the pregnancy to keep using the bleach to get rid of it. Now we are renting, but already have seen an improvement in our health just in the two days we have slept in our new home. Life is hard, this is hard, but when you have to choose between the life of your children and a moldy house . . . there is no choice.

Mold stories are horrific. The microorganisms in mold and Lyme routinely destroy health, degrade function at home and work, and can have devastating effects. Some of these exposures can actually kill, but only after a long protracted battle with these deadly organisms. You can get exposed to spores carried throughout your home from a faulty air conditioner or from a pond, lake, or an estuary.

Or maybe a Lyme tick will bite you. It's biotoxic as well.

When biotoxins act without control, they interact with and disrupt our immune system, causing an inflammatory response. That is why both conditions are so confounding. Often, chronic fatigue, fibromyalgia, irritable bowel syndrome, anxiety, and depression are misdiagnosed and instead you may have mold toxicity. The same is true for biotoxin-induced Lyme disease, which is often diagnosed as myriad other ailments. Biotoxins are the cause of so many different illnesses, and many of the biotoxins can't be measured by blood tests.

People often say they tested negative to mold, but they know they don't feel right. Listen to your gut; despite its difficulty to measure, mold toxins easily do damage to our bodies. An experienced doctor can see the signs. Some people can get exposed and not be bothered by it; others who are genetically susceptible do not have that built-in protection and may become unable to function.

Just because you don't see molds in your house doesn't mean you don't have them; they can be hiding, munching away at your drywall, insulation, and plywood; these are mold toxin "happy foods."

Some people report that despite twelve hours of sleep, they spend their days exhausted, dizzy, and out of sorts. They claim that everything hurts, and occasionally they feel stabbing pains. If you haven't been able to source why, it could be mold.

Dr. Ritchie Shoemaker, whom you'll hear more from later, describes mold under magnification: "I couldn't get around the images from old sci-fi movies; the fungi were like something from *Little Shop of Horrors*."

How about that? Like little monsters reproducing and wreaking havoc in your body, mold keeps reproducing unless stopped like mold on your bathroom tiles.

Stachybotrys is an especially nasty fungus, a moisture-loving, poison-manufacturing organism that thrives in indoor places where leaky roofs, trapped condensation, or porous basements allow water to seep into a building's structure, permitting mold to grow. It damages drywall, insulation, and wood. If a building part has cellulose, the mold will eat it; but mold can also thrive on metal air ducts. Mold likes to live in the same temperature that we do; all it needs is plenty of moisture and food. Its favorite food in your GI tract is sugar. Mold loves it. But in your home, it loves drywall, air-conditioning ducts, and any warm, damp place in which to procreate.

By not understanding molds' ability to harm us and our homes, we neglect to take small leaks seriously, and then we turn on the heat or an air conditioner and they go on a rampage. That's what happened to us. As my husband, Alan, mentioned in his story, we leased a beautiful home after our house in Malibu burned to the ground. In this new leased home was an unfinished room under the house. I never even went down there, but unbeknownst to us it had standing water that grew dangerous black mold that found its way through all our air-conditioning ducts; it also made its way throughout all the dry-wall in many of the rooms. We were literally swimming in mold, but because it was *invisible*, we lived with, breathed, exercised with, and were surrounded by spores.

Four years into it I began to notice my husband had chronic red, watery eyes, and a sinus drainage problem. There were times it was so bad we couldn't go out. As you've read in Alan's story, the symptoms progressed from there. Around the same time I was misdiagnosed in the hospital and put on six days of IV antibiotics with no probiotic. The combination of the antibiotics, which seriously disrupted the health of my GI tract, coupled with mold in our home, made my quality of life very uncomfortable. We finally left the beautiful home two weeks after we realized the depth of the mold and the damage it was doing to our health. We have been on a long journey ever since. I embraced a serious detox program that I will lay out for you in the upcoming pages.

Detoxing our mold required many different protocols because the mold simply was the starting point for many different issues of environmental illness. I am finally free of these biotoxins and pathogens, and Alan is getting better but is not all the way "there" yet. This is what I mean by needing "patience."

HOW MOLD TAKES HOLD

When I write here about biotoxins, it's just another word for mold organisms. The body acquires mold biotoxins or toxin-producing organisms from food, water, air, or arachnid (bug) bites. In genetically susceptible people, biotoxins bind to fat-cell receptors, causing continuing unregulated production of cytokines (important for cell signaling); if the cell isn't getting its signals correctly, it doesn't know what to do. Now you're in trouble. In most people, biotoxins are removed from the blood by the liver, or attacked by the immune system, then broken down and excreted harmlessly. People who carry the HLA gene are extremely susceptible to chemicals and toxicity of any kind. They are the canaries in the coal mine. These "carriers" are usually English, Irish, French, German, Spanish, but not exclusively, as my husband is Eastern European and carries this gene. This doesn't mean that the rest of the population is not susceptible, it's just that the HLA carriers are the first to go down. (For gene testing on this, see the back of the book.) If these biotoxins are not cleared from the body, they can remain in the body indefinitely and cause lifelong trouble. Mold can seriously affect vision; if you suspect this is happening to you, it can be tested with a contrast sensitivity test (CST), the most widely used measure of functional vision in the world.

The effects of toxicity are different in each body; one person may have vision impairment; another, tremors and tics (like Alan). Often these tremors and tics are diagnosed as Parkinson's disease. Think of all the people diagnosed with Parkinson's and put on harsh drugs when the problem might be mold. Mold also can create serious forms of brain dysfunction; other people will gain tremendous amounts of weight because the mold induces their fat cells to produce more leptin. This is why a person can become obese, a condition that doesn't respond to exercise and diet. How exasperating to be eating less yet getting fatter.

The Mold Pathway

• Excessive cytokine levels can damage leptin receptors in the hypothalamus (hormone central in the brain) so production of melatonin is reduced, leading to insomnia because the cells are not receiving their proper signals. Also, endorphin production is suppressed and this can lead to chronic, sometimes unusual pain.

• Lack of MSH (melanocyte-stimulating hormone, a small peptide that regulates aspects of the immune system) can cause malabsorption in the gut, resulting in diarrhea. This is another form of "leaky gut" and resembles (but is not) celiac disease.

• Colonies of *Staph* bacteria with resistance to multiple antibiotics may develop in mucous membranes. The bacteria produce substances that aggravate both the high cytokine levels and low MSH levels.

• High cytokine levels in the capillaries attract white blood cells, leading to restricted blood flow and lower oxygen levels. Reduced VEGF (vascular endothelial growth factor) leads to fatigue, muscle cramps, and shortness of breath.

• Damaged leptin receptors also lead to reduced production by the hypothalamus of MSH.

• White blood cells lose their ability to properly regulate
the cytokine response. Then recovery from other illnesses, including infectious diseases, may be slowed.

• Reduced MSH can cause the pituitary to produce lower
levels of antidiuretic hormone (ADH), leading to thirst, frequent urination, and susceptibility to shocks from static electricity. MSH can cause the pituitary to lower its production of
sex hormones.

• The pituitary may produce elevated levels of cortisol and
ACTH (adrenocotrophic hormone) in early stages of illness,
and then drop to excessively low levels later. (Patients should
avoid steroids such as prednisone, which can lower levels of
ACTH.)

That's the mold pathway. Scary, huh?

High levels of cytokines as a result of mold exposure can
produce chronic flulike symptoms such as headaches, muscle
aches, fatigue, unstable temperature, and difficulty concentrating. High levels of cytokines also result in increased levels
of several other immune-response-related substances affecting your brain, nerves, muscles, lungs, and joints. Those who
carry certain HLA genotypes (immunity-related genes) may
develop inappropriate immunity.

Clearly, mold is no joke.

TOXIC THREAT #4: THE OVERUSE OF PILLS

As Americans we have been brainwashed into believing the only way
to treat a disease or a condition is with a pill. So many individuals
wake up each day and start with a bagel, or toast, or a muffin with
margarine, served with processed, packaged breakfast cereal. And
then they grab their antacids, statin pill, diet pill, diuretic, diabetes
medication, synthetic hormones, antidepressant, and more. And they
wonder why they aren't feeling well?

We have to ask ourselves, how is the allopathic approach working
out? Are people better off as a result of taking the billions of dollars'

worth of pills we collectively take yearly? Are people cured as a result? An honest assessment would be: no.

Pills don't cure. Pills are for the most part a Band-Aid, requiring in many cases a lifelong addiction to "maintain" your status quo. Now, granted, I would not want to live in a world without pharmaceuticals, in particular for pain, infection, mental illness, and other things outside my scope. But the point of this book and all my other books is to encourage people to find the holistic reason for a condition; where did it originate? Then look *first* for a natural remedy to truly heal, before resorting to a pharmaceutical bandage.

Why would it be important to avoid pharmaceuticals and over-the-counter medicines unless absolutely necessary? Every time you take a chemical pharmaceutical pill, you are now compromising your GI tract and weakening the integrity of your intestinal barrier wall. Since your gut is your first line of immune defense, this comprises most of your immune system.

The pill actually masks the symptom, while doing damage to the body. In allopathic medicine the focus is on treating the symptoms. If your symptom is, for instance, high blood pressure, you get a pill to lower it. As I said, allopathic medicine is exactly that, a pill for every symptom. Rarely does orthodox medicine dig deep to find what is *causing* the symptom. As we'll learn from Dr. Garry Gordon, most often high blood pressure is an overload of accumulated lead in your bones and the solution is not a dangerous drug you take for life, but instead chelation, which will over time remove the lead from your bones, allowing your body to dramatically lower your total toxic body burden.

Doesn't this make more sense than to keep putting the high blood pressure pill (Band-Aid) into your body for life? How can you expect the outcome of this to be anything but negative to your health? New medicine, alternative medicine, fills that gap.

Every time you go for a pill you might want to think about this: Is there a better way? And if you're a parent, you really need to pause and read the next section . . . because what orthodox medicine is prescribing for many children is even more shameful.

Toddlers are being medicated? In reading the most recent research, I've become baffled about why we are not alarmed and horrified that such a large percentage of children in America are on amphetamines.

Is no one questioning why so many children are being diagnosed with ADHD? This is a new phenomenon, conditions that did not exist in our own childhoods. What has changed? Of course we all know. But it gets worse.

> According to CDC officials, more than 10,000 American toddlers—children who are just 2 or 3 years old—*are being medicated* for alleged attention deficit hyperactivity disorder (ADHD).
>   —National Alliance for Health, June 3, 2014

OMG! What are we thinking? What are we doing? These are innocent children just doing what they are told to do, and their caretakers unknowingly (I hope) are risking the physical and mental health of these children and most likely shortening their lives in the process. I am stunned by the lack of creativity of the orthodox medical community.

How We Got Here

I once asked a doctor I was interviewing, "How did it come to be that Western medicine has become 'allopathic only'?" and he said, "I'll tell you exactly how. At the turn of the century there was a guy by the name of Abraham Flexner, who was hired by the two richest families in America, the Carnegies and the Rockefellers (who owned pharmaceutical companies), to go to the institutes of higher learning, Mayo Clinic, Johns Hopkins, etc., and offer funding in *perpetuity* if they would teach only allopathic medicine. From that time on, all the 'pathics'—homeopathic, naturopathic, and specialties like chiropractic—became regarded as 'wacky' and 'not real medicine.'"

Now, as a businesswoman I admire the creative thinking of these two pharmaceutical giants, but . . . at what cost to us in the big picture? We are seeing the effects in our present world. People loaded up with pills. Our seniors are so "pilled up," they have no thoughts left, and then sadly we warehouse them in nursing homes, drugged up even more to live out their last pathetic days not knowing who they are or who they were. The tragedy is that as a result we are not only losing them but we are also losing our wisdom pool.

Alternative medicine is composed of mostly Western-trained doctors and naturopaths who look for a real cure. Pills don't cure. Pills are a Band-Aid designed to take away immediate discomfort, but in most cases they assure that the condition most likely will return. Instead, alternative medicine doctors ask themselves, what natural substance or technique does this patient need to make him or her better? Is it a vitamin or mineral deficiency? Is there an herb that works especially well for the problem? Does he or she need a spinal adjustment, acupuncture, or a homeopathic remedy? As Dr. Jonathan Wright (the father of bioidentical hormones) so often wisely says, "using Nature's tools to heal."

It's a lot of work to be healthy in today's world, but it's a lot more work to be sick. Health is all there is, and the environment has presented a major challenge for all of us. No one is escaping this. Some are more sensitive than others to the toxic assault, but eventually everyone will be affected to some degree.

Like the Carnegies and the Rockefellers paying to fundamentally change medical information in our universities, the food manufacturers have also brainwashed the public into believing that chemicals are nutritious.

We are trying to *detoxify* our *tox-sick* bodies. It makes sense that the fewer drugs you need to take, the healthier you will be; and best of all, through detoxification, your need for drugs will diminish.

The answer to toxicity is FOOD, not drugs! The right foods can actually heal conditions caused by chemicals and eliminate the need for drugs.

Antibiotics: Another Threat Within a Threat

More than half of adult Medicaid patients with colds or respiratory tract infections *were prescribed antibiotics in 2007*—although antibiotics are not recommended in these cases and such inappropriate prescribing directly contributes to the global antibiotics resistance crisis.

This is crazy . . . antibiotics for a cold? A cold is a virus, not an infection. Antibiotics can only kill infection. To jeopardize your stomach and intestinal tract by taking an antibiotic that will do nothing for your cold but wreak havoc on your GI tract is, frankly, insane, and lazy on the part of our professionals.

Mothers need to know the truth about antibiotics; they have been overused to the point that, as just stated, we have reached a global antibiotic resistance. They don't work anymore because they have been used recklessly and without caution. When a serious infection comes along, what are we going to do? Today's hospitals are infected with *Staph*, a deadly infection that causes many people to have extended stays in hospitals, not because of the original reason for entry but because of staph infections that sometimes take months to heal and often kill the patient.

Again, the laziness and lack of creativity on the part of the professionals prescribing makes them suspect. Is there an incentive to do something so reckless to a patient? Could bonuses be part of the incentive? And why are the poor so much more likely to be prescribed dangerous drugs?

I came across research recently that shows that overall Medicaid patients don't fare much better than those without insurance. Here's why:

> Medicaid often reimburses doctors much less for nondrug interventions like counseling and therapy than it does for drug prescriptions.

Think about the wisdom of this: Instead of drugs, how about encouraging communities to use vacant land to allow people to grow their own high-quality organic food? Community leaders could teach the benefits of having your own garden. The community could spend its dollars on starter plants, seeds, gardening tools, and available instructors to teach how to successfully grow your own food. The difference this would make is incalculable. But society has gotten lazy, government is so often uninformed, and the pharmaceutical companies have gotten greedy. It's just easier to drug people; then they stop asking questions. We become complacent. Adults become children, doing whatever the doctor tells them, too drugged up to question, with one drug creating a side effect that causes a need for another drug and so on. This continues in today's society until one day the patient hits the tipping point, so drugged and *tox*-sick that the only place left to go is the nursing home.

DON'T ACCEPT THIS PARADIGM!

TOXIC THREAT #5: GMOs (GENETICALLY MODIFIED ORGANISMS)

> Control the oil and you can control entire continents. Control the food and you control the people.
>
> —Henry Kissinger

This is perhaps the most frightening toxic threat of them all. And one of the most distressing new changes hijacking our food supply is genetic modification.

While watching the documentary *Genetic Roulette* I was struck by one sentence in particular: "GMO foods create an 'insecticide factory' in your intestines." Let's factor that into your bloating, constipation, cramping, and overall stomach discomfort. But even worse, consider the results in a study of lab rats fed exclusively GMO foods for two years: all of them had organ failure or organ damage; half of them were sterile; the other half that didn't die had strange aberrations like hair growing between their teeth and hair growing around their organs.

Talk about confusing the nature in YOU! And this is the food designed "to save the world."

GMO foods are a new form of food manipulation, and no one has any true idea of the additional implications down the road for human physiology. The ramifications could be disastrous. GMO food manipulates the natural essence of these food substances by altering their DNA. When we incorporate these foods into our bodies, this altered DNA now becomes part of *us*. The alteration now has the potential of damaging, or even worse, becoming incorporated into our own genetic code. Anything foreign to the body is an antigen to which the body will make antibodies, potentially giving rise to a host of new autoimmune diseases. Dr. Nicholas Gonzalez, whom you'll meet later in this book, told me the following:

Twenty years ago, I never heard the phrase "leaky gut syndrome," but it's become epidemic and been complicated by GMOs. Big business is saying that GMOs are safe, that GMO foods are the answer to end hunger, but they compromise our gut. Certain bacteria produce molecules that function as natural herbicides and pesticides. In addition, some bacteria produce substances that actually block the action of synthetic herbicides. But now molecular biologists who are working for these major companies have learned how to insert these bacterial genes *into* the cells of the seed of food plants so the crops will in turn produce these herbicides and pesticides, allegedly protecting the crop. In addition, those bacterial genes that provide protection against synthetic herbicides allow the farmer to use high doses that theoretically will kill the vulnerable weeds, but not harm the useful crop. But now thanks to GMOs we have a little insecticide factory in our gut and that can be disastrous for our health. I've read about places in Asia where they've experimented with GMOs, where entire villages are getting sick because the normal flora in their intestines has been completely disrupted; these people now have pesticide factories within their guts. These molecules can poison our gut, our liver, and eventually the rest of us. Left unprotected the liver can't do its job because our livers were designed to process the nutrients from normal, healthy food, and the normal breakdown products of metabolism. But now those of us whose livers have been exposed to GMOs have the added unnatural burden of dealing with the barrage of herbicides and pesticides being produced right within us.

In the last ten years, the proliferation of GMO foods has compounded the disruption of the normal gut flora (as if we didn't have enough to deal with, with antibiotics, poor-quality food, and too much sugar). And the chemical companies have everyone believing their big lie: "This is how we're going to feed the world." Whenever I hear that, I think, *No, this is how we're going to end humanity.* Sadly, this is the infatuation with "chemistry as the answer to all our problems." It's not; it's a real problem, and it's the "arrogance of science" rather than what it should be, the "humility of scientists."

The idea that man knows better than nature is absurd. These GMO food crops now contain bacterial genes that produce natural toxic herbicides and pesticides. The problem begins because when we eat these GMO foods, the abnormal bacterial genes *transfer* to our normal bacteria that inhabit our gut and now we end up with bacteria-producing herbicides and pesticides right in our own *intestines*. And it's catastrophic!

Most of us feel that the FDA approves drugs, products, and food through rigorous, in-depth, long-term studies. This is a myth . . . nothing could be further from the truth, especially as it pertains to GMOs.

You must understand the severe ramifications of ingesting this lab-created "food." As Dr. Gonzalez explained, the lab process of artificially inserting genes into the DNA of food crops or animals can be engineered with genes from bacteria, viruses, insects, animals, or even humans. The primary reason the plants are engineered is to basically allow them to drink poison, aka pesticides. They are inserted with foreign genes that allow them to survive what would otherwise be deadly doses of poisonous herbicides, fungicides, and insecticides.

No kidding. Our grandmothers would never recognize what we call "food" today as food: Cheetos? Ho-Ho's? Funyuns? Our grandmothers fed us real food: grass-fed meat and vegetables and potatoes that were never sprayed with pesticides and herbicides. We didn't have freezers full of frozen foods; we didn't have six-packs of sodas hanging around. Desserts were an occasional "treat," and we drank whole milk and ate full-fat cheeses. We also ate eggs and bacon (that wasn't filled with nitrates). Refined carbohydrates were few and far between, and pasta was what you had occasionally at an Italian restaurant, a treat that happened maybe twice in my childhood. Also, it wasn't so long ago that people didn't eat the bulk of their meals in restaurants. Our small town had a coffee shop and no places for dinner. If we did go out for a meal, which was rare, we drove to San Francisco to have a dinner at the steakhouse. This was usually reserved for a big occasion like a wedding in the family.

> Don't eat anything your great-grandmother wouldn't recognize as food. . . . You may need to go back to your great- or even great-great-grandmother.
> —Michael Pollan, *The Omnivore's Dilemma*

Those steaks we were eating were not from cattle fed GMO corn and soy. They ate grass as nature intended. Think about how much GMO you are getting from corn-fed beef.

In the United States, incidences of low-birth-weight babies, infertility, and infant mortality are all escalating. Could GMOs be a culprit? Very possibly. Especially knowing what GMO foods are doing to many animal populations in recent studies. It seems clear from them that they are particularly dangerous for pregnant moms and children.

In one clinical study, GMO soy was fed to female rats, and most of their babies died. Those babies that didn't were smaller and possibly infertile. Testicles of rats fed GMO soy changed from their normal pink to dark blue. Mice fed GMO soy also had altered sperm. Embryos of mice fed GMO soy had changed DNA. And mice fed GMO corn had fewer and smaller babies. In Haryana, India, most buffalo fed GMO cottonseed had reproductive complications such as premature deliveries, spontaneous abortions, and infertility. Many calves died. Thousands of pigs across the globe have been reported to have become sterile from certain GMO corn varieties. Some had false pregnancies; others gave birth to bags of water. Cows and bulls also became infertile. In 2013, a Texas farmer came out to find fifteen of his nineteen cattle were dead. The reason? Grazing on GMO alfalfa.

> It has been noticed that animals when offered GMO or non-GMO foods avoid the GMO one.
>
> —Dr. Joseph Mercola, Mercola.com

The animals are smarter than us! Why isn't all of this more commonly known? And the only "testing" required for proving safety is for the GMO producer to submit a self-authored report. Michael Taylor, a former FDA lawyer, established the "not testing" policy, reasoning that GMOs are "substantially equivalent to food and have been deemed safe." By the way, Mr. Taylor is notorious for his revolving-door employment between the U.S. government and Monsanto and was chosen by President Obama in 2009 as the FDA deputy commissioner for foods, our "food safety czar." Monsanto is the corporation largely responsible for the introduction of GMO to our food supply. Monsanto also gave us Agent Orange and dioxin and is currently pushing GMO crops on the American public, touting them as safe. Currently, Monsanto's mutated seeds comprise over 93 percent of the U.S.'s soy crops and 86 percent of the corn crops, and next they are going after the wheat market.

And here we are . . .

Our immune systems are so damaged as a result of hijacked food, GMOs, pesticides, and herbicides that they can't do their jobs.

Sadly, our food sources have been dealt a death blow. Genetically modified foods offer little to no nutrition and carry chemicals that can destroy the immune system and digestive tract. Our cattle have been switched from their natural evolution of eating grass to a diet of corn. Usually this corn is also GMO, shown to irritate the intestines of the animal.

Nice, huh? Our fragile GI tracts are being exposed to damaging biotoxins, leaving our immune systems without defense. Undefended! This is not good.

Feeding cows GMO corn (or any corn) goes against the natural evolution of the cow, and can cause infections like *E. coli.* Then we consume this damaged meat, and we in turn get stomach issues, impaired digestive tracts, and immune systems that are not firing. This is indeed "dangerous meat," but not because of the fat content. Consuming beef from cows fed GMO corn is inviting that insecticide factory into our own intestines. Grass-fed beef is the only way to go.

The body in its wisdom has had to scramble to figure out a way to keep us alive in this toxic environment. To keep the toxins and chemicals away from our precious organs and glands (namely, your liver), the body has been conveniently storing chemicals in your fat cells, trying to protect you. That's why you've put on unexplained weight while you "thought" you were eating healthy low-fat and processed foods. Diet foods . . . dissect that word, *DIE-IT*!

This is the way it works: the more toxins you take in and are exposed to, the more fat you need to store them. I'll say it again, the more toxins you take in, the more fat is needed for storage. It's a merry-go-round. Is it truly any wonder obesity is an epidemic?

Look at what we have come to think of as normal:

- Epidemic of obesity
- Epidemic of diabetes

- Epidemic of Alzheimer's
- Epidemic of brain disorders
- Epidemic of "initials": ADD, ADHD, OCD
- Epidemic of digestive tract disorders
- Epidemic of cancer
- Epidemic of heart disease

This is the new normal! Our bodies are groaning under toxicity, and nowhere are we getting more of it than through our foods. Yet you can't "not eat," can you?

Certified organic products are not allowed to contain any GMOs. Therefore, when you purchase products labeled 100 percent organic, organic, or made with organic ingredients, then you don't have to worry about eating these lab-produced dangers.

To start protecting yourself today, avoid nonorganic versions of these foods, as these crops have been taken over by GMO versions:

Soy	93% are GMO
Cottonseed oil	93% are GMO
Canola oil	93% are GMO
Corn	86% are GMO
Beets and their sugar	95% are GMO
Hawaiian papaya	80% are GMO
Zucchini, crookneck squash	More than 25,000 acres in the United States are now GMO

TOXIC THREAT #6: EMFs AND CELL PHONES

Did you ever think that knowing about EMFs (electric and magnetic field frequencies) would be something of concern to you and to your health? How about the simple ER (electromagnetic radiation) that comes from your cell phone? There are many invisible pollutants in your home, including these EMFs and ERs; another is the Wi-Fi you're likely hooked up to right now. Yep, it's emitting harmful "rads" (radiation).

EMFs have severe biological impacts on your health, and the spectrum includes wireless devices and frequencies, cell phones, Bluetooth, cordless phones, microwave ovens, computers, laptops, tablets, and Wi-Fi. This could be one of the biggest "oops!" of our century.

Your health may be affected in the following ways:

- The possible EMF effect on the brain can be severe and catastrophic, including the risk to a child's not fully formed teenage brain. Why take that chance? EMFs may impact Alzheimer's, and have effects on the spinal cord, MS, the immune system, and cancer, including brain cancer. There have been no long-term studies on EMFs and the human brain. With the toxic assault everyone is already experiencing, why add to the problem?
- EMFs affect red and white blood cells and platelets, even the skin.
- EMFs affect sleep and insomnia, fertility, fetal development, immature versus mature cells.
- EMFs may affect asthma incidence in children and promote obesity, diabetes . . . and the list goes on.

Excessive chemical and electromagnetic radiation burdens have resulted in symptoms of multiple chemical sensitivities (MCS) and electromagnetic sensitivity (EMS). Studies are showing that EMF exposure opens the barriers that are designed to protect the vulnerable areas of the brain, gut, and placenta from toxic chemicals and pathogens. People who are already on toxic overload are being additionally burdened by EMF radiation that is further altering their biochemistry, resulting in their experiencing symptoms unique to this generation.

Have you heard about smart meters? Well, beware, your electric company is going to come calling and hopefully (from their perspective) you will be another "dumb consumer" and you will allow the meter man inside your property so he can install the new meter. Smart meters are on twenty-four hours, seven days a week, 365 days a year and collectively add to the massive amounts of electro-smog created by TV, radio, Wi-Fi, and cell-phone and cordless-phone frequencies that are already bombarding and microwaving us. In addition to the frequencies that smart meters emit, officials have had to boost the cell towers' power capacities to be able to read the meters.

CALLING OUT DANGER: CELL PHONES AND THEIR HARMS

Cell phones are not safe . . . research now shows the connection of cell phones' electromagnetic rads to brain tumors. Consider the following information.

After an extensive eleven-year report came out squashing the link between mobile phone usage and cancer, a new report from French scientists may turn that on its head. However, although it may raise a specter previously thought banished, the emphasis this time is on cancer and heavy use. In the *British Journal of Occupational and Environmental Medicine* researchers write that people who used their mobiles for "more than 15 hours each month over five years on average had between two and three times greater risk of developing glioma and meningioma tumors compared with people who rarely used their phones." The link between glioma—a type of tumor made from glial cells that account for 80 percent of all brain tumors—and long-term mobile phone use has been hard to prove, but the new study aims to tackle that. The new study looked at 253 cases of glioma and 194 cases of meningioma from four French departments between 2004 and 2006. Scientists then compared these to 892 healthy people from the same local population. "The comparison," reported the *Guardian,* "found a higher risk among those who used their phone intensively, especially among those who used it for their work, such as in sales. The duration of use in this category ranged from between 2 and 10 years, averaging at five years."

In the twentieth century, thousands of man-made chemicals were introduced into our environment. Now in the twenty-first century, excessive EMF radiation is bombarding our already chemically burdened bodies. These two assaults are creating a perfect storm challenging our bodies' defense systems. We know that our immune systems are already seriously compromised from toxins entering the GI tract and the liver; now we have to contend with this as well.

The new smart meter records when you are home, when you are not, and tracks your usage. An EMF "grid" covers your entire home once a smart meter is installed, emitting electromagnetic frequencies and radiation throughout your home and your body nonstop and with no escape.

Utility companies began installing these in 2009. The new technology allows the energy company to wirelessly transfer customers' energy use back to the utility company. EMF frequencies are classified as nonionizing radiation. So they have been thought to be safe compared to the ionizing radiation that is utilized in atomic bombs and nuclear power plants; however, research is showing that EMFs are now being revealed as biological hazards also.

If your neighbor allows for the smart meter to be installed in his home, you will also experience his EMFs radiating into your home. If, God forbid, your neighbors on both sides have smart meters, you get a double whammy even though you refused to have the smart meter installed. I can feel your frustration through the pages! But there is hope and there are answers. Don't forget that!

You have power with your vote. Next time it comes up, just say no! In the meantime, refuse to have a smart meter installed in your home and explain the dangers to your neighbors. It's time for communities to have meetings to discuss the dangers of today's exposures and toxicants. Working together you can help one another. Education is power and discussion is how it happens.

However, there may be a very simple low-tech way for people to filter out EMFs from their home. Philip S. Callahan is a scientist well-known for his discoveries in paramagnetism. Dr. Callahan has stated that incorporating highly paramagnetic magnetite (an iron oxide) into paint would filter EMFs and reduce a person's exposure. His book *Paramagnetism: Rediscoverng Nature's Secret Force of Growth* goes in depth into how it works. You can also order a sterling silver pendant to protect you from EMFs.

Also, as stated earlier, the nanotechnology company LifeWave makes an inexpensive chip to insert between your cell phone and your cell phone case that protects you from ER (electromagnetic radiation) by 98 percent.

"They" say that the smart meter is a money saver, allowing for the electrical company to eliminate home visits by the "meter reader." If you refuse to have a smart meter installed in your home, expect to have a fine attached to your monthly electrical bill for as long as you hold out. The very thought of this imposition gives me shivers down my spine.

Studies to date have been conflicting. It's difficult to measure what you cannot see with the naked eye. Without information on the health hazards, no self-respecting biochemist or human physiologist would ever have approved installing these grids over entire states, as is slowly being done all over California. Whatever the research uncovers in the future, it clearly makes little sense to install technology that radiates electromagnetic radiation twenty-four hours a day, leaving people with nowhere to go to get away from it. Not even out in public.

Public transportation is subjected to much more radiation because of the tremendous use of cell-phone and Wi-Fi devices by passengers. This has been proven in a study conducted across five European countries. Radiation abounds in trains, buses, and now airplanes with Wi-Fi (plus the added radiation from flying due to the closer contact with the sun and the radiation that is emitted).

As for hybrid and electric vehicles, hybrids that use rear wheels to generate power are small generating plants and create an EMF electrical energy field within the vehicle. Also, solar panels being placed on the car roof to generate power for the car's air conditioner create EMFs. (Those who bought these for the right reasons, protecting the environment, can protect themselves by using grounding pads on the floors and eliminating the use of electronic devices within the car.)

Elizabeth Plourde, Ph.D., in her book *EMF Freedom,* says, "Having been a health consultant for 15 years, I began hearing health complaints from people in Northern California of migraines, insomnia, heart palpitations, and shortness of breath. Then in 2011 after they began to install electric SMART meters in Southern California, the same pattern of symptoms emerged: migraines, insomnia, heart palpitations, shortness of breath, as well as itching skin and rashes."

How will EMFs affect our hearts? How are they affecting us now? We don't know enough to take this collective chance with our already compromised health and overwhelmed planet.

According to renowned cardiologist Dr. Stephen Sinatra, whom you'll hear from later, "EMFs can drive your heart out of rhythm. SMART meters can cause you to go into atrial fibrillation; plus they're very toxic and they destroy DNA. I write letters all the time for patients to get them out of their house, because they're having problems with their hearts."

Then factor in Wi-Fi, the cordless phone, the cellular phone, the cell-phone towers. Experts now think EMFs may open up the blood-brain barrier. We're being bombarded and we've no idea how disastrous that can be to our brains, and to those of our children. Add to that the crappy food everyone is eating and all the toxins and other irritants in the environment that are going right to our brains. It's the perfect storm.

We don't know anything about long-term effects of EMFs, but one can only connect the dots and conclude the effects are not going to be good. So how do we protect ourselves? Keep reading.

CHAPTER 2

OUR BODY'S PROTECTOR SYSTEMS—AND SIGNS THAT SOMETHING IS WRONG

HEALTH BEGINS AND ENDS WITH THE GI TRACT. IT IS OUR FIRST and most important protector. If your gut is inflamed, then you are not healthy. As a result, you will be lacking energy, as well as more susceptible to disease, including autoimmune diseases that will now have the opportunity to flourish. This toxic GI distress will affect every part of your body, including your bones, joints, organs, glands, skin, hormones, and, most important, your BRAIN!

THE FIRST PROTECTOR: THE GI TRACT

As human beings, it behooves us to educate ourselves as to how our body works. In this next section, we will begin that process. Our bodies are incredible machines. Yet to understand the harm that has been done to our digestion from the toxins in the environment and our damaged food supply, it is imperative to know how the internal body mechanisms operate and what they need for optimum performance. Think about this:

> Did you know that if you laid out the GI tract from end to end, it would be approximately the length of a tennis court!

No wonder so many are plagued by stomach problems. That's a lot of distance to cover and keep healthy.

Nature truly is a miracle worker and nowhere is this clearer than in the digestive system. The design is magnificent. The entire length of the digestive (GI) tract is coated with a bacterial layer (like a mucus) surrounding the gut lining that provides a natural barrier against harmful invaders such as undigested food, toxins, and parasites. If this protective bacterial lining gets damaged, your gut wall suffers. This physical barrier is essentially your immune system; 65 percent of your immune system is in the intestines in the form of this "mucus." In addition, a healthy immune system produces organic acids, the beneficial (good) bacteria to reduce pH near the wall of the gut to 4.0 to 5.0, making a very uncomfortable acidic environment for growth and activity of the bad pathogens, which require more alkaline surroundings. Wondrously, this (mucouslike) physical barrier works against invasive pathogens (bad guys) by producing

- Antibiotic-like substances
- Antifungal volatiles (protection from molds, fungus, yeast)
- Antibacterial substances
- Anticancer substances such as interferon

These substances make up the mucous-protective barrier that is your immune system. They act as "guards" to your health. You want to protect these valuable assets.

How does the stomach lining get damaged? Toxins.

A poor high-carb diet of processed, sugar-laden, nonorganic food; the overuse of pharmaceutical drugs (especially antibiotics); as well as the toxic environment and the switch so many have made over the years to chemical household toxic cleaners, fluoride, and chlorine . . . all contribute to digestive tract damage.

These toxins "eat" away at the mucus lining.

When this happens, your health degrades. Think about this with every food choice you make. It doesn't take much in the form of toxins to reach the tipping point, because you, like the rest of us, most likely are already toxic to some degree. Sadly, it's inevitable due to the planetary environmental assault, especially if you already have a chemical belly.

The gut lining also gets shredded from toxic mold exposure, which often takes up residency in the intestines, sinuses, and organs (in particular the brain). When Lyme and/or mold damages the intestinal lining, the first indicators are often food allergies and food intolerances, which is what happened to my granddaughter Violet (you'll read about it in the next chapter).

It Begins with Balance

Balance in the GI tract is essential for good health; that means an equal balance of the good pathogens and the bad. We need both. The good guys (gut flora) neutralize toxic substances like nitrates, indoles, phenols, skatols, antibiotics, and lots of other toxic substances. These "good guys" inactivate histamine and chelate heavy metals and other poisons. The cell walls of beneficial bacteria absorb many carcinogenic substances, making them inactive. They also suppress hyperplasic processes in the gut, which is the basis of all cancer formation.

Good Flora Is a Very Good Thing

If the beneficial bacteria in the gut are imbalanced from a lack of probiotics, then the gut lining gets damaged and stops functioning as it should, because the "barrier" has been compromised. Now, it can't do its job and that's when that nasty chemical belly emerges.

A damaged gut wall allows for viruses, yeast, and fungus (like *Candida albicans*), bacteria, parasites, and toxic substances to leak out and invade the bloodstream. Then the bad guys start roaming around looking for opportunities to attack. These "bugs" are all capable of damaging our digestive system and causing chronic inflammation in the lining. (Here's your bloating, constipation, intestinal pain, etc.) They then go on to attack your organs. (Here's your brain diseases and autoimmune diseases, plus seemingly unrelated conditions like eczema, rosacea, and the like.) When this imbalance happens, the opportunistic (bad) pathogens, which are normally tightly controlled by the good flora (probiotics), are sitting there and ready to cause trouble. But to holistically try to decipher the source of your unique damage to the intestinal lining, we need to look deep. Where and when did it begin? We have to look to that blissful time we spent inside our mother's womb.

Yes, we have to go that far back . . .

It started with your mother! And her mother . . . and her mother.

Nature is perfect, and in that perfection, nature figured out how to colonize our digestive tract from the moment we enter the world. Our very first "swallow" as human beings as we emerge from the birth canal is from our mother's microflora. This important function upon entry into the world provides a perfect environment for a well-functioning GI tract. That vital-for-life journey we each take through our mother's vaginal canal is how nature planned for us to colonize our own GI tract to have a healthy, well-working digestive system and thus immune system. Now factor in that over one million babies are born by cesarean birth each year in this country. That means that those babies never get that first colonization from their mother's vaginal flora as nature intended. This lack of colonization explains why so many children today have intestinal problems. Then factor in all the toxic exposure bombarding our babies, when these children have no intestinal balance to fight the pathogens. It's a setup that medicine is slow to realize. A simple flooding of that baby with probiotics would offset the missed flora; but how many doctors prescribe that in the delivery room?

Here's another little-known fact . . . and this is important, if a mother does not have balanced microflora in her own GI tract, then that's what the baby will inherit (only worse). Balance is the intended plan of nature; lacking it, things start to go awry.

Looking at the GI tract of a pregnant mother is a big step in solving the puzzle of imbalance we see so ubiquitously. It wasn't so long ago that most everyone had a healthy GI tract. But several factors have interrupted the process. The toxic environment and all that entails is a huge component, but so is the ingestion of birth control pills (BCPs). It is thought that the chemicals inherent in these BCPs eat away at the gut lining, upsetting the microflora balance. Here's where ignorance, or plain deceit, comes into play: I remember in the '70s, the freedom and thrill of the new birth control pill. We all thought it was great. I never gave chemicals a thought. Our periods were predictable. We could manipulate them for a "hot date" by continuing to take the pills when we were supposed to be bleeding, to have sex without worrying. Imagine what that kind of interference did to the "nature in us" for those who used them? No one has ever done a study on how many (me included) got breast cancer as a result of this chemical interference in our bodies. But I have to say, when I was diagnosed, it certainly came to my mind as an *I wonder if?* And now, I wonder if these chemicals haven't upset the microflora of a generation of women and their offspring. We know antibiotics upset the GI ecobalance; why wouldn't these BCPs?

My son, Bruce, started his little life with me, a teenage mother. I was a child myself and had no idea how to mother, other than to go by instinct. But Bruce also had a distinct advantage; due to my young age, I had never had a drink of alcohol, never smoked a cigarette (still haven't), never had an antibiotic, and hadn't yet taken BCPs. He was born to a mother with a perfectly healthy functioning body and a perfect GI tract of balanced flora. That's the GI tract he inherited from me.

But unfortunately no one mentioned nursing during my pregnancy, not my doctor, not my mother; I didn't realize my body was even capable. At that time if a teen was pregnant we "had" to get married and that marriage and birth was all wrapped in the shame of that time. I went through an entire nine-month gestation asking as few questions as possible, not wanting to bring attention to my growing stomach, so a query like *Should I nurse?* was never brought up.

As all mothers know, birth is truly a miracle. Nurses put Bruce in my arms, and I instantly fell in love looking at his worried little face. When I was asked by the attending nurse, "Are you breast feeding?" I said, "I don't know." The nurse said, "Well, mother's milk has germs, and baby formula is much better for the baby." Naively, I said, "Well, I want to do what is best for the baby," and before I realized it, I was given a shot that dried up my milk, and all nursing options were off the table. Two weeks into his life I had an overwhelming urge (nature) to nurse, but of course by then, I truly wasn't capable. It's my only life regret.

Baby formula at that time was a racket supported by big government lobbies to get all new mothers to feed their babies formula instead of breast milk. They were hugely successful. Women were deeply involved in women's liberation at that time, wanting the equality and freedom afforded men, which included working full-time in traditional men's jobs. They burned their bras (I couldn't afford to burn my bra!), prevented pregnancy by taking birth control pills, and eschewed nursing for the convenience of baby formula that could be given by the mother or the babysitter or caretaker. They had freedom! But at what cost?

Without the protection of the *high-fat* mother's milk, my baby and all the others of that era were denied a chance of having a perfectly functioning GI tract. The digestive lining requires healthy fats to form the protective barrier that keeps the gut lining intact, as well as to continue aiding the formation of the baby's brain by providing needed fats.

Another contributing factor to our collective GI woes was the low-fat craze (Toxic Threat #2 that you just read about), which was beginning to take hold around that time. If low-fat was good for adults, then the thinking of that time was, it had to be good for babies, so the formula given our babies was low-fat. The train had left the station; by now in the general public, the low-fat myth was well under way. We mothers felt we were doing a good thing for our babies. As a result, many of our babies inherited a poorly functioning digestive system. Now studies are connecting this lack of fat and its resulting GI effects (along with toxins) as key factors involved in autism, ADHD, ADD, OCD, brain fog, asthma, eczema, allergies, dyspraxia, dyslexia, hyperactivity, inability to learn, and mood and behavior problems. (My son, Bruce, had severe asthma for the first thirty-five years of his life. Knowing what I now know, I feel that had I breast-fed, he likely would never have developed it.)

Like you, I did the best I could with what I knew at the time.

But wait, you say . . . what about the children who are lucky enough to be breast-fed? They are fine, right? Well, not so fast. Certainly breast milk is the first, second, and third choice for a new and growing baby. It is protective in so many ways: the prolactin released in breast feeding calms the mother and is protective for her in the future from breast cancer and also protects the child from the same.

But if the mother's gut flora is imbalanced, then that breast milk is not going to be of top quality.

Hopefully, new-thinking doctors understand that when a woman becomes pregnant, or plans to become pregnant, stomach testing for pathogens is vital and a regimen of pre- and probiotics should begin immediately. Making sure a mother's ecosystem is in balance is an essential assignment for all pregnant mothers. It also helps if upon fertilization the father has a GI tract that's in perfect condition; two good stomachs will produce a new, perfectly primed GI system in the next generation. It's that simple.

Probiotics: The Key to Restoration and Balance

I have come to believe that probiotics are the most important supplement one can take, more important than a multivitamin or any other supplement (and you know I am a big believer in supplementation), due to environmental toxins, the damaged soil, and the resulting degradation of our food supply. Probiotics provide balance, allowing for an equal distribution of the good and the bad, and the necessary ecobalance in the human system designed by the Master to protect us from all disease. Dr. Gonzalez is a big believer in probiotics and considers them an important part of his cancer-fighting regimen for his patients.

"When I was in medical school, the word *probiotic* was never once mentioned, ever. The term *normal flora* was never mentioned. I learned about these things on my own and found data going back a hundred years on the value of probiotics. Metchnikoff, the great Russian researcher and Nobel laureate, was the first person to talk about what we call probiotics. He showed that certain bacteria in the gut are critical for normal health, and that disruption of the normal flora could lead to disease. He studied the long-lived people living in isolated areas of Russia at the time, and he realized they always had a source of natural bacteria in their fermented foods like sauerkraut or yogurt, which are nature's own original probiotics.

When you ferment a vegetable, you're actually producing all kinds of healthy bacteria, like the *Lactobacillus* bacteria that is so important for a healthy gut. Metchnikoff came to believe that health and disease both begin in the gut and began recommending yogurt for everybody. If the gut isn't healthy, then *you* aren't healthy. But when I was in medical school, it was like Metchnikoff never existed. I never heard his name, and yet he was a very brilliant conventional researcher. He wasn't some crazy guy, but he was ignored, like he didn't exist, because our medical schools are owned by the pharmaceutical industry. You see, probiotics have nothing to do with pharmacology."

Knowing the answer, I asked Dr. Gonzalez if a person should take probiotics daily. He said, "Well, a person *should only* take a probiotic if he or she wants to maintain good health." I asked him how much probiotic should the average person take for balance, or is there no set amount? He said, "There's no set amount; it depends on the history of the particular person, but for my average patient, I use a Klaire Labs product, which is a basic probiotic with ten strains. But for more therapeutic indications, there are different formulations out there. I like the Ohhira product."

If you don't like "taking" any type of pill or supplement, even though it is highly recommended, I'll show you how to make your own probiotics in Part III of the book. I don't care how you take them, just that you do!

Your Genes or Your Environment?

Think of what people write off as genetics: "My mother had stomach problems; my grandmother had stomach problems. It's part of our genetic makeup." What if you understood that it wasn't genetics but instead was a poorly functioning GI tract passed on for generations? A GI ecosystem that is then being further compromised by poor dietary and lifestyle choices because of a lack of knowledge?

Knowledge and understanding is how *you* become in control of your health and a well-functioning immune and GI system. The choices you make relative to your diet and lifestyle habits determine if you will be in good health or poor health.

Sounds impossible, right? Who among us has a perfect ecosystem in our polluted toxic world? That is why there is an epidemic of GI gut wall problems. We have been hit and hit hard. The fragile but perfect design of the human body and nature in general has been bombarded. Add in all the misinformation about cholesterol and no-fat and low-fat diets, foods sprayed with poisonous chemicals, and being told that certain levels of chemicals are "safe" by the agency formed to protect us, the FDA, and we find ourselves in this catastrophic place.

But you can turn it around. Each one of us can regain our good health through dietary changes and detoxification. Keep reading.

> The use of pesticides has increased exponentially over the past fifty years and continues to increase. A great number of independent studies have shown a link between a number of human health problems, including cancer, allergies, autoimmune disorders, infertility, liver and kidney failure and the use of these products. When combined with the trans generational harmful effects of GMO foods, pesticides represent one of the major risk factors for human disease. With the widespread use of glyphosate-containing herbicides (such as Roundup) in cities and suburbs these pesticide/herbicide toxicities are no longer limited to agricultural lands.
>
> —Dr. Russell Blaylock, neuroscientist

IDENTIFYING THE SYMPTOMS OF BEING *TOX*-SICK

But how do you know if toxicity is truly affecting you? What signs are there to look for to see whether your body's functioning has been compromised or is holding up under the onslaught? I've identified three of the most common and discuss them next: if you're experiencing these, then your body is shouting out to you to make some changes.

Common Symptom #1: A Chemical Belly

> All diseases begin in the stomach.
>
> —Hippocrates

Frankly, it's no surprise that Hippocrates was correct: all problems stem from the gastrointestinal tract, and the GI tract is degraded and made "sick" from toxic exposure. Every doctor in this book will validate Hippocrates's theory. My readers and fans have also validated it through their questions. The biggest one: "What's wrong with my stomach?"

Yes, the question I am asked most often is about the dreaded "chemical belly." If you are plagued by bloating, headaches, digestive problems, unexplained weight gain, chronic fatigue, constipation, brain fog, sleep issues, or autoimmune diseases, you are *tox*-sick, meaning your stomach and your entire GI tract are not functioning correctly due to imbalance and massive chemical exposures. As you are learning, most all of these conditions affect hormonal output, too. The human body is a system; when one part is "off," the rest of the parts lose their abilities to send the correct signaling. If your gut is not healthy, your entire system is not working correctly, and therefore you are not healthy. This common complaint is an indicator that most everyone is experiencing, and it's their first "wake-up" to their individual toxic burden.

Look around you—chemical bellies are affecting most everyone: children (even babies), teenagers, women, and men. No one is exempt. The phenomenon knows no economic or cultural barrier. If you are human and alive, you need to be concerned. A bloated, aching, cramping, or swollen stomach are the symptoms, and they are your body talking to you, screaming at you.

This is your body's language; your stomach is talking to you. It's important to learn to listen to this language, just as I have told you throughout my other books about listening to your body's signals of hormone decline. These symptoms are so pervasive, so widespread, that they have become normal. How often are you hearing people say they are allergic to gluten or some other food? Restaurateurs are tearing their hair out trying to accommodate the new growing demands of their patrons: no dairy, no gluten, no soy, no eggs.

Most people are not connecting the dots. You walk into a freshly cleaned area and your eyes water or your nose starts dripping. What is that about? How many times have you said upon walking into a room, "I'm allergic to something!" Why are we accepting these allergies as the new norm and making excuses for our stomach upset, drippy noses, sneezing, coughing, or red eyes? Why? Here's the deal:

By the time you become symptomatic, your body is on overload. Your liver is groaning. These accepted everyday symptoms are your body's way of finally saying, "I give."

You aren't alone. Most everyone is experiencing to some degree or another reactions that have been accepted as normal.

How is your belly? Have you found it doesn't matter how much you work out or how little you eat, you just can't contain it? You suck it in, but it's still there. And it's uncomfortable; do you always have slight cramping, discomfort? Can you not depend on being able to wear that favorite dress because you might be bloated that night?

Men experience it, too. When you see a guy in an unbuttoned sports jacket, you can bet your belly it's because he has a chemical belly. Personally, I've had a terrible bloating problem. I had all the tests (blood, stool, etc.), checking for every possible scenario in my quest to find the culprit. I am not fat. I was eating (as far as I was concerned) perfectly. I grow my own vegetables; I cook most of our meals at home. I have good diet and lifestyle habits, but I had this stomach I couldn't count on. Sometimes in the morning I would wake up and it was nearly flat, then by the end of the day something happened and I looked like I was about to deliver a basketball.

It got noticed in candid paparazzi photos, which was humiliating, but most of all it was very uncomfortable (and, I now know, dangerous). Clearly something was wrong. I didn't know I had mold fungus in my GI tract. But it's not only me; I'm hearing this from women all over this country and in other parts of the world. My tests said bacterial overgrowth and high toxicity. How did that happen? I wondered. Where did the bacteria come from? Why was my digestive tract unable to manage the toxic load in my body, which is the job of the gut wall? Why was mine damaged?

What happened to me, as well as to my family, drove me to take on this subject. Our GI tracts get imbalanced, and all that most doctors do is throw pills at us. This is not the solution.

Discovering the reasons for your stomach discomfort takes detective work. For starters, any of you who have read my book *Knockout* know from the opening chapter about my being misdiagnosed with inoperable full-body cancer (the doctors were wrong). In my distress at being diagnosed, and also being in anaphylactic shock, I found myself in a hospital room with IVs in both arms that, unfortunately, I did not question. (Fear does that.) I was on IV antibiotics for six days straight, day and night, antibiotics pouring through my body, killing *everything,* and that means the good and the bad. My stomach was never "right" from that time on. At that time I did not understand the *crucial* role of probiotics. Had I understood, I might have been able to offset the damage the antibiotics were doing by replacing probiotics to rebalance the gut microflora. The antibiotics essentially "sterilized" my GI tract. Without the presence of good flora, the bad pathogens took over and had a field day. The bad guys "ate" through the wall of my GI tract and caused leaky gut, allowing the entire load of bad flora (pathogens) to leak out and start attacking other parts of my system.

This is how food allergies and intolerances begin, along with autoimmune diseases. It all starts with a disrupted gut wall. Think how many have been diagnosed with MS, or fibromyalgia, or lupus when in fact it's actually a result of an imbalanced GI ecosystem. A *qualified* doctor who has chosen to step out of the orthodox allopathic box would understand what to look for. The GI tract has a direct link to the brain; in fact, the GI tract is called the "second brain." For my condition, correcting the damage to my gut wall was imperative, before I became another of the many people experiencing brain deterioration as in brain fog or worse. (You'll read about that next.) That's what an imbalanced ecosystem can do. I needed to find out what and why this phenomenon was happening to not only me but to so many of us. I've spent the last three years researching and interviewing, and it thrills me to pass on this information to you.

Common Symptom #2: Foggy Brain

> Unfortunately, I predict disaster in the next twenty years for today's children who are so widely and intensely affected now by toxins that when they reach thirty and forty they are going to be sick and dying . . . in much greater numbers than today. So I pray that people start paying attention.
>
> —Dr. Russell Blaylock, neuroscientist

Foggy brain is a new phenomenon in recent years. Yes, there have always been crazy people and dementia, and women have been made fun of for who knows how long for being "scatterbrained." But this is something new. The GI tract speaks directly to the brain at all times; when the tract is off and not working properly, it can explain away a lot of the forgetfulness, depression, and hormonal deficiencies that plague so many. How would hormones be affected by the GI tract? you ask. It's all about the gut/brain connection. Some of the important "feel good" hormone, serotonin, is made in the intestinal tract. The rest is made in the brain. Serotonin "speaks" to the epicenter of the hormone system, the hypothalamus, which resides . . . you guessed it, in the brain. If the GI tract is distressed and not working properly, then serotonin does not get delivered to the brain, so the HPA axis, (hypothalamus/pituitary axis) does not get the proper signals to activate the hormonal system through its conductor, the thyroid. If the thyroid is not activated properly, the rest of the hormones in the body don't know what to do. Now you've got chaos, mood swings, fatigue, no libido, depression, and a body out of control. All because your stomach is in distress. You have bloating, constipation, and more. It's that simple and it is that complex.

Common Symptom #3: Unexplained Weight Gain

My daughter by marriage is Leslie Hamel: I love her as my own; we work together, play together, and have a deep connection. She is beautiful, talented, and lovable. Her story is one of frustration and confusion, and resonant with the toxicity of today. She eats right; she takes good care of herself. Yet out of the blue she experienced unexplained weight gain, chronic stomach distress, and devastating fatigue that was alarming and depressing. Read about it in Leslie's own words:

> It all started ten years ago when I found myself looking swollen, my face and my body. I was constantly tired and constantly bloated, even if I hadn't eaten anything. By 10 a.m. every day I would start getting a terrible stomachache, and by 3 p.m. I felt exhausted. I was working out with a trainer and eating well: high protein and veggies, low carbs, almost no sugar. Yet I was gaining weight and felt awful.
>
> All of my doctors told me to "cut down on the goodies," but there were no goodies to cut out of my diet—I didn't realize that the very small amounts of sugar I was eating could possibly be a problem. I felt so help-

less, and as a last-ditch resort, I went to a nutritionist, outlined all of my symptoms, and gave her my food diary. She suggested that I take a food allergy test. The test results showed that I was highly allergic to eggs, which I had been eating daily.

I stopped eating eggs and took digestive enzymes and HCL with my meals and continued my low-carb/almost-no-sugar regimen, along with working out . . . Still, nothing changed. My nutritionist told me to stick with it, that it would take time for my cells to release the toxins I'd built up from the eggs. After about a month, I started looking and feeling much better, but the weight loss was slow and discouraging. Finally, after three months, the weight literally melted off me very quickly and I lost twenty pounds. I went back to normal.

About a year ago, though, the bloating and stomachaches started coming back. Soon after, I began gaining weight—the progression was fast and I gained twenty pounds almost overnight. My face and body became chronically swollen, my eyes were bleary, and I didn't look like myself anymore. Even the way the fat felt on my body was not like regular fat; it felt like swollen tissue. It was very obvious that the weird, firm fat on my body wasn't normal fat.

I couldn't gain control of what was happening to me.

One morning I woke up and my eyes were almost swollen shut. I thought that I might have a terrible disease that had gone unchecked; my doctor suggested that I start doing IV infusions of vitamin C and glutathione, which helped somewhat, and my extreme swelling seemed to go down a tiny bit, but not much.

I called Suzanne, who called Dr. Gonzalez; he spoke to me about everything that was going on with me and asked me to come to him for a physical exam. After, he looked over all my blood work and suggested that I aggressively start detoxing my body.

He said that my body was so toxic that it couldn't process anything; my liver was kicking out the toxins into my bloodstream, so it was all building up and essentially "overdosing" me with chemicals.

It has been about two months that I have been doing all the detox stuff. I have lost seven pounds (with twenty to go) and I look and feel better, but not all better. The swelling in my face has subsided, but not all the way; my eyes are finally clear, and the fat on my body is changing and seems less swollen, but I still have a ways to go with this; still, there is finally a light at the end of the tunnel. I may never know what in particular caused this toxicity to build up in me, but it is clear that my body has reached a saturation point when a single tiny bite of sugar causes a huge setback and throws everything off. My little bite of Halloween candy made me gain two pounds overnight and look and feel terrible the next morning.

Regular dieting cannot help me. I have to be vigilant about everything I put into my body and continue doing my detox regimen. Even though the progress has been slow, I finally feel that I have found the way to regain my health.

It is important to keep in mind that many of today's toxins are stored in the fat tissues of our body and can remain there for a lifetime. Studies have shown that many people have over one hundred such toxic chemicals stored in their fat tissues for decades or even a lifetime. Suddenly losing a lot of fat weight can release these toxic chemicals into the bloodstream, redistributing them to such tissues as the brain and heart. With a sudden loss of body fat (as with dieting) such a massive release of multiple toxic chemicals and toxic metals from the fat tissue can occur as to cause one to appear as if they were acutely poisoned. While death would be uncommon, significant sickness probably occurs much more often. This can manifest as debilitating fatigue, clouded thinking, confusion, difficulty concentrating, heart problems, infertility, a loss of sexual drive and a number of other symptoms that can be difficult for the average physician to diagnose. Many toxic metals, such as lead, fluoride, and mercury, are stored in the bones in very high concentrations for decades. With aging, one frequently experiences a loss of bone, which releases these metals into the bloodstream, and again, are redistributed to other tissues, such as the brain, kidneys, liver and heart. Fracturing a bone can also release these metals. Unless your doctor measures blood levels (and RBC levels) of these metals, he or she will not appreciate the real cause of your sudden illness. In fact, in most such cases the doctor adds a number of toxic prescriptions to the brew in a vain effort to make you feel better.

—Dr. Russell Blaylock, neuroscientist

My heart broke for Leslie during this time. Clearly her toxic burden was overwhelming her body. The bad pathogens in her GI tract were standing by, just waiting for even the teeniest amount of sugar in order to start reproducing again. They don't need much when you are as toxic as Leslie. Was it restaurant food (she dines out often) or a leak in her home causing undetected mold, or was it just years of toxic exposure building up to where finally her body reached a tipping point?

Are you experiencing anything similar, but hopefully less drastic? Have you been eating less and working out more and getting fatter? Sadly, that is the new phenomenon. After reading Leslie's story, you may now realize that perhaps your unexplained weight gain is a result of your own personal toxic burden. The more chemicals you take in or are exposed to, the more fat you need as storage. It's your body's way of saving your life in the meantime.

The wisdom in *you* knows the human body was never meant to handle this massive toxic assault, so to protect your precious organs and glands, the brain has creatively directed your chemicals to your fat for storage. That's your cellulite. People often remark that at my age I have no cellulite, and it's because I consciously go out of my way to avoid chemicals whenever and wherever I am, and I believe that has made the difference. So it's a good news/bad news scenario; until you reach your chemical tipping point, the poison is still in your fat. Your organs and glands are protected (for now); the bad news is that you have all this extra weight.

How to get rid of it? Here's the real good news: You don't have to diet!

Imagine losing weight without dieting, and imagine achieving your perfect natural body composition eating healthy fats and high-quality great-tasting organic protein. You are in control of your health and weight by simply reincorporating the foods you've been warned to avoid (healthy dietary fats) and most important eliminating all chemical so-called foods, including sugars. By now I hope you are convinced that healthy dietary fats are not the enemy. The weight that has stubbornly refused to leave the premises will slowly melt away by emptying out your fat cells with a change in *what* you eat and the *way* you eat. This change in diet will naturally begin the detox process of the chemicals that have taken up residency in your digestive tract and your fat cells.

The world has changed. Toxicity is slowly killing us in a variety of ways. These changes in the environment as well as to our food supply, compounded by everyday stress (which is at an all-time high), are the reasons we've hit a wall not only in our wellness but in trying to lose weight. Toxicity is not going away, so how do we survive and how do we lose weight?

As a general rule, we don't understand how to eat. For the most part we don't understand nutrition as fuel, the gasoline that makes the body work. We all know that high-octane gas makes cars work better. But we give our cars (i.e., our bodies) sugar instead; and you know what that does to an engine. If you have yeast, candida, fungus, mold, and other bad pathogens in your GI tract and you feed yourself sugar in any form, you are going to have problems. Until you clean out your body, the combination of toxins and sugar are a "happy meal" for your gut. Until you are detoxed and you reestablish your ecobalance with probiotics and strict adherence to a no-sugar, no-carb diet, you will likely experience the same scenario as my daughter, Leslie. It's that sensitive at this point.

Obesity is a problem with today's children; let's look at the typical school meal provided in elementary school. For breakfast they are offered pancakes, for lunch it's macaroni and cheese, a white flour roll, and apple juice. Consider what these meals are composed of:

Pancakes: trans fats, white flour, and sugar (no nutrition)
Macaroni and cheese: white flour (no nutrition); cheese, man-made chemicals (toxic)
Apple juice: no fiber plus pesticides and added sugar (toxic)

As you can read, this menu is not food. Yet these are typical meals for so many in this country, not just our children. Our palates have become used to the taste of chemicals, which have been designed to taste scrumptious and cause addiction. Sadly, but predictably, these poor eating habits easily explain the epidemic of obesity and poor health we are currently experiencing.

Our bodies have wisdom; innately our body "knows" that these chemicals are dangerous to our health, so the brain takes over help-

ing us by *storing* the toxins for us. In order to keep the dangerous toxins away from our precious organs and glands, the toxins instead get
stored in the fat! Here's the equation and the answer to the puzzle:

The more toxins you take in through your skin, lungs, or stomach
(eating), the more fat you need for storage.

- The more toxins, the more fat.
- The more fat, the more toxins, and so on and so on.

This is the obesity problem.

If you are holding excess weight (unless you are overeating an excessive amount of sugar and carbs), you are fat from toxins.

Did you realize the higher the pesticide levels in your blood, the
slower you burn calories while you are sleeping or sedentary? If you
have a slow metabolism, you have more body fat. The effect chlorinated pesticides have on metabolism was revealed in a study that
gauged how efficiently mitochondria (energy center of your cells)
used fatty acids for fuel. The higher the blood levels of pesticides and
PCBs, the fewer fatty acids were burned. This means that besides
burning fewer calories, a person will be more likely to gain weight
and have a difficult time losing it.

The point is, toxins make you fat and sick.

If this resonates with you, I highly urge you to read my book *Sexy
Forever*. It is an in-depth look at the toxic burden that is making people
fat and will give you every tool necessary (including recipes) to shed
the fat and shed the toxins. It is loaded with information that took me
years to compile and was the missing piece to my own issues with
unexplained weight gain.

THE SECOND PROTECTOR: YOUR LIVER

Let me explain the importance of a healthy well-working liver in addition to a well-functioning GI tract.

The liver, which deserves great respect, performs over a thousand
tasks daily and filters every drop of blood that flows through it. The
liver produces chemicals to combat viruses and bacteria, supports
phagocytosis (cell-eating), and produces antihistamines to neutralize

substances that promote the growth of cancer. It is such a powerhouse that scientists estimate that up to 80 percent of the liver can be damaged without producing any symptoms! Plus, the liver regenerates itself every six weeks. This is truly amazing! In his 1994 article entitled "The Liver, Laboratory of Living," Dr. Leo Roy states, "No disease, especially degenerative diseases including cancer and AIDS, could survive longer than a few weeks in the presence of a healthy liver." In his book, *The Liver and Cancer*, Dr. Kasper Blond refers to the liver as the "gateway to disease." In that book, he states, "No other stimulus is necessary (for the growth of cancer) than a metabolic toxin which has not passed the liver filter or has not been neutralized owing to liver failure."

The liver processes nutrients coming in from the intestines and neutralizes toxins from food and anywhere else in the body. The pancreas, like the liver, is another accessory digestive organ that secretes both insulin (which manages sugar metabolism) and pancreatic enzymes. These enzymes not only are necessary for the digestion of proteins, fats, and carbohydrates, but researchers now understand that these enzymes are also crucial as a defense against cancer. A defect in any of these digestive organs can ultimately have catastrophic effects, such as cancer. It's important to consider that the intestines are not only a digestive organ but a critically important immune center. The basis of Dr. Nicholas Gonzalez's protocol (which you will read in an upcoming chapter) is taking pancreatic enzymes and liver flushes daily. His patients get well and stay well by utilizing this daily regimen.

The liver is key for detoxification, but with the onslaught of chemicals from the environment almost no one has a well-working liver. Yet as stated above, the liver can be 80 percent toxic without your feeling any symptoms. I suspect this was also the problem with Leslie.

Now that you are starting to see the importance of a healthy liver for overall health and functioning of the human body, you can understand that this is why when the liver is malfunctioning, among many other problems, your hormones will be out of balance. More on that in a minute. Just know, it's all connected; the human body is an entire system. Each subsystem (e.g., the GI tract, the liver, the pancreas) depends on the health of the other subsystems for your entire body to be well.

The liver will work overtime for you until it becomes chronically fatigued; then the body starts experiencing an array of negative side effects. Since the liver has had to do much more than its share, most likely because of toxic blood caused by a clogged large intestine, the liver now has to pass on this burden to the kidneys. But your kidneys are weak from the added pressure of your colon being dysfunctional prior to your sluggish liver situation. Chronic low-back pain can set in due to all the unwanted toxic poisons, and then other symptoms appear: sweaty palms, bags under the eyes, frequent urination, and bladder infections. When the kidneys can no longer handle the toxic load, the bladder gets stressed. This is the domino effect. It starts with a toxic colon, then the blood gets "dirty" from toxemia, then the liver is affected, then the kidneys, then the bladder, and then the lymph system becomes toxic.

At this point the only thing you can do is cleanse and detox. And eliminate fast foods, processed foods, sugars, and all avoidable toxins.

Hormone Imbalance and the Liver Connection

Dr. Nick Gonzalez speaks in depth about the importance of optimum liver function in his interview (page 88). The liver is responsible for using metabolic enzymes to properly handle all the chemical compounds we are exposed to, which include hormones, medications, environmental toxins, and the natural beneficial phytochemicals in foods. The liver also has to metabolize estrogens.

A healthy woman with a low toxic burden won't have the same uphill battle in balancing missing or declining hormones as a woman whose body is environmentally poisoned with an overload of toxins. If your liver is toxic, you will have a difficult time (among many other problems and bodily complaints) absorbing and metabolizing hormone replacement, too. Also, many people can't get on top of their health (or their weight) due to thyroid imbalance. Thyroid is an important hormone and when it isn't functioning properly, the whole body becomes discordant. Thyroid and toxins do not go well together.

In today's world, most everyone has a sluggish liver. Not paying attention to the symptoms of a dysfunctional liver can create a "perfect storm" of illness for a person who requires hormone replacement for optimum quality of life. He or she cannot feel the relief of symptoms that accompanies hormone balance because the liver is so toxic it literally kicks the hormones out into the bloodstream. At this point the liver is groaning, overloaded with chemicals, pesticides, and other toxins and now cannot handle even one more molecule, including hormones. The glass is full. One more drop and it will spill over. The severity of contamination will determine the time it takes to clean out your liver. If your liver is not functioning at optimum, you will not ever get well, feel good, or be able to benefit from hormone replacement.

So many women write me and tell me that "hormones don't work for me." I took this concern seriously and discussed it with my top doctors. It's clear from those discussions that in reality it's their livers that cannot tolerate BHRT (bioidentical hormone replacement therapy). So they should focus first on detoxification of the liver, so they can benefit and tolerate hormone replacement. Hormones are metabolized in the liver, but if your liver is damaged, toxic, or sluggish, as was said before, your hormones don't get metabolized and then they back up into the blood; then, of course, you can end up *overdosed* and toxic from excessive hormones. That explains why some women start on hormone replacement and freak out because they suddenly feel worse, or they gain weight and suffer a myriad of other symptoms. Again, a toxic liver won't metabolize hormones when it is full up with contaminants. It's overworked. It can't do the job. It's not that these women don't need BHRT; it's the state of their toxic livers "talking" through these symptoms. You can't be deaf to the "language" of the liver.

When the liver kicks out these hormones, it puts the body into a toxic state, causing many terrible effects: tremendous weight gain (even if you are eating almost nothing), puffy face, swollen eyes, lower back pain, thyroid disruptions, brain fog, depression, inability to sleep, and even chronic fatigue.

You are also playing with fire because toxins are not being filtered and can now roam freely throughout your bloodstream looking to cause trouble. When the liver kicks out the "junk," those toxins can back up into the portal vein and then go directly into the GI tract, creating leaks in the intestines. Those toxins then sneak out looking for organs of opportunity. Now you are in a dangerous place, cancer being one of the dangers.

That's how important it is to get your liver working right. The only way to rectify the problem is to clean your liver. Otherwise, you will never be truly well.

My book *I'm Too Young for This!* is my most comprehensive book on hormones of all my hormone books. If hormones are a mystery to you, if hormones are not understood by your doctor (they don't teach BHRT in medical school), then I strongly urge you to read that book. It will answer all your questions about replacement, symptoms, what they mean, and how to find the right doctor.

For those of you who have already experienced the joys of hormone replacement and the glorious return of quality of life, but have reached this toxic crossroad, here's what you need to do: To get the relief of hormone replacement that suddenly just isn't working for you, it's time to look at cleaning out your liver. (The "recipes" for cleaning out your liver are on page 263.)

PART II

BULLETPROOFING YOUR BODY AND HOME

INTERVIEWS WITH DOCTORS
WHO ARE MAKING A DIFFERENCE

CHAPTER 3

THE GUT

The interconnectedness of your gut, brain, immune, and hormonal systems is impossible to unwind. The past few years have brought a scientific flurry of information about how crucial your microflora are to your genetic expression, immune system, body weight and composition, mental health, memory, and minimizing your risk for numerous diseases.

—DR. JOSEPH MERCOLA, MERCOLA.COM

DO YOU HAVE ANY OF THE FOLLOWING?
fatigue and low energy
fungal or yeast infection
unexplained weight gain
diarrhea
constipation
frequent urination
stress
anxiety
joint pain
skin problems
blurry vision
brain fog
acid reflux
hemorrhoids
gas/bloating
poor immune function
acne
eczema
rosacea

If you check even one of these symptoms, then you need probiotics daily, and most likely for the rest of your life. Everyone alive needs the proper balance of gut flora for optimal health. This is achieved by replacing the missing good bacteria.

When you heal your gut, then the rest of your organs (including the liver) will follow suit. A balanced GI tract will affect the health of your entire body, and as I have discovered, you most likely won't need to take any pharmaceutical drugs to stay well. Wisdom says this can only be a good thing. When you heal your gut and all is working well, you can also easily be thin for life. Isn't that a dreamy thought?

Turns out the most essential building blocks for our gut are healthy dietary fats, as discussed earlier. These healthy fats create the protection for the GI barrier wall, keeping the immune system working optimally and locking toxins inside to eventually be neutralized and then eliminated. Without dietary fats, the toxins are free to roam in our bloodstreams, damaging our health, our livers, and our GI tracts.

> Imagine a swimming pool. When its sides are intact all around, it holds the water. But if the pool has cracks, the water will then leak out. This is exactly the example to explain your GI tract. The healthy fats create the mucus walls (also 65 percent of your immune system) of the swimming pool as a barrier. If toxins eat through the mucus fats, then the toxins leak out into the bloodstream. That's where your problems are coming from.

Bring on the butter! Organic healthy fats are not only delicious but perform vital functions of human health. A lack of healthy fats is one problem plaguing people's health, but there are also so many things that are working against us in today's world, for instance chlorine. Chlorinated water kills harmful bacteria in drinking water, but it also kills the good bacteria in your digestive tract. Chlorine is one of the toxins in today's environment that are responsible for the massive assault on our gut.

Toxins running rampant in the GI tract overtake the good flora and then problems begin. Probiotics are your "good flora" replacement. Each *body* is different and an imbalance in gut flora manifests in different ways for different people. But it all comes back to the same thing. If your GI tract is distressed and the microflora are imbalanced, you will suffer with one or all of the symptoms listed above. Several factors, both internal and external, can cause a dramatic impact on the overall level of health and well-being of your beneficial (good) bacteria. They include over-the-counter and prescription drugs (including antibiotics), as well as cortisone and birth control pills, all of which wear down the normal levels of good bacteria in your intestines. Also, radiation and chemotherapy treatments, environmental pollutants, food additives, alcohol, tobacco smoke, and stress (big one) all negatively impact good bacteria. What you eat or don't eat is another critical factor. And unfortunately, a lot of the good bacteria is lost as part of the natural aging process (aging is about worn-out parts).

Probiotics need mentioning once again. They are health-promoting bacteria that, when introduced into the intestinal tract, replenish and help the body digest and absorb food as well as fight off illnesses and disease. Most friendly bacteria come from

- *Lactobacillus*: guards your small intestine
- *Bifidobacterium*: protects your large intestine
- *Lactobacillus bulgaricus*: found in yogurt and is a transient bacteria that aids the first two as it passes through your body
- Soil-based organisms, or SBOs

SBOs are beneficial bacteria that live in the soil. Until the nineteenth century, SBOs formed a regular part of our diet. But food processing has replaced eating real food like healthy fruits and vegetables (if you can pick it, pluck it, milk it, or shoot it—eat it), and our health has diminished as a result. Today's food supply and modern agricultural practices include powerful pesticides, fungicides, and germicides, as well as chemical and heat-based food processing, which are all toxic to SBOs. The soil has been raped of its health. But don't let that deter you; nutritional supplementation beyond probiotics is essential to live healthy today. (More on supplementation in Part III.)

Our gut contains about three and a half pounds of beneficial bacteria and these bacteria produce essential vitamins and hormones. SBOs are a vital source that help your digestive system to break down fats, proteins, and carbohydrates as well as to digest wastes such as toxins that enter the body through your food and breathing.

Did you know that both good and bad bacteria have the ability to divide every twenty minutes to form two new microorganisms? This means by the end of an eight-hour period, one little microorganism can produce about 42.5 million microorganisms.

Now imagine your GI tract is already imbalanced and then you eat a bag of sugary chemical cookies of some sort. The bad guys jump for joy. Yippee! What a bonanza! A happy meal! This is what happened to Leslie. For her, even a bite of sugar started the process. If in your GI tract there aren't enough "good guys" on patrol to overtake and wipe out the growth of negative organisms, the bad guys win this one. Now you have a big mess to deal with. This is exactly what would cause my stomach to blow up like a basketball for what I thought was no reason. Giving up sugar and taking daily probiotics changed this scenario for me, but it took ten months of restriction to accomplish. I will never go back to my other way of eating. I'm thinner and healthier and have lost the constant discomfort of "chemical belly." Remember this: Whatever progress you have made with your dietary restrictions trying to create balance in your gut to get rid of the bloat, cramping, gas, constipation, and unexplained weight gain will be given a setback if you lose control and indulge in sugar and processed foods. Don't worry, eventually when you achieve healing, you will be able to reincorporate certain foods in small amounts, but you might (as with me) no longer desire sugar or carbs. My cravings have gone away and now I "get off" on healthy fats. They satiate me. Ironic: I started eating fats, gave up sugar and carbs, and got thin.

GO PRO, NOT ANTI

It's worth repeating: the overuse of antibiotics has been a disaster for the GI tract and is also problematic due to lack of understanding on the part of most orthodox doctors that probiotics are a necessity to offset an antibiotic.

- *Anti*biotic takes away.
- *Pro*biotic puts back.

Probiotics were around long before modern medicine but are just being recognized by modern scientists to maintain or restore health. Probiotics are the beneficial bacteria taken by capsule or powder, or obtained through fermented foods, to repopulate that which is missing in your GI tract to have gut health.

Antibiotics not only kill off and sterilize your enemies (bad pathogens) but also kill off the good guys, leaving us defenseless. The bad guys can replenish more quickly than the good bacteria, and when that happens, all toxins and good food alike entering your stomach get absorbed into your bloodstream and then are turned into dangerous toxic pathogens. That's when digestion begins to suffer; that's when leaky gut gets activated; that's when your food allergies are triggered; and that's when your autoimmune disease gets the green light.

It's no mystery where autoimmune problems originate. Scientists keep "looking for the cure," but it's simple. Forever Health doctors understand that the cure is not more pharmaceutical drugs; the cure comes from diet and a balanced ecosystem free of toxicity. That's why probiotics are so essential. Without supplementation of probiotics you can expect to live with and create a chronically unhealthy condition in your GI tract and brain. Without a healthy GI tract . . . *YOU* are not healthy.

LAXATIVES AND ANTACIDS: WHY YOU SHOULD AVOID THEM

Laxatives

Bowel movements depend on peristaltic action to move things along. The contraction of these muscles that line the walls of the small intestine prevents bad bacteria from setting up residence. These muscles (peristaltic action) coupled with lots of good bacteria (found in probiotics) discourage bad bacteria from setting up house. When this peristaltic action slows down (with laxatives), overgrowth of the bad guys is not only possible but probable.

Overusing laxatives is why your peristalsis stops. Here you are taking laxatives to move your bowels, but the laxative itself is inhibiting the body's ability to move your bowels easily the next day. Now you are hooked. Some people use laxatives their whole lives. So you are saying to yourself, *Then I'll just take laxatives forever!* Well, it's not so easy; dependence never allows your intestines to heal and then your peristaltic mechanism stops working forever. Your intestines will become "lazy" and then "forget" their responsibilities. The result will be chronic stomach pain, discomfort, and weight gain.

If you are guilty of overusing laxatives, you can strengthen your function by taking probiotics to keep the microflora in your intestines balanced so the bad bugs can't find any place to attach themselves. Laxatives are good for extreme constipation when even enemas won't help, but you should discontinue them as soon as possible, to get your body to start working on its own. And of course, a correct diet is imperative. You have to give yourself the right food and enough good fats to aid and assist in this mechanism of peristalsis and its wondrous ability to function properly. A person who is not constipated feels good and light and energetic and loses weight, has better hair and skin and glowing eyes. Constipation creates the opposite. It's worth it to tackle and heal your situation.

Antacids

People pop antacids like candy. Go to any drugstore and the shelves are lined with different brands. What you must know is the relief you get is momentary, which accounts for repeated use throughout the day. But the most important takeaway is that antacids exacerbate your problem . . . they ultimately make it worse.

Antacids are designed to neutralize and absorb the acid secretions of the digestive tract, but hydrochloric acid is a major player in your gastric juices. These juices are vital for proper digestion of food and destroy harmful bacteria that would otherwise impair your digestive tract.

Your GI tract must have hydrochloric acid for proper function. Antacids actually "take away" more acid from your GI tract, which is the opposite of what your body is asking for; you momentarily get relief because that burning feeling goes away. But your burning feeling is actually the language of your body telling you that your body isn't making *enough* hydrochloric acid (HCL) and what your GI tract actually wants is *more* acid in the form of HCL. So by taking *ant*-acid (as in *anti*-acid), you take away more acid, which is the exact opposite of what you need. Instead, purchase supplemental HCL, which is available in most drugstores (I order mine from the Tahoma Clinic in Washington State; it's called Betaine HCL). Take one with every meal. If there is no burning, then take two; your body will tell you when you reach a "tolerance point." Burning is the indicator. If you start to feel the burn, then eliminate one capsule at a time. It is also important to take HCL only during meals (not before, not after). You are trying to mimic what your body once did on its own. HCL is naturally released in the body when a person consumes food. This is how we digest our food. Without it, the acid will "back up" into the esophagus, causing discomfort. The throat and esophagus were not designed to handle any acid.

Note: If you have had radiation treatment for breast cancer, it eliminates your body's ability to make hydrochloric acid FOR LIFE! (This is one of the things they don't tell you when you have radiation.) That's why you have reflux and chronic indigestion. In that case, you, like me, might need more per meal. I find to eliminate reflux and stomach burning, I need to take four capsules per meal. It's a lot of pills, but I am preventing esophageal cancer, which comes from irritation to the esophagus from reflux, and I'm also keeping my GI tract lining healthy by giving it what it wants. Prescription drugs like Nexium, and so on, are a Band-Aid and never heal or cure. Most drugs are designed to keep you on them for life.

Probiotics will be as life-changing to medicine in the twenty-first century as antibiotics were when they came on the scene in the twentieth century. Today's doctors who are on the front lines of medicine are recognizing the limitations of conventional medicine, and in particular the overuse of antibiotics. In many cases, these drugs have been rendered ineffective just when they are needed most. A number of harmful bacteria, such as certain strains of *Staphylococcus aureus*, are becoming resistant to them.

Antibiotics kill the bad guys and, unfortunately, the good guys. When the good bacteria are weak or in small numbers or nonexistent, the field is left wide open for microbes. That is what happened to me after six days in the hospital for a minimally invasive biopsy (it turned out to be a misdiagnosis). Six days of IV antibiotics (which in retrospect I did not need) left my stomach in shreds. I did not understand the need for probiotics to offset the antibiotics at that time. This was the beginning of my stomach problems that then became compounded by mold and toxins. If you have yeast, mold, or a toxic gut, you will most likely have developed *Candida albicans,* a nasty yeast that, when given the opportunity, proliferates and transforms into a dangerous fungus that can wreak havoc with your immune system.

BYE-BYE SUGAR AND CARBS

Right now you must know:

> If you want to heal your gut, you cannot have sugar and you cannot have carbs! (For now.)

There; I said it. Sorry. This is the magic combination for winning your health back: no sugar and no carbs until you are healed. During this time you will consume plenty of healthy fats and animal protein, and plenty of delicious vegetables, along with probiotics and this detox program. You will not be hungry.

If you only take away one thing from this book, take this. This simple message is the most important change you can make: **No sugar, no carbs (until you are healed)**. You will see and feel a tremendous difference in the first thirty days. But total healing will take time, maybe a year or two depending on your damage. It is worth it to give up these foods while you are bringing your body back to health.

I realize giving up these foods is a hardship, but if you don't bite the bullet at some point and do this, your stomach issues will never go away and you will keep on getting fatter and sicker and your stomach will keep on being a gas machine. It's that important.

A CAUTIONARY FAMILY TALE:
INTERVIEWS WITH VIOLET AND CAROLINE

Sometimes the best way to really identify with a condition is to hear a personal story. It's hard to connect the dots that your bloating could affect your brain, but reading my granddaughter Violet's interview will help you to understand how it can take a perfectly healthy and happy person and degrade her life until it is no longer recognizable.

It happened to her and took away her quality of life during fun childhood times when all her fourteen-year-old friends were enjoying normal lives. Instead, Violet was battling an enemy she could not understand. It was heartbreaking to watch and not be able to help. I have asked Violet if she could tell her story in her words, of her journey and the cascade of bodily discomfort and brain disruption that resulted. To say I love Violet is an understatement. I was anguished watching her go through this horrific ordeal. To hear her tell it will help you to understand what you might be experiencing, or perhaps what someone in your family is going through.

SS: Thank you, sweet Violet, for sharing your story. You are sixteen years old, but because of what you've been through, you have the wisdom of someone twice your age.

How old were you when you realized that something just didn't feel right in the way your body was working?

VS: I was around thirteen; I only remember that it was an age where I didn't feel like I could eat anything I wanted anymore and look the same way every day. I couldn't depend on my body feeling right and I couldn't depend on my stomach not being bloated. I was also starving . . . I would be so hungry. As soon as I stopped eating, I would be starving again. It would happen after every meal. It was an insane feeling. I didn't seem to be in control of myself; I could never get enough. For me it felt like the world was ending. I felt like I wanted my life to be over. I didn't know what I was going to do, but I was filled with the feeling that everyone was going to hate me and that the worst thing in the world was going to happen. It's a horrible and awful way to feel. I felt completely out of control.

SS: Did you talk to anybody about it?

VS: I was too embarrassed, because I felt it was something that I did to make this happen. I was embarrassed that I couldn't function normally and I didn't want people to know that I was having trouble thinking. So I withdrew because I didn't want to see anyone until I looked and felt the way I wanted to. I stayed home and slept all the time.

SS: You must have felt so despondent. It's a lot of stress for a teenager to handle. I remember you were so concerned about your looks changing. What were you seeing?

VS: When I would look in the mirror, it looked like my face had turned gray. My face was puffy. I also gained a lot of weight. I could put on fifteen pounds so easily. When I would starve myself, I could lose it, but then when I went back to eating I would put on ten pounds in a week. That's why I got so scared of food.

SS: So now you've discovered that you not only have food issues and food allergies, but then you found out you also have Lyme disease. How do you think you got Lyme disease?

VS: I went on vacation with my friends to their house in Nantucket. One day I noticed a mark on my leg. It looked like a bull's-eye.

SS: You mean kind of like the Target brand logo?

VS: Yes. They took me to the clinic and called my mother and told her it was a Lyme-tick bite and that the only treatment was antibiotics. So I took them. A couple of months after the Lyme diagnosis, I started noticing that my face was very oily, which was extremely embarrassing. I would go to class and at the beginning of the class I would go to the bathroom to blot my face, and then two minutes later it was really oily again. It was just another part of my body that was out of control.

SS: Who could you talk to about this?

VS: I could talk to my mom. We talked a lot about my depression. That's all I wanted to talk about . . . Why did I feel so sad?

SS: Of course. You went from an idyllic life, a safe life, with perfect health and a slim, trim dancer's body; and then everything changed. Suddenly you are never feeling well, you are having trouble thinking, plus you have unbelievable fatigue, your face is like an oil well, and you are gaining weight at an alarming weight. I'd feel sad too.

Then I told you about the Sponaugle Wellness clinic in Florida. Doctors there seemed to be dealing with your type of issues, so your mother decided to call and find out what they were doing for people like you. Was that the turnaround?

VS: Yes. Dr. Sponaugle sent lab forms and after he had all my lab work back, he kept e-mailing my mom and saying all these things about my condition. We both thought he was crazy because we had never heard of this syndrome before. He would use huge words when talking about Lyme and say that it wasn't gone. In fact, it was nowhere near gone, even though they had already given me antibiotics. He suggested that I needed to come to his clinic for a few weeks.

SS: How did you feel about that?

VS: Well, it was hard. I had to leave school and my friends and be gone for several weeks. But I wasn't happy at school; I kept feeling sick and I didn't want my friends to see me. So it seemed like the only thing that might help me.

SS: Tell me about being in the clinic and what that was like on a daily basis.

VS: We stayed in a hotel and went to the clinic every day like a job. And it was. My job was to get well. I started getting IV drips of different natural detox substances: glutathione, vitamin C, and a lot of other things. Dr. Sponaugle also gave me a drug to help replace the dopamine in my brain that my brain wasn't making because of all the toxins in my system. I learned about my syndrome, that the toxins were leaking out of my weak digestive system and making their way to my brain, upsetting and stopping my hormone production; these things that were causing the cravings I had been having for food and the binge eating were because my brain was wanting to get a "dopamine hit." Also, as a result, I was not making serotonin and that was what was making me depressed.

SS: That makes sense. Serotonin is your feel-good hormone, and if you weren't making hormones, that would also add to your depression. You had a real whammy: no dopamine, no serotonin, food allergies; you didn't even know about mold allergies yet, and then the big one, Lyme!

VS: Right. On the second or third day I was there [in the clinic], all of a sudden I started talking to my mom saying things like: "Mommy, how was Catholicism formed? Maybe we should go to church Sunday. Want to go on a hike? Can we go to the beach tomorrow?"

SS: You mean you were starting to be able to think again and these were the first questions popping into your head?

VS: Yes. I realized that for two years, I couldn't think! I had thought I was losing my mind.

SS: So what did that mean to you that you were asking these questions?

VS: I don't want to analyze it too much, but in that moment it felt like the best feeling of my life. Just to experience normalcy again. I didn't realize I had been in this kind of space without thoughts. I was starting to feel normalcy again. Then I got scared.

SS: Why?

VS: I had the feeling of fear that this normal feeling was going to go away. When I was at the clinic, I found I not only had Lyme but also I had mold. I now know that mold is what made my digestive system inherently weaker, which is why I had food allergies in the first place.

SS: The puzzle was starting to piece together?

VS: Yes. And then when I found out that it was the antibiotics that could destroy my digestive system and make it even weaker, it was hard.

SS: Well, yes, you are a kid and when a doctor tells you this is the treatment, you do it.

VS: Right. But for me antibiotics were ultimately the wrong thing. I didn't know that I already had mold and food allergies and that the antibiotic was going to make it so much worse.

The first three weeks at the clinic I just felt that I was trying to heal. That wasn't too horrible of a feeling, but it definitely took a lot of determination to wake up each day and focus on healing. I just wanted to get better.

SS: Of course, you wanted your life back again.

VS: Yes. I told Dr. Sponaugle to do as much as possible with as much power as he had in his arsenal because I wanted to get better as fast as possible.

SS: So you decided, as they say, to "bite the bullet."

VS: I guess so. But it created a lot of anxiety. We were bringing up the toxins and it made me feel crazy. But I kept on . . . I embraced as much detox as he could give me because I wanted to get well. I wanted to be well more than anything, and it was the only thing that mattered.

SS: Did you miss your friends?

VS: Yes, but not like you would think. I missed them but didn't want to see anyone until I was all better.

SS: That's so sad. I feel so badly for you. What did you feel like physically when you were going through all of this detox?

VS: I felt like I had the flu: I had headaches, the nausea was real bad, I threw up in the car on the way there a couple of times. I had unbelievable fatigue and deep depression. The depression and the anxiety made me so scared; I talked to Dr. Sponaugle about it. He reassured me that this was supposed to be happening and it was part of the detox. He also explained that the mold allergy had made me much more susceptible to the Lyme. Like a person who didn't have mold or allergies wouldn't have been hit so bad by a Lyme bite. A person without these issues might have a much lower chance of having such a severe reaction. Because of the mold, the food allergies, and my already weakened digestive system, I also found out another thing; I carry the gene for the mold allergy and that made me much more susceptible to all of it. Some people get Lyme and it doesn't bring them down like it did for me, but I had all these other things going on.

SS: Right. Our family carries the HLA gene, which heightens people's responses to toxins. So how long did you stay in the clinic and what was it like when you went back to school?

VS: I stayed in the clinic for six weeks, although the doctor wanted me to stay longer. He said I was much better but I wasn't well. But I wanted to go back home. I was so happy to see everyone and so happy to be feeling better than before when I left school.

SS: I love you, Violet. Thank you for sharing your story. Today when I am with you, my heart soars with happiness to see you well and functioning normally. I am very proud of you, and I also think you are very brave. Your story is going to help so many.

VS: I hope so. I now know, if I choose the wrong food, I am going to have a setback. I look at food as the battery for my body; it's what makes it run. If I want it to run in top form, then I have to put top-quality food in it . . . getting well just takes a lot of patience. I love you, Zannie.

As you've just read, the journey to wellness not only involves the affected child but also the entire family. I have asked my daughter-in-law to explain the trauma and unbelievable stress placed on parents trying to unravel the puzzle of fixing and healing a child or children made ill by today's mystery illnesses that are chemically induced. Caroline is a magnificent woman: unbelievably smart and capable, beautiful, and an incredible wife, mother, homemaker, and businesswoman. She is also executive vice president of our company. I love her like my own and also have a fantastic mother/daughter/business relationship with her. But over the years while going through this horror, it was painful to watch Caroline change from an upbeat, happy-go-lucky, positive person to a mother in constant distress. Her mood changed, her face became serious, and no one was able to comfort her. Her focus, and all she wanted, was wellness for her girls. *Tox*-sickness is a family disease and has serious ramifications for the whole household.

A MOTHER'S SEARCH: CAROLINE'S STORY

I feel like I've been at the heart of a mystery for the last seven years. Both of my amazingly healthy daughters, who danced three hours each day, became ill in their teenage years. I have been chasing the cure ever since.

Camelia's trouble began when she was thirteen. Migraine headaches, stomach cramps, unexplained weight gain, and facial swelling were the key indicators that something was definitely not right. A food allergy and intolerance test was the first piece of the puzzle: she was allergic to gluten, dairy, eggs, soy, beans, most nuts, mushrooms, pineapple, peaches, and many more. She cut out these foods, but her symptoms persisted. How could this poor kid who was not eating any processed food still be bloated? On top of dancing three hours every day? Simultaneously, her anxiety was through the roof. People told me it was normal for teenage girls to gain weight and have anxiety. This was NOT normal. I knew we were missing something . . . it was like she was allergic to all food.

Two years later, Violet began experiencing similar symptoms—also at that critical age of thirteen. Food allergy and intolerance tests revealed similar foods that needed to be eliminated—gluten, dairy, eggs. Allergies can be consistent in families, we were told. Violet was diligent—and yet the unfair bloating began to plague her the same way it had with Camelia. Violet took to eliminating most food as the only way to control her body. While it helped with the inflammation, this created new problems with lack of nutrition, fatigue, and depression. So I had one with anxiety through the roof and the other who was retreating and depressed. They were both hanging on by a thread. I needed more answers.

In the summer after her fourteenth birthday, Violet took a trip to Nantucket and almost immediately called to tell me she had a bite on her leg that had been identified as Lyme. A course of strong antibiotics was recommended. I knew this would wreak havoc on her already sensitive intestines, but even my antiaging doctors told me not to mess with Lyme and that she needed the antibiotic. By the end of the six weeks of antibiotics, Violet's body was not able to digest food. She would be swollen and bloated, even when she was only eating foods to which she was not allergic. She was despondent, trying so hard and still not able to control her failing system. We met with several specialists, but none could help her. I was out of options . . . but held out hope for one more doctor I had been speaking with about Camelia's ongoing issues. He was recommended to Suzanne by Brenda Watson, and Brenda thought he could unravel Camelia's intestinal issues along with the anxiety. But he was in Florida and I wasn't ready to pull Camelia from school. He was also a Lyme specialist. So when Violet's Lyme treatment failed her body, we packed our bags for Florida.

Violet spent six weeks with Dr. Rick Sponaugle at the Sponaugle Wellness Institute. When she arrived, he said her immune system was ravaged. She still had Lyme, and he uncovered the core of the health issues for both of the girls . . . a genetic allergy to mold. The mold allergy eats away at the intestinal lining, creating holes in the intestines until you have leaky gut syndrome. This allows *all* food to enter the bloodstream undigested, which is viewed by the body as an enemy. All of your body's resources go to fighting this enemy, leaving your immune system depleted. They really were allergic to all food, because their intestines were in such bad shape. And in the process, you may experience high levels of inflammation. Bingo! No wonder eliminating the allergy foods was still not eliminating the inflammation! Their leaky gut syndrome was not healing because of the mold allergy. He also explained that having the mold allergy made Violet more susceptible to Lyme. Many people may get tick bites and never have symptoms of Lyme because their immune system is strong enough to keep the Lyme suppressed, but Violet was in such a weakened state, the Lyme took hold of her immediately.

Dr. Sponaugle was the first doctor to explain the connection of the damaged intestine and how it had blunted Violet's hormone production and created neurological issues. She has none of the hormones a girl her age should have to regulate her moods. No wonder she was so depressed. And the intestinal damage had also blunted her production of neurotransmitters—she was not making serotonin, dopamine, or taurine—none of the feel-good neurotransmitters for contentment, happiness, or joy. In addition, she had developed ADD (quiet type) so she had a very hard time focusing (and Camelia has ADHD-hyperactive type, which explained her anxiety). The mold created leaky gut, which created leaky brain, and the Lyme shut down the rest of her immunity and neurological function—so much brain fog. He said that had it gone untreated, she would likely have been diagnosed with MS within the year—and no one would have known the source.

The treatments at the clinic were not easy, but Violet wanted to accomplish as much as she could in the time we were there. As they undergo the process of extracting Lyme and mold from the body, patients range from extremely anxious to extremely depressed. Watching her go through this was excruciating, but she had a singular focus to get well. And at least we now knew the enemy! Violet asked Dr. Sponaugle to give her as much treatment as she could handle. On some nights the anxiety was so bad she was raging and suicidal. Then we would back down. On other days her depression was so bad I could barely move her from bed. Removing the host of toxins from her system was very hard on Violet, but once they were gone, she would feel relief and clarity, until the next treatment.

At the end of six weeks, she was a different person. Her moods were much more even. She was in control of her body. She was eating very carefully—100 percent organic and had decided to go vegan to assist in digestion.

Over the course of the next two years, she has been in and out of school. We decided her health is most important—and ended up placing her in a homeschool program so she could focus on her health. Her body's normal functions are returning. She started eating meat again, which increased her energy level and brain function. Her intestine is dramatically improved so that she no longer experiences inflammation, except on rare occasions. If she gets a moment of anxiety or depression, she knows how to push it away.

While these debilitating issues tried to bring her down, the creative artist in her spirit emerged. Violet is finally back in school, at Los Angeles County High School for the Arts—a brand-new building (no mold!) and a place where she is free from the anxiety of overwhelming academics. She spends time with her friends, creating art, smiling, and laughing along the way. And she can study and focus! She's finally in charge of her health now. Camelia is off at her first year of college. She is also in charge of her health. Her intestines are greatly healed and rarely have bouts with inflammation. We even convinced the cafeteria in her dorm to prepare organic meals for her. Her life depends upon it!

Lyme and mold are never really gone from your life. You learn to manage them. Healing the intestines takes time, months and months, but with healing comes mental clarity and happiness. The Lyme ended up being a great gift. It led us to the root cause of the mold—and gave us the information to heal both of the girls. If you or your children are having mystery illnesses, bloating, depression, anxiety, OCD, ADD, ADHD, symptoms of arthritis, chronic fatigue syndrome, and more, I highly recommend you visit SponaugleWellness.com. Don't expect miracles in a couple of weeks. These are chronic illnesses that take a lifetime of management . . . but Dr. Sponaugle was the one who connected all the processes of the human body—how the intestinal system is connected to the hormonal system to the neurological system. I am forever grateful to Suzanne and Brenda Watson and Dr. Sponaugle for helping us unravel this mystery.

As you can see from my own family's struggles, adults and children alike are being affected by the great environmental assault of toxins in our world today, and the price has compromised health, happiness, and quality of life.

Interesting to note, both Camelia and Violet were born by cesarean. Camelia's birth was difficult and the attending doctor recommended it. As is common in gynecology these days, Caroline was encouraged to give birth to Violet by cesarean because the scar was already there. This scenario is commonly repeated, with over one million cesarean births performed yearly in this country. It's tragic that doctors are not savvy to the ramifications of missing that vital-to-life journey through the vaginal canal where the very first swallow we take is our mother's vaginal flora. This is how nature provided for the colonization of our GI tracts. It is likely that unbeknownst to the birth mother, this decision results in a GI tract that begins life unbalanced and is a setup for problems down the road.

Today, younger and younger people are reported to be contracting cancer. The childhood cancer rate has risen 67.1 percent since 1950 (the United States has the fourth-highest rate in the world). Kids are even *born* with a toxic burden! As discussed earlier, toxins are passed from mother to child in utero, just as an imbalanced microflora system in the mother is passed to the newborn.

We know what happens once the body loses its ability to process all the toxins and pollutants we are bombarded with every day: the body's oxygen supply dwindles, the liver loses its ability to process any more toxins from the overload, the immune system begins to collapse, the body's pH becomes more and more acidic, and now you have a perfect breeding ground for deadly microbes, parasites, and disease. Microbes are the end result when your body's immune system has lost its ability to protect its cells from carcinogens.

Unfortunately, these viruses, bacteria, parasites, and fungi act as the actual catalyst for cancer and nearly all diseases. Viruses exhaust a cell's oxygen and energy supply until the cell withers, dies, or mutates into an anaerobic cell . . . this is not good. This anaerobic (i.e., cancer) cell now relies on fermenting sugar to produce energy.

The battle with cancer is fought at the cellular level in an effort to cleanse the body of microscopic invaders, while radically changing the body's internal terrain back to a healthy one. This is why cleansing is so vitally important for most everyone.

THE GUT-CANCER CONNECTION:
AN INTERVIEW WITH NICHOLAS GONZALEZ, M.D.

Dr. Nicholas (Nick) Gonzalez practices in the heart of Manhattan and is my personal cancer doctor. He is the premier Western-trained alternative cancer doctor in this country, maybe the world. But his healing ability is far broader than just cancer; it includes the GI tract, environmental diseases like Lyme and mold, and the new conditions affecting the brain such as ADD, ADHD, and OCD. Most orthodox doctors are stymied as to what to do for the toxin-related conditions plaguing the health of people today. Dr. Gonzalez explains in this interview how we get cancer, its connection to a damaged GI tract, and how to reverse even the most traumatic illnesses. Do not miss reading this interview.

SS: Thanks once again, Dr. Gonzalez, for your time. The deeper I get into writing about the intricacies of a distressed gastrointestinal tract, the more it appears to be the root of all diseases. "If the gut isn't healthy, you aren't healthy" goes the saying. I'm trying to establish if there is a connection between GI distress and cancer. You are a cancer doctor; what do you think is the answer?

NG: Unquestionably, there is a connection. The twentieth-century Viennese researcher Kasper Blond made the case that all cancer has its origins in malfunction of the liver, one of the *accessory digestive organs.*

SS: There's that liver connection again.

NG: You are right, the health of the liver is crucial. The digestive system consists of the stomach and intestines that assist in the breakdown of food and the absorption of nutrients. All this is critical for life and health—and for protection against cancer.

The liver processes nutrients coming in from the intestines and neutralizes toxins from food and from anywhere else in the body. The pancreas, like the liver, is an accessory digestive organ that secretes both insulin (which manages sugar metabolism) and pancreatic enzymes. These enzymes not only are necessary for digestion of proteins, fats, and carbohydrates, but we believe they also represent the body's main defense against cancer. A defect in any of these digestive organs can ultimately have catastrophic effects, such as cancer.

It's also important to consider that the intestines are not only a digestive organ but a critically important immune center. They're filled with immune cells like the various lymphocytes that produce cytokines and immunoglobulins. These molecules protect us from pathogenic bacteria in the gut but also help regulate our overall systemic immune function. In this capacity, the immune cells lining the intestines contribute to our defense against cancer.

SS: So toxins are disrupting the immune systems of so many and leaving us defenseless against cancer?

NG: Yes. Carcinogenic molecules come into our bodies any number of ways. We can breathe in toxic substances that go from our lungs into our bloodstream and eventually get processed in the liver. Or fat-soluble toxins like hydrocarbons in the air or in body-care products and cosmetics can then be absorbed through the skin. The skin is very high in fat and cholesterol, so fat-soluble toxic molecules dissolve very quickly and then are absorbed into the bloodstream, eventually ending up once again in the liver.

Toxic molecules such as preservatives and additives in our food are absorbed by the intestines and end up in the liver, but if the liver is overloaded, they leak into the bloodstream, or flood back into the intestines. All these chemicals can have devastating effects locally or systemically, including ultimately cancer. So I believe the connection between toxic molecules and cancer is pretty straightforward.

SS: I know this is not an easy answer, but how exactly does cancer begin?

NG: This is as simply as I can put the explanation for how cancer begins. Traditionally in medical school, they taught that cancer develops from mature normal cells in whatever organ they appear, be it the breast, liver, colon, pancreas, etc., that suddenly go berserk and lose all their regulatory control. Now there's a new trend replacing the old theory that instead cancer develops from stem cells, primitive, undifferentiated cells that already exist in every tissue and organ in our body. Under normal circumstances these cells are absolutely critical for maintaining life, providing replacements in whatever organ they appear for those mature cells that are lost due to normal turnover, such as in the intestinal tract, or from disease, injury, or aging. For example, the lining of the intestines turns over and completely regenerates every five days, a remarkable feat possible only because of stem cells. In the case of cancer, these primitive undifferentiated stem cells lose their normal highly regulated life-sustaining function; they start growing without restraint and start spreading throughout the body, invading other organs with deadly effect. In our polluted world of today, toxic molecules can serve as irritants to stem cell DNA, causing these cells to start growing wildly. Remember: under normal circumstances stem cells already have enormous potential to replicate, so it doesn't take much to get them going. Today all the abnormal irritants that shouldn't be in our body can cause stem cells sitting in some organ somewhere to go berserk (molecularly speaking) and turn into cancer.

SS: I figured you would say that toxins are the body's enemy, most likely leading to cancer. What is the trigger?

NG: *Inflammation* is the trigger, disrupting stem cell DNA, and here's the connection to *toxicity*; we are awash in a sea of toxic chemicals. I've read there are approximately 79,000 synthetic chemicals being released into the U.S. environment, most of which have not been tested for safety. Even if we eat organically (which is crucial), things like heavy metals can be taken into the body through the air itself. In New York City there is mercury and aluminum dust in the air coming from China, and other toxins from their unregulated factories, which circulate everywhere. There are pesticides in the air pollution in New York City, even though we're not agricultural; they come in on the wind currents. Eating organically is extremely important, of course, but unfortunately doesn't protect anyone from breathing in toxic chemicals in the air.

SS: So these toxic irritants then create inflammation in the body and disrupt the stem cells, and this ultimately can cause cancer?

NG: Yes. Not only toxic chemicals, but infection can do it too in certain cases such as in Burkitt's lymphoma, though I believe it's usually the toxic heavy metals, synthetic hydrocarbons, and pesticide residues that disrupt the DNA in these stem cells.

So yes, in summary, cancer develops by stem cells getting irritated by the toxicity we take in from the environment.

SS: It seems we are sitting ducks. We have to breathe. To say this is a dilemma is an understatement. Can you explain the pathway?

NG: To understand the process, you need to think about the liver, a most remarkable organ, which is a storehouse and processing center for nutrients. All the protein, fats, and carbohydrates taken in from your food first go through the liver via the portal vein, and then the liver decides what needs to be done with them; it can send them into the bloodstream for use in a distant organ or put them into storage. It can also change them into another form. For instance, amino acids can be converted into other amino acids, and fatty acids can be turned into triglycerides or cholesterol.

The liver is also the body's main filter for toxic chemicals; it's very effective at filtering and neutralizing toxins coming to it from the gut or from the circulating blood. Once the toxins are neutralized into harmless substances, they are released via the common bile duct into the intestines for excretion.

SS: That's provided your liver is in perfect working order. But in today's world, it's a lot of work to keep the liver clean and healthy.

NG: Right, and if the liver gets overloaded, as it commonly does in this day and age, you get a backup of toxins like mercury into the portal vein, which leads from the *intestinal tract* directly into the liver. It's like a beaver dam that backs up. There are connections between the portal vein and the bloodstream, so instead of being excreted harmlessly, the toxins end up going back into the general circulation or into the intestinal tract. Now you have this toxic load floating in the bloodstream where it doesn't belong, and overloading the *intestinal tract*.

SS: So toxins ultimately wind up in the gut?

NG: In the bloodstream and in the gut. Food is another way our GI tract gets exposed to toxins. For example, GMOs (genetically modified organisms) and pesticides have a direct effect on the gut.

SS: It makes sense. Today, everyone's got bloated bellies; even the skinny people have bloated bellies.

NG: There's no question that even in my professional lifetime, I've seen an explosion of gastrointestinal problems. Even from ten years ago there's been a big change. Our overuse of antibiotics contributes to the kind of symptoms you are describing. Antibiotics knock out the normal healthy flora in the gut, and this leads to all kinds of symptoms.

It's been estimated there are well over three hundred different species of normal bacteria that should occupy the small and large intestines. There are up to five pounds of bacteria in our gut at any given time. We all grew up thinking bacteria are the enemy of mankind, but these normal gut bacteria are essential for a healthy life. First, they synthesize nutrients like B vitamins and also help metabolize nutrients, like proteins, fats, and carbohydrates. These beneficial bacteria also have antibiotic effects; a normal, healthy balance of flora will block pathogenic microorganisms like candida.

The ecology in our gut is very complex, and entire textbooks have been written about the importance of the flora to our general health. It's a very delicate system in which certain types of bacteria should inhabit the small intestine; others should live in the large intestine. But very few of us are walking around in the twenty-first century with normal gut bacteria, due to the overuse of antibiotics and exposure to toxic substances like mercury.

SS: And it's very easy to disrupt the gut from all the various toxic chemicals coming from the environment, overuse of antibiotics, and processed poor-quality food?

NG: Many toxins are poisonous to normal bacteria in the GI tract and made worse if we include antibiotics in the mix. Our current generation has been raised on antibiotics. These drugs were touted as a miracle after World War II that was going to eliminate infectious diseases. Instead, different types of infection, like Lyme, are flourishing, and the overuse of antibiotics has led to resistance, while also disrupting normal gut bacteria.

SS: When I was a kid, we were given penicillin for everything. My doctor didn't know anything about probiotics. Explain how an antibiotic disrupts the gut?

NG: It kills the normal, healthy gut flora, and in its place pathogenic or toxic microorganisms take over. Like you, I remember that any time any of us in my family had a cold, the flu, or just sniffles, we would get an injection of penicillin. In retrospect, not only did penicillin disrupt the gut flora, but it was useless most of the time because many of the common kinds of infections, like bronchitis, are viral anyway and don't respond to antibiotics.

Normal gut bacteria are phenomenal in what they can do, but they're very susceptible to antibiotics; even one course of antibiotics can knock out your normal flora. When that happens, the ecology of the gut is completely disrupted, and pathogenic bacteria take over and can make you sick.

SS: So swollen bellies and candida can be a result of this imbalance?

NG: Yes. Candida is yeast, a type of fungus, that's a normal inhabitant of our gut. We all have it, but it's meant to be kept in check in the ecological balance created by the bacteria that normally live there. But when you destroy the bacteria that keep candida under control, it grows without restraint and starts causing trouble.

SS: And candida loves sugar, so sugar is part of the problem?

NG: Yes, absolutely. I've read that the average American eats a hundred and sixty-four pounds of white sugar a year. That's an issue because like any yeast, candida thrives on sugar and with the typical American diet loaded with sugar, candida has a great opportunity to grow like crazy. Then add in antibiotics, which knock out the normal flora that suppress candida, and you have a major problem.

SS: Then what happens?

NG: When candida starts growing, it metabolizes sugar into alcohol in a fermentation reaction. That is why people with an over-growth of candida often walk around feeling like they're hungover. In fact, they will use those actual words: "I feel hungover, I feel toxic, like I had too much to drink."

Bloating also comes directly from this fermentation process, which produces gas. One of the classic symptoms of yeast overgrowth in the intestinal tract is gas, both burping and rectally, and it can be uncontrollable.

SS: Well, there it is; if you have candida overgrowth, and you eat sugar in any form (refined or concentrated carbohydrates also), that yeast will ferment the sugars and quickly produce a huge amount of gas and that is why we are bloating?

NG: Yes. As you've mentioned to me, you used to wake up in the morning and not be bloated and then eat a meal that includes sugar of any kind and suddenly you're bloated out a foot. That's because of the quick action of the yeast on these concentrated carbohydrates. It's an insidious process resulting from a two-pronged attack; antibiotics knock out the normal flora (which normally would control yeast), then add in a daily intake of white sugar and refined carbohydrates, which are the ideal fuel for these yeast cells, and the yeast is able to grow like crazy and take over the gut.

SS: Is a coated tongue an indicator of a yeast infection?

NG: It can be. It often indicates that our gut is overloaded with candida. But it can also indicate other things such as liver stress.

Candida fermentation of sugar in the intestines produces a variety of toxic molecules that end up in the bloodstream, where it can cause all kinds of havoc. And then if the liver gets overloaded with this constant barrage of toxins from the overgrowing yeast, the liver stops working efficiently. Once again, the portal vein backs up and the toxins that should be neutralized in the liver end up floating around in the bloodstream and in the gut itself.

SS: Will this lead to leaky gut?

NG: Yes, when you have abnormal bacteria coupled with an overgrowth of yeast (and the toxins produce both), the gut lining gets inflamed.

The intestinal lining is a very sophisticated tissue, normally capable of determining what it should absorb and what it should reject.

But when you have abnormal bacteria and yeast overgrowth, the molecular connections between the cells lining the small and large intestine (the epithelial lining) start breaking down. Normally these cells are held together by what are called tight junctions, literally molecular bonds between the cells that prevent toxic molecules from getting through. It's a pretty tough barrier. In the presence of this toxic load from abnormal bacteria and yeast, this barrier breaks down. In turn, you start absorbing complex molecules and toxins that normally should be kept in the intestinal lumen, and these molecules end up in the bloodstream causing all kinds of problems.

SS: Periodically there are studies attacking organic food, in particular a study last year that got a lot of press publicity: "Organic doesn't make any difference." What do you think about that?

NG: There are well-done comprehensive studies going back ninety years conclusively documenting that organic food is not only more beneficial in terms of nutrient content, but healthier because you don't have the residues of herbicides, pesticides, and toxic fertilizers. Pesticides are neurotoxins. No one should be ingesting neurotoxins. There are studies that show children raised with organic food do better in school, are healthier, and can get along with each other better than kids eating the pesticide-laden, neurotoxic food. And very recently there was a well-done study showing organically raised produce does indeed have a higher nutrient content, and lower pesticide residue, than conventionally raised produce.

SS: Also a factor in cancer . . . toxins disrupt the ecobalance in the gut lining; yet didn't nature provide a natural cancer protection called interferon in that lining to keep us protected?

NG: Yes, a healthy intestinal lining is protective against cancer. In the research world we continually underestimate the importance of the gut for immune function, and even for normal nervous system activity. The intestines contain not only a good portion of our immune system but a good portion of our nervous system as well. It's been shown that 95 percent of all the serotonin in the body is actually found in the GI tract, and not in the brain. This reference is from Dr. Michael Gershon at Columbia, the expert in the gut-brain connection. His book *The Second Brain* dealt with this very issue and I believe he may actually have made the discovery about serotonin.

The gut has its own active nervous system and also has an active immune system. Scientists never used to think of the gut as an immune organ, but now we know it is, and a very sophisticated one at that. That horde of immune cells like lymphocytes and neutrophils in the intestinal lining help protect us against pathogenic microorganisms by producing molecules like interferon.

Our intestines utilize a variety of methods that protect us from the toxins we take in with food. For example, with cholera, people get terrible diarrhea, which, as dangerous as it can be, is actually a protective mechanism. The cholera bacteria produce a very deadly toxin, and when exposed to this, the intestinal lining secretes large amounts of electrolytes and water to try and flush out these toxins. That's what diarrhea often is, the body's protective mechanism against toxic substances coming in with our food.

The immune system of the gut is very efficient under normal circumstances, but when it gets disrupted through endless poor-quality food, overuse of antibiotics, too much sugar, too much candida and abnormal bacteria floating around, then you add in GMO translocated bacterial genes producing pesticides, you get a breakdown of the immune system in the gut so it can't do its job. Then the weakened gut immunity allows abnormal bacteria to start taking over with impunity.

SS: I'm trying to make a link between toxic exposure intake and cancer; so many people have these bad pathogens roaming around the bloodstream looking for areas of opportunity, especially fatty organs, like the brain. These toxins also attack the skin.

NG: Yes. If the gut breaks down, you're headed for trouble. For example, you mention the brain, which is 60 percent fat; fat-soluble toxins like hydrocarbons accumulate in the brain, other fatty tissues, and in the liver. So yes, many chemical toxins tend to gravitate toward fatty tissues.

SS: So, when you put it all together—how toxins enter the body (lungs, skin, poor-quality food), how these entities try to be processed into an overloaded liver, which then shunts the toxins out and into the portal vein so that they finally end up in the gut—can we conclude that cancer *originates* in the body from the toxic overload in our GI tract?

NG: Yes, many cancers originate in the GI tract from the overabundance of toxicity that breaks through the gut barrier. In addition, the brain is a magnet for toxins because toxins love to live in fat. So the brain is also especially vulnerable.

SS: That's quite a statement and makes perfect sense; think of all the people who essentially have said the same thing starting with Hippocrates in 460 BC: "All disease begins in the stomach." This information finally connects the high incidence of ADD, ADHD, OCD, and others, as originating from the gut "leaking" toxins into the bloodstream and making their way to and affecting the brain.

NG: The brain has more fat and cholesterol proportionally than anywhere else in the body and these fat-soluble, toxic chemicals circulate and can end up in the brain. True, there is a blood-brain barrier that under ideal conditions will function to keep out unwanted chemicals and toxins. But the blood-brain barrier breaks down just the way the gut lining breaks down in "leaky gut," and you get a "leaky brain" syndrome.

SS: Leaky brain? What is that?

NG: It's my term. I use it to describe the situation in which toxic molecules like pesticides and hydrocarbons get into the brain and accumulate because they're lipophilic, meaning they move into fatty tissue. In a worst-case scenario, these chemical irritants affect the stem cells in the brain, which can then start growing uncontrollably.

Conventional experts are totally confused as to why rates of brain cancer are rapidly increasing; to me, it's perfectly predictable when you have the body awash in toxic fat-soluble chemicals. The toxins float around in the bloodstream and gravitate to the brain, which is largely fat. Once there these chemicals can cause damage to the brain's stem cells, and I believe that is how you end up with terrible brain cancers like glioblastoma. So absolutely, you're right . . .

SS: That cancer originates in the gut as a result of massive chemical assaults on the GI tract. This is explosive information that should alarm all people who are walking around with distressed, sick, and damaged gastrointestinal tracts.

NG: By not taking it seriously, by eating poor-quality diets, consuming processed foods, and not limiting toxic chemical intake, people are simply "asking for it." As a start, unless you become vigilant about your diet—which all of us can control—you're asking for trouble. But even people who eat organically are at risk because we're still breathing in toxicity. We have to breathe, and the air everywhere is loaded with junk. But at least if you're eating organically and properly—not eating white sugar, white flour, white bread—and limiting your exposure to synthetic chemicals and GMOs, you are minimizing the toxic assault in your gut and in the rest of your body.

Our bodies are really quite remarkable; they have an enormous capacity to regenerate, repair, and rebuild, and the gut lining can repair, regenerate, and rebuild also. But there's a point of no return. There's a threshold beyond which the toxic junk from the bad food and bad bacteria, along with GMOs and the abnormal bacterial genes, the overuse of antibiotics, and too much sugar (which feeds the bad bacteria) all overload the gut. In turn, carcinogens end up in the bloodstream and circulate everywhere, including the brain.

This can lead to cancer anywhere.

SS: So what you are saying is, we are in control for the most part. I mean, if you live next door to a chemical plant, the odds are against you . . . but if you go out of your way to clean up your GI tract, you have a good chance of avoiding the diseases that are killing everyone today?

NG: That is correct . . . every food I eat, every food choice I make, I do based on what's best for my body. People are more concerned about the fuel they put into their cars than they are about what they put into their own bodies. It astonishes me. Not many think about food as a fuel, yet our body "engines" are so much more sophisticated than the most sophisticated cars, and food is its fuel. Our bodies are the most extraordinary engines on earth, yet people in general still do not make the connection between the fuel we put into our mouths as food, and how well or poorly our bodies will function.

SS: So the general public needs to be educated to understand that every food choice makes a difference, right?

NG: If not, they will end up sorry. Particularly in terms of our thinking, our emotions, our personality. We've been talking about the brain. Well, the brain weighs only two and a half to three pounds, which really isn't much compared to the weight of the body. Our feet weigh more than that. Yet our brains use 25 percent of all the body's energy, so the first organ that's affected by imbalances in nutrition is going to be the brain. And often the first organ affected by systemic toxicity is the brain because it's so delicate, sensitive, and metabolically active; it's not like a lump of clay but very metabolically active.

The body needs a steady supply of good-quality nutrients to operate at maximum efficiency, and it needs to be clean. When you're not eating properly, when you're ingesting a steady supply of sugar and junk food, nutrient-depleted foods that have little value, you are actually starving your brain, which demands all the various nutrients all the time.

SS: How do we clean out a toxic gut and protect our brains?

NG: I keep going back to the liver; the first thing you have to do is get the liver to work better. If the liver is not working, the gut's never going to work, and that will affect everything, every organ, including the brain. As I said earlier, the intestinal blood supply, carrying breakdown products from digestion along with whatever toxins are in the food, empties into the liver directly through the portal vein. If the liver isn't working correctly, toxins are going to back up into the bloodstream without being neutralized in the liver, then they back up into and overwhelm the gut.

You have to get the liver to work!

I can't tell you how many cancer patients we've had with leaky gut or gut problems, who when we did the liver detoxification procedures like the "liver flush" and the coffee enemas (which help the liver to work better) had their "gut" problems resolved. We also address the gut issues directly with a variety of tools, including *probiotics*. Every patient who walks into my office, whether the problem is toenail fungus or brain cancer, we just assume the person has abnormal gut flora and recommend probiotics. That's everyone.

SS: What kind of probiotics do you give them?

NG: We use different forms depending on the situation. For example, if a patient has a serious gut problem like IBS (irritable bowel syndrome), I get more aggressive with the probiotics. We also recommend for all of our patients colon cleanses, which are very effective to flush out the junk in the gut.

SS: Colon cleanses as in colonics or enemas?

NG: Coffee enemas do help clean out the gut, but we have procedures such as the "Clean Sweep," which involves ingesting a combination of fibers including psyllium, ground flax, and ground pectin, along with bentonite clay, a special clay that absorbs toxic junk wonderfully. It's an absorbent for toxins in the gut. Pectin also absorbs toxins like a magnet, as does psyllium.

I've had patients with food poisoning that I've turned around in six hours with bentonite taken orally. It absorbs bacterial toxins, even *Salmonella* and *Candida* toxins, and you just poop them out harmlessly. So if someone has gastroenteritis, an acute example of intestinal toxicity, I recommend bentonite clay liquid, a quarter cup three times a day, up to half a cup three times a day. This can knock it out. I myself take a tablespoon of bentonite every morning and have done so for twenty years just to help protect myself against the world.

SS: You're saying we must be proactive to prevent toxic distress?

NG: No one else is going to help you; people have to take charge of their own bodies. You have to because by the time you're sick, it's already late in the game. As you know, we treat many very sick patients, and many do well, but it's always better to prevent a disease from occurring in the first place.

SS: When did you get interested in nutrition? I mean, it's not usual in the doctor's arsenal.

NG: I got interested in nutrition when I was in my twenties, when I was still a journalist before going to medical school, and I've been eating organic food for thirty-five years. I changed careers and went to medical school because of my interest in nutrition.

When I was a medical student, I did have some solid support for my interests. As you know, my research career got started with support from the man who was at the time president of Sloan Kettering, one of the teaching centers of Cornell, where I went to medical school. But the consensus among a number of my professors who knew me well was that my interest in nutrition was almost like being a pedophile. Actually, they would have been more forgiving if I were a pedophile. They'd say, "This intelligent young man who's got all this promise academically is interested in nutrition?" Horror of horrors.

SS: Remember Schopenhauer's quote on the three stages of truth? The second stage is violent opposition. A new idea usually garners that response. You have a unique cancer protocol. I've been practicing your protocol for a few years for preventative reasons, and my husband practices your protocol for mold. You said something very interesting to me a year or so ago: that you treat your mold patients in the same way that you treat your cancer patients.

NG: In my approach we don't treat the disease; we treat the person with the disease. So we have to figure out, regardless of whether it's cancer or toenail fungus, what the patient is lacking in terms of diet and nutrition, and what the patient needs. If you do that, if you provide the things that are missing, the body usually can get rid of the disease. You have to realize, in terms of cancer, for example, if the body is smart enough to create cancer, it's certainly smart enough to get rid of it.

Our bodies just need to be pointed in the right direction. You have to correct the metabolic imbalances that led to the body going off track, in the wrong direction. The same is true with mold as with cancer. The body can deal with mold. The body can deal with just about anything. With good nutrition and good detox (detox is critical)—and that's what our conversation is about, the importance of detoxification—the body can get over just about everything. In our office, we have people who were diagnosed originally with advanced cancer who have been with me twenty-seven years. You and I were just talking about one patient we both know who's been with me twenty-two years with stage 4 ovarian cancer; she's doing fine and is a glowing example of how our bodies can overcome just about anything, even advanced cancer.

In terms of mold, which you mentioned, this is much easier to treat than cancer. As a first step, you have to reestablish the normal gut flora. The three hundred different species of bacteria that should be living in our gut amount to trillions of living cells. We have more cells in the gut, in terms of the quantity of healthy bacteria, than all other body cells combined, counting from the brain to the toenails. And these healthy bacteria know how to kill mold. Their job is to keep things like mold under control. So if you reestablish the normal ecology and normal flora of the intestines, miracles can happen.

A lot of patients coming to me for mold exposure, like Alan, all have terrible symptoms, and they've been to fifteen doctors trying to figure it out. Unfortunately, most conventional doctors are only recently acknowledging that something as toxic as black mold may be a problem.

The first thing you do to attack mold is reestablish gut flora and this will help enormously. If it's systemic, if it's through the body, then we use things like Candex, as well as our detox procedures. I have to go back to the liver (because the liver filters out everything). We detox junk in the liver whether it's toxic chemicals or mold toxins. The liver can detoxify those mold by-products if it is working efficiently. Often our patients with mold toxicity have livers that are not working properly and cannot get rid of the toxins being produced by the mold. The liver can't filter them out—it's overworked, it's shut down—so the toxins float around in the bloodstream and then get into the brain, causing a variety of neurological symptoms.

When the liver works better, the body gets rid of the junk more effectively, be it mold or dead cancer debris, and then people feel better. But most importantly you have to get the gut flora reestablished or nothing's going to work. Nothing!

SS: Do you think it's important for every single person today, in today's damaged environment, to be on probiotics daily for the rest of their life?

NG: Absolutely. If I was going to be stranded on a desert island and had a choice between a ten-year supply of probiotics or a ten-year supply of multivitamins and minerals, I would take the probiotics. Without normal bacteria you are not going to utilize nutrients sufficiently anyway. Second, these healthy bacteria produce B vitamins like biotin, B_1, even B_{12} to some extent, as well as vitamin K, which is produced right in our gut if you have the right bacteria present. And while probiotics can't create minerals, they help the body utilize minerals more efficiently. So when you take probiotics, you are actually taking a multivitamin and a multimineral in effect, directly or indirectly.

SS: The master design is rather wondrous.

NG: You can't improve upon nature.

SS: You are known for your coffee enema protocol as a major way of detoxing the liver. Clearly the liver is a major player in the master design; can you explain why a coffee enema is such an excellent way to detox the liver?

NG: Coffee enemas are the single most effective way of detoxing the liver. My mentor Dr. Kelley was famous for prescribing coffee enemas for all his patients, whatever their problem.

Dr. Kelley had collected scores of studies from the mainstream medical journals, going back to the 1920s, 1930s, and 1940s, when doctors weren't so fussy or beholden to the pharmaceutical companies, and when they routinely used coffee enemas and enemas of various types to treat a host of different syndromes.

For instance, in 1941 a group of scientists in Uruguay reported on a number of hospitalized patients near death from advancing metabolic shock whom they treated with coffee enemas, with dramatic reversal of the situation. These patients were coming out of comas with the enemas, when all other pharmacological interventions had failed.

The enemas got these patients' livers to work better, and when the liver works better, miracles happen. Now, oddly enough, when you drink coffee, we find it tends to suppress the liver. When you take coffee rectally, it works through a spinal reflex that within seconds causes the liver to release all its toxins. Basically, coffee taken as an enema—but not drunk—stimulates the major detoxification systems in the liver, so it can efficiently neutralize and excrete this toxic waste into the intestine and then you poop it out. Patients feel better, whatever the problem. I've done them myself for thirty-three years, since July of 1981 when I first met Dr. Kelley.

SS: So the not-so-big secret to health is detoxing the liver?

NG: Absolutely, and I stress once again:

When the liver works better, the gut works better!

SS: And enemas help the liver work better?

NG: Yes, and when the liver works better, everything else works better, particularly in this toxic world. Until the environment is cleaned up and the world is remade perfect, as the Bible says it someday will be, I'm going to do coffee enemas.

SS: It seems radical that we have to go to such lengths to get and remain healthy.

NG: Critics have stated that coffee enemas are abnormal. Of course no one should *have* to do coffee enemas. But we now live in an imperfect world that gets worse every year; the levels of toxicity get worse. We now have GMOs. We didn't have GMOs ten years ago. We have so many levels of toxicity that stress the liver. Our livers, in the healthiest of us, are working beyond their designed capability.

SS: It's amazing that people still can walk around and function.

NG: It is amazing, and a credit to the wonderful design of our bodies, that so many who are eating poorly and living in a toxic world still have jobs and function. But we've reached a critical point where pollution, overuse of antibiotics, poor diet, overuse of sugar, and GMOs are pushing people's health to the limit.

Dr. Kelley used to say he'd rather treat an eighty-year-old than a twenty-year-old and the first time I heard that I said, "Why?" That made no sense to me. He said, "Each generation gets weaker, the food gets worse, the pollution gets worse." He explained that the eighty-year-olds when he was in practice grew up in a cleaner world and on cleaner food than younger patients. The heavy use of pesticides didn't really begin until after World War II. These older folk were just made of better stuff and easier to treat than the kids raised on junk.

SS: Now, sadly, the younger generation is going down with the prevalence of ADD, ADHD, OCD, autism, bipolar disorder, dyslexia, and schizophrenia. It seems like half the children in today's schools are on mood-stabilizing drugs.

NG: Only half, that's pretty good actually.

SS: What's this going to do?

NG: It's just terrible because the drugs are toxic in and of themselves; they blow out the nervous system.

SS: Are these drugs wreaking havoc on their delicate immune systems and GI tract linings?

NG: Absolutely. In fact, some of these amphetamines that are prescribed we believe can stimulate solid tumors to form and grow— tumors of the breast, lung, stomach, for example—and we believe there is going to be an epidemic of cancer with these kids who are on these drugs in ten, fifteen years.

SS: What are the names of the amphetamines?

NG: Adderall, Vyvanse, Concerta; these are the most popular drugs used for kids and adults with ADD and ADHD. Doctors prescribe these amphetamines that stimulate the sympathetic nervous system, and patients become more alert and focused. The Japanese gave amphetamines to their factory workers during World War II because with amphetamines these people could work twenty-four-hour shifts and not be tired. But when you chronically overstimulate the sympathetic nervous system, through a complicated series of reactions, people tend to get the solid tumors like those of the breast, lungs, stomach, pancreas, colon. So in my opinion it's a real time bomb ready to go off.

The idea that you can overstimulate any part of the nervous system without having any effect long term is itself just insanity. It's not natural, it's not normal. It isn't an appropriate way to deal with these problems.

SS: Are there natural alternatives to these amphetamines for patients with ADD and ADHD?

NG: There certainly are. For example, the amino acid tyrosine is a precursor to the neurotransmitters dopamine and norepinephrine, which both stimulate sympathetic nerve activity. When you take tyrosine as a supplement, it is absorbed through the gut and gets into the brain, where it can be converted into these molecules. The effect on the sympathetic nerves is gentler than the drugs, but it works. We also find the old Vermont country doctor remedy, apple cider vinegar, two tablespoons in a glass of water with some honey, also stimulates the sympathetic nerves, increases energy, and improves focus and concentration.

SS: We presume everyone *has* a healthy immune system, but that isn't necessarily the case anymore, is it?

NG: That's certainly true. But the current population of young adults who are overvaccinated, in my opinion have immature immune systems. For example, something like chronic fatigue, which didn't exist when I was growing up, is rampant today, particularly with people in their twenties and thirties to the point that they can't function; these are people with MBAs, yet they can't go to work because they're so tired.

SS: Do you think this is because of vaccinations?

NG: They are part of the problem that is keeping the immune system immature and not able to function effectively. We're witnessing the first generation of kids who were overvaccinated and now their immune systems don't work very well. They contract an infection like Epstein-Barr, which causes mononucleosis, and ten years later they still can't get out of bed because their immune systems can't fight it. I saw my first case of chronic fatigue–Epstein-Barr when I was an immunology fellow; the patient was a nineteen-year-old girl who had gotten mononucleosis a year earlier and hadn't been functional since.

SS: Hmm, compromised immune systems, messed-up guts, mercury poisoning from vaccines, bad food . . . this is all very alarming.

NG: Yes, and these vaccines don't allow for normal illnesses to occur in the normal way, illnesses that teach our immune systems to work in a natural, helpful fashion.

SS: So if this produces a generation of people whose immune systems are immature, isn't this going to cause havoc as they get older?

NG: Everything is accelerating the damage: the bad food, eating too much sugar and refined carbohydrates (which feed the bad bacteria), stress, GMOs, toxins, overuse of sophisticated antibiotics, and overuse of vaccines. Mix it all together and you have a catastrophe in the works.

I have patients who come to me who've been on antibiotics four, five years for acne, and now their flora are a mess. My patients come in with their livers so overwhelmed from environmental toxins, their livers are barely functioning. In this situation you end up with the backup of the toxins into the bloodstream and the gut, then the gut breaks down, its barrier mucosal wall breaks down, more toxins seep into the bloodstream, then they get into the brain and people start going nuts.

SS: It's the food, it's the drugs, and it's even the over-the-counter drugs. It's what's in your water. It is pervasive. It's everywhere. You can't change the whole world, but what about a total cleanup of your own personal sphere?

NG: I have patients who have never had an antibiotic in their life and they come in with dysbiosis, abnormal gut flora, with all the signs of leaky gut: depression, fatigue, malaise, bloating, and candida. They've never had an antibiotic and have never been on birth control pills (which can cause candida to grow), but they drink tap water. As you know, most municipal water systems use chlorine, and chlorine comes with two risks. First, it's carcinogenic. All the scientists at water treatment facilities know that, but they can't stop using it because they have millions of dollars of technology set up to put chlorine into a city's water supply.

Second, they put chlorine into water supplies because it's a natural antiseptic; it kills bacteria. Guess what happens when you drink the recommended six to eight glasses of tap water a day with chlorine? You are on a daily basis poisoning your normal flora.

SS: Here we go again. . . . Why are you the only doctor I've come across who has had such remarkable success with pancreatic cancer? Most everyone dies from it (and quickly) except your compliant patients. Is it the coffee enemas?

NG: We could not get pancreatic cancer patients well if they weren't doing the coffee enemas. There's nothing more toxic to the body than dead tumor wastes, and in these patients as their tumors die, the toxic tumor debris can overload the liver. That's when people tend to get sick on our therapy, and we have to manage them through those episodes with the coffee enemas and other detox procedures. In those patients with pancreatic cancer, this is a particularly serious problem because their livers are already stressed out by the nature of the disease. If these patients don't do the enemas and other detox procedures, they will not survive.

Usually we start at four pints a day and then we'll vary it, depending on how the patient reacts.

SS: When the patient gets sick from detox, what form does it take? Is it similar to flu?

NG: Yes, usually it's flulike; patients feel tired, fatigued, lethargic, and headachy, and they complain of joint aches and pains. They can get fevers and skin rashes. Remember, the skin is a detox organ, so if you've got dead tumor cell debris floating around, it can start coming out of your skin, and you may get skin rashes. To avoid too much toxicity, we have all our patients stop the enzyme and supplement capsules for five days periodically so they don't get this overload, but if the detox is severe and they feel sick, we increase the enema dose until we see improvement.

SS: I am one of your patients practicing prevention because I don't want to ever get cancer again. For someone reading this book and concerned about the toxic assault on humanity, what would they do to live a Gonzalez cancer-preventative kind of life?

NG: Well, clearly, as you know, disclaimer, I can't prescribe for individual patients I have not personally evaluated, but I can certainly speak generally. First, everyone should eat organically. You can't control the toxins in the air; if you walk down the street, even if you live in Alaska, you're going to breathe toxins coming in from China. So at least you can control your food; you have to eat organically, and if you do, you won't be eating GMOs. Minimize the pesticide intake. Minimize the synthetic herbicide intake; minimize or preferably eliminate synthetic and nutrient-depleted junk food. Get the cleanest food you can get and eat it.

SS: So first and foremost, it's about the quality of food?

NG: Yes. Now in terms of diet, we use ten different basic diets that range from raw plant-based food to largely red meat, and everything in between. The point is, everyone needs a diet designed for his or her particular needs. How can you tell what diet an individual should follow? Well, people usually should be eating the foods that they like. Everybody likes chocolate, that's not what I mean, but in general, if you like eating meat, that's probably what you need. Genetic vegetarians don't like eating meat. If you don't want to eat meat and you like fruits and salads and those kinds of things, you're probably a genetic vegetarian. If you like a variety of foods, you need to be on a variety of foods. So go by your own instincts. It sounds simplistic, but that's actually the best general test. Make sure the food is clean and organic and don't eat pounds of sugar and chocolate a day. Clean whole food is absolutely critical.

Second, even if you eat clean food, the world is floating in toxic chemicals in the air and in the water and everywhere. You have to detox and the best way is with coffee enemas. I'm a firm believer that everyone on earth should do coffee enemas.

Coffee enemas are the single most important healing technique that you can do. The enemas get the liver to work better, and when the liver works better, as we've been discussing, everything else works better. Third, you have to be on a probiotic. That's been an emphasis in this discussion. Without a good probiotic, I don't care how many vitamins and minerals you're taking, you're not going to utilize them properly. You need to be on a probiotic. There's nobody walking around today who wouldn't do better with a probiotic. Such a person in my experience doesn't exist.

In choosing a probiotic, each of the many normal gut bacteria has a different purpose and function; for example, *Bifidus*, which is a normal inhabitant of the colon, helps block allergies and helps heal leaky gut. *Saccharomyces* is useful for treating *Clostridium difficile*, the bacteria that creates deadly types of colitis you get after overuse of antibiotics. So with some knowledge you can use probiotics therapeutically. Often health food store owners will have that kind of knowledge.

I'm also a big fan of pancreatic enzymes, which we use to treat cancer. But I know this isn't a book about cancer.

SS: Actually, this discussion is about toxicity as the pathway to disease, and cancer is one.

NG: Well, relative to *cancer* there are four things you need to do: you need to eat organically and minimize toxicity; you need to regenerate your normal bacteria with probiotics; you have to take pancreatic enzymes; and you need to do daily coffee enemas.

Why pancreatic enzymes? They were first identified around 1858 in Europe and were known as essential for normal digestion. By 1900, the three classes of pancreatic enzymes had been identified:

- the amylases that break down complex carbohydrates
- the lipases that break down triglycerides into fatty acids
- the proteolytic enzymes that break down proteins into component amino acids

John Beard was the eminent professor at the University of Edinburgh who in 1902 first suggested that the proteolytic pancreatic enzymes, in addition to breaking down protein in the gut, have a powerful anticancer effect. He maintained that they are the body's main defense against cancer, and he did animal studies confirming his hypothesis. He then worked with human patients diagnosed with cancer a hundred years ago who experienced total regression of their disease.

A hundred years ago was not the dark ages in cancer medicine; Sloan Kettering already existed, and scientists knew what cancer was, how it behaves, where it forms. They didn't know the molecular biology of the disease, but they certainly knew what cancer was and how to identify benign versus malignant tumors. And Beard was getting many of them well.

SS: Do you take enzymes between meals? Or with meals? There's a lot of discussion about that.

NG: When you take them with meals, they're used as digestive enzymes to break down food. And that's important, of course. In this sense, they certainly help the gut work better. When you take them on an empty stomach away from meals, they get absorbed into the systemic circulation and selectively destroy cancer cells that might be forming. So I take them with meals for digestion, as well as away from meals to kill any cancer cells that might be daring to pop up in my body.

SS: When you say you take them between meals, is that so they can eat (for lack of a better term) debris?

NG: Yes, exactly; they basically chew it up like a Pac-Man; they just chew up cancer. But these proteolytic enzymes don't affect normal tissue at all. They only selectively destroy cancer cells.

SS: That is quite amazing. And to think of the simplicity of this protocol as opposed to chemical poisoning. If I hadn't personally spoken with so many of your long-term patients, so many with stage 4 pancreatic cancer who are alive seventeen and twenty years later, I would have found this hard to believe, but their stories made a believer out of me.

NG: Yeah, they're quite amazing. In Dr. Beard's book from 1911 called *The Enzyme Treatment of Cancer*, he pointed out that he believed cancer cells have the opposite electrical charge of normal cells. Pancreatic enzymes themselves have an electrical charge that is repulsed by normal tissue, but creates an attraction with cancer cells. So he believed cancer cells are like a magnet for the enzymes; they draw them in and then the enzymes can chew up the cell membrane. As a result, the cancer cells die.

SS: So if a healthy person doesn't want to get cancer, he or she would take about twenty-five pancreatic enzymes throughout the day, eat organic, do coffee enemas, and take daily probiotics?

NG: I take twenty-five enzymes daily, but I lead an abnormal life. As you know, I work twelve, fourteen hours a day, which is abnormal and not recommended. But for someone out there who's healthy, in their twenties and thirties, who is interested in nutrition, I would say take enzymes, four or five, three times a day. As you get older you want to take a little bit more.

SS: And with the prevalence of children and adults with brain disorders—ADD, ADHD, et cetera—would coffee enemas and pancreatic enzymes be a formula for them also if you could convince them to do it?

NG: Absolutely.

SS: So that is your formula for prevention. That doesn't sound difficult to me.

Once again, I want to thank you, Dr. Gonzalez, for your time and sharing insight on your life's work. Making the connection between cancer and a damaged GI tract puts a whole new spin on "What's wrong with my stomach?" I believe once my readers understand and make the connection between our toxic lifestyles and poor health, it will be the impetus for many lives to be changed. We are the first generation to experience this toxic assault. But the good news (as you say) is, we are in control and you have given the tools for prevention.

I always enjoy interviewing you, a Western-trained doctor, who has stepped outside of the orthodox box to have real results. What you have laid out for those who *are* ill and those who want to *prevent* illness is sound and makes sense. It puts the body in a balanced state, and nature requires balance.

NG: When that is achieved, we do well.

SS: Thank you.

GO FROM *TOX*-SICK TO NOT SICK

To prevent disease and to heal your gut and your liver, the remedies are:

1. Eat clean good-quality organic food for life.

2. Avoid all chemicals as best you can.

3. Take coffee enemas daily for life.

4. Take probiotics daily for life.

5. And for cancer prevention, take daily pancreatic enzymes.

CHAPTER 4

THE BRAIN

One of the most ignored aspects of toxicology (the study of poisonous substances) is toxin synergy. Synergy is the interaction of one or more toxins that when combined have a much more powerful toxic effect than would be expected by just adding together their individual toxicity. This is a common phenomenon. What this means is that if you add one toxin that is known to be rather weak as a toxin to another weak toxin, together they can be highly toxic to humans. (Most of these toxic chemicals are not tested for synergy by the regulatory agencies such as the EPA.) We see this not only with exposure to toxins of a similar class, for example the more than 1,000 pesticides/herbicide and fungicides in common use, but also when different types of harmful environmental substances are combined—such as industrial chemicals, prescription medications, toxic metals, microwave radiation, and even infectious organisms. Even stress, when combined with toxic substances, can have a synergistic toxic effect—that is, it will magnify the toxicity of the chemical. Our world is now filled with so many toxic substances and harmful events that the risk to our health is greatly magnified over that just forty years ago and continues to increase.

—DR. RUSSELL BLAYLOCK, NEUROSCIENTIST

WE JUST DISCUSSED THE GUT: HOW IT WORKS, HOW IT GOT TOXIC, the damage that toxins have done, and the connection of chemical toxins in the GI tract to cancer. Now we go to the second half of the equation, the brain.

The gut/brain connection is essential to understand, especially in how one affects the other, how these organs talk to each other, and the signaling that goes on between them.

When the gut is working right, then so too is the brain; in reverse they both take the hit. That was the essence of Violet's story. When her GI tract became toxic and compromised, it then affected her brain and her ability to process. The two are inextricably intertwined. Have you noticed the epidemic of brain-related conditions, diseases, tumors, and cancers?

We have to ask ourselves why.

The answer is clear . . . we are bombarded by toxins, and they are making their way up to our brains, usually starting in the gut. The very young and the very elderly are the first to succumb; the young because their brains are not fully formed until ages twenty-five to twenty-seven, and older people because they have been under toxic attack for over fifty years and the chickens have finally come home to roost. It isn't natural to lose your brain as we age, but under the circumstances, is it any wonder that our brains have not done so well under this assault?

The brain is the most complex tissue in the human body. It weighs about three to five pounds and is the most oxygen-demanding organ, as well as using up to 30 percent of the body's glucose supply to function. The brain allows us to sense our environment, move with purpose, feel emotions and interpret them, operate all our bodily functions twenty-four hours a day with no conscious effort, think, and ultimately become who we are with our various personality traits, habits, and quirks.

Dr. Datis Kharrazian, neuroscientist and author of *Why Isn't My Brain Working?*, writes: "It's always important to address the fundamentals of brain health. Are the neurons receiving enough oxygen (exercise), glucose, and stimulation? Are blood sugar issues, poor liver function, inflammation, hormonal imbalances or lack of neurotransmitter activity promoting brain degeneration?"

Look at the words he is using in reference to the brain: blood sugar, poor liver function, inflammation, hormonal imbalances. All these issues begin in the gut and then affect the brain, which we now know is also taking a huge hit. The liver is affected by toxins; inflammation is caused by toxins, hormone imbalances are due to natural aging or toxins.

Starting to see the connection? Toxins are wreaking havoc in the stomach, the GI tract, the bloodstream, the essential organs, and the BRAIN!

WHEAT BRAIN: IS GLUTEN SENSITIVITY REAL?

I think it's important to discuss the role gluten plays in a healthy brain and gut. If your brain is not working right, it's most likely due to toxic exposure and toxic burden; and if you have ADD, ADHD, OCD, autism, bipolar disorder, or even schizophrenia, it's likely that sensitivity to gluten could be causing an immune assault on your brain and creating symptoms or worsening an existing condition. This will lead to brain inflammation and increase the risk for an autoimmune attack on your brain tissue.

Many doctors do not understand the concept of gluten sensitivity. I've even heard it mocked and dismissed on TV as "the latest fad," but today's gluten is not the gluten of yesterday. There used to be eighty different strains of wheat. Today those eighty strains have been "engineered" to five strains, and their gluten content is now off the charts.

If you suspect that you have a sensitivity to gluten, you can get tested (Forever Health offers both a gluten sensitivity as well as a food safe allergy test at ForeverHealth.com). The gluten sensitivity screening test is for anyone who suspects that grains like wheat, spelt, rye, and barley may be affecting their health. It is also suggested that the food safe allergy test be done as well since a person can react to wheat/grains in different ways. Gluten sensitivity testing looks at the autoimmune mediated reaction component, while the food safe test looks at a delayed food sensitivity reaction. A person can react in both ways or just one or the other.

The fact is many people today are allergic to many foods that might never have bothered them fifty years ago, and many people cannot tolerate even one bite of gluten due to their severe reactions. Eating foods to which you are intolerant is like consuming poison for your particular body. My husband, my daughter, and our two granddaughters are severely gluten intolerant. As I've said, our girls have ADD, ADHD, OCD, and food allergies, and as you've read, one has mold exposure and Lyme. It's been tragic to watch them suffer. My heart has ached for them.

Sadly, until you do the detective work (blood tests) to find out, there is a lot of suffering involved. These "initials," as I call them, create a very painful existence for so many and they are yet another of the new conditions that get easily mocked. Many gluten-intolerant individuals are told, "It's all in your head."

My husband had digestive issues for years before he discovered he was gluten intolerant. He had severe fatigue during the day, weight gain, constipation, bloating, and moodiness. He would take two or more naps a day from sheer exhaustion. I didn't understand but just figured it was part of the deal. Finally, when writing my book *Sexy Forever*, about how the toxic burden is making us fat, I urged him to take the food allergy test along with me. His results showed severe intolerance to gluten, and he was advised to "avoid it forever." My test results showed severe intolerance to eggs and I was told to avoid them forever. Good-bye cakes, cookies, and all things made with eggs. For me this was ultimately a blessing in disguise, the precursor to my living a sugar-free/carb-free life. For Alan, when he was exposed to black mold, his GI tract had already been weakened from years of gluten intolerance. The black mold put him over the top. It was his tipping point. Then the mold found its way to his cerebellum, the base of the brain, and attacked his central nervous system, which is what produced the facial spasms. I thank God every day for Dr. Gonzalez; he helped Alan clear the mold toxins from his body and has gotten him almost to the point of being well again. I know we will achieve total wellness, but as I have said again and again, clearing toxins takes time. The operative here: recovery is possible, but it takes diligence and patience.

So what do gluten intolerance, food allergies, mold, Lyme, and GI problems have to do with the brain, you ask? Just about everything.

We have discussed the gut/brain connection. For those who are intolerant, consuming gluten causes leaky gut syndrome, allowing for the bad pathogens to make their way up to the brain, causing brain fog and worse. The high gluten content of today is caused by engineering. Often the chemical process of making the wheat or soy "Roundup ready" (a chemical weed killer in most all GMO foods) is enough to put anyone's body into a sickly tailspin.

Also, many people with gluten sensitivity have silent celiac disease, meaning their symptoms are not intestinal. Instead they experience reactions to gluten in the brain, thyroid, joints, skin, or other tissues. The most common area of nonintestinal manifestation of gluten sensitivity is the brain and nervous system. One study of patients who manifested gluten sensitivity in the brain found that only a third of them also suffered from gastrointestinal disorders.

The journal *Neurology* showed that out of 10 participants with headaches, abnormalities in how they walked (hence mimicking Parkinson's), and elevated antigliadin antibodies (gluten sensitivity), 7 of the subjects experienced complete resolution of symptoms on a gluten-free diet. The interesting part of this study was that 6 out of the 10 subjects had no intestinal complaints.

So what has this got to do with toxins? Again, just about everything . . .

For instance, transglutaminase is used by the food-processing industry to tenderize meat and as a meat *glue* to hold processed meats together in distinct shapes. Transglutaminase creates a chemical process (toxins) that, when in the human body, seeks out the central nervous system. Gluten triggers immune reactivity to TG6, leading to autoimmune destruction of brain and nervous tissue.

Pesticides like organophosphate are used on vegetables and fruit. Unless you wash the poisons off the nonorganic produce, you are having pesticides for dinner (and they will make you sick and fat). Indoor and outdoor pesticides are hard to avoid. I often comment when I am in hotels that even though food service trays are left in the hallways, I *never* see rats, mice, or cockroaches sniffing around. Hmmm . . . why would that be? Perhaps it's that more toxins are sprayed to keep the little critters away? Or maybe they know better than to eat these foods?

Clearly pesticides are everywhere, and they are wreaking havoc on our systems.

As we just learned from Dr. Gonzalez, we breathe in these toxins and they go into our lungs, or through our skin, then they try to get into the liver to be filtered, but if the liver is overloaded with toxins, they back up into the portal vein, and then wind up in the GI tract. Toxic gut makes for a toxic brain. See the connection?

No single dietary protein is a more potent trigger of neurological dysfunction and neurological autoimmunity than gluten, the protein found in wheat. By hybridizing and creating a "new" wheat, we've triggered severe immune reactions, especially in the brain and nervous system. Deamidation, a process used to by the food-processing industry to make wheat water soluble, has been shown to cause a severe inflammatory reaction in people.

> I'll say it again. They are messing with the food. We believed.
> They told us it was safe. It's not true!

Another mechanism is that immune reactions to gluten can break down the blood-brain barrier (the thin lining that protects the brain) and this leads to what Dr. Gonzalez called leaky brain. You need a healthy blood-brain barrier to prevent pathogens from getting into the brain, but at the same time to allow in necessary compounds, such as precursors for neurotransmitters. A leaky brain can allow in pathogens that increase the risk of autoimmune reactions in both the brain and nervous system.

The initials (ADD, ADHD, etc.) are the by-products of brains under attack. Doctors are stymied and the only thing in their arsenal is to give yet more drugs. As you just read in Dr. Gonzalez's interview, the drugs being given to children, teenagers, and adults to treat these issues have the potential to be addictive, and withdrawal is very difficult. But worse, the long-term potential for solid tumors of the breast, prostate, lungs, and liver again make you wonder: What are "the experts" thinking?

Diet is a better place to start. If the brain is composed of 65 percent fat, then to deprive it of its most important ingredient (fat) is to weaken and make the brain susceptible to inefficiency from many sources.

The other huge component in your not being able to get well and thrive is sugar consumption. The American diet is composed mainly of nonfood, manufactured, processed chemicals. High-fructose corn syrup (HFCS) is used in virtually all packaged and processed food in America today. In essence, it means we are eating huge doses of sugar, most often in the form of HFCS. In recent history, we've gone from 20 teaspoons of sugar per person, per year (in the form of fruit), to about 150 pounds of sugar, per person, per year. That's a half pound a day, for every man, woman, and child. In addition, we stopped eating essential healthy fats. See the picture?

Sugar at that dose is a toxin. And HFCS is the worst toxin. It is the real driver behind our current epidemic of obesity, type 2 diabetes, fatty liver, heart disease, cancer, and dementia. It contains mercury and other contaminants and is a marker of poor-quality, processed food.

As a whole we are lacking nutrition, even though we are obese and eating more than ever. A quart of ice cream and two bags of cookies loaded with trans fats, HFCS, and sugar is not fuel!

The brain needs a healthy diet of healthy fats, vegetables, fruits in moderation, eggs, nitrate-free bacon, grass-fed beef, pork, lamb, wild-caught fish (especially salmon), and organic butter, cream, olive oil, flaxseed oil, and coconut oil. These foods are brain fuel and excellent sources of nutrition.

> You will heal your GI tract, your brain, and your heart with healthy fats!

Today's health requires a shift in your thinking. If you are not feeling well, if you don't like your nude body, then you have to make some changes. You *can* get your health back and your beautiful body will return (with patience) if you truly grasp the concepts in this book.

The free ride of chemical food is over. Those who don't make the shift are most likely not going to have a good outcome. Whenever I visit a nursing home, I am struck by the lifeless bodies tied to wheelchairs, and I know they never thought (back then) that this is how it would end up. Was the fast food worth it? Was the sugar binging worth it? Was the careless lifestyle worth it? Nature is kind in that most of these people no longer have working brains, so they don't have to live out their last days in remorse. That remorse happened along the way when their bodies and brains started betraying them. You inherently know midprocess when your lifestyle is doing you in.

Many people heed the wake-up call and make serious life changes. The others toss it off, saying, "It'll never happen to me." Then, when it's too late, they realize the consequences of their choices.

You *can* survive in this toxic soup, and your body will begin to operate at optimum again.

AND DO IT FOR YOUR CHILDREN, TOO!

Research shows a well-functioning digestive system holds the key to a child's mental development. It's that serious. So serious that Philippe Pinel (1745–1826), who worked with the mentally ill for many years, concluded in 1807 that insanity resided there.

> The primary seat of insanity generally is in the region of the stomach and the intestines.
>
> —Philippe Pinel

Insanity?

When you factor in the poor diets of most young people of today—bags of chemicals, diet sodas, trans fats, processed food, fast food, drinks in plastic bottles leaching chemicals—then try to track what is happening to their GI tracts, and then imagine these harsh toxins invading their young undeveloped brains, you'll see a recipe for disaster. Sadly, for these generations, this is the new normal.

I think of this every time I see a young person wig out and go on a horrifying shoot-'em-up. I'm not forgiving their actions, but I can't help but wonder, knowing everything I do about the gut/brain connection and the *tox*-sick assault, could it be that these perpetrators are actually victims of toxicity and severely damaged gastrointestinal tracts that have been leaking harmful toxins into the brain, making them feel "crazy"?

Look at the foods of today; look at our toxic houses. Could these elements be culprits, or at least possible causes, for the insane actions of individuals? Certainly, it's food for thought. Though I've been ridiculed for suggesting this in the media, I still stand behind it.

It is possible that the hormonal turmoil of puberty in some way
interacts with the toxins in the child's body and tips the child
into a psychotic state. It is also possible that the hormones open
the blood-brain barrier for some of the toxins, which were in the
child's body all his/her life, but could not get into the brain before.
Apparently through different stages of growth the brain prunes its
receptors. The most active pruning goes on around two years of
age and at puberty. It is possible that at puberty, opioid peptides
and other toxins escaping the gut of the youngster interfere with
this natural pruning process and tip the brain into psychoses.
—Dr. Natasha Campbell-McBride, author of
Gut and Psychology Syndrome

It bears repeating: Dr. Nick Gonzalez says, "My patients come in
with their livers so overwhelmed from environmental toxins, their livers are barely functioning. In this situation you end up with the backup
of the toxins into the bloodstream and the gut, then the gut breaks
down, its barrier mucosal wall breaks down, more toxins seep into the
bloodstream, then they get into the brain and people start going nuts."

I asked him about the fact that there are a lot of people going crazy
these days, and that it seems to have started with Columbine. I wanted
to know if our brains are on fire. As in environ-*mental*? His response:

A lot of these kids, like the Columbine kids, the Gabby Giffords shooter,
the Colorado theater shooter (who ironically was a student of neuroscience), and the Sandy Hook shooter, were on antidepressants and antipsychotics. The dark underbelly of these drugs is that they can provoke
violent behavior and mood disturbances, though they are supposed to
cure mood disturbances. A doctor at Harvard wrote a book about the dangers of the overmedication of people with these antipsychotics, which he
claims are not miracle drugs. First, I know they don't work that well, and
second, they can cause and provoke violent behavior. I have read that the
recent shooter in Santa Barbara had been treated much of his adult life
for mental illness.

Think about the eyes of these people; think about the Gabby Giffords
shooter's eyes. As the media puts their pictures up, you'll notice they all

have "bug eyes." That look can be an out-of-control thyroid (not all people with bug eyes are crazy, but it is often an indicator of Graves', a thyroid disease); people can feel "crazy" when their thyroids are on super overdrive. If antidepressants are affecting their brains and in addition they are eating a lot of sugar and carbohydrates, it would affect their most likely already damaged gut lining. This would allow the toxins to travel to the brain, affecting the HPA axis; HPA axis is the hormone control center that speaks directly to the thyroid. It makes sense that all of this creates a perfect storm of out-of-control behavior, right?

Antipsychotics and antidepressants will affect thyroid function, so that goes along with what you're saying; there's no question these people have been affected by their prescribed medication, in addition to the junk food that starves the brain, and toxins like mercury that poison the brain. All these things together disrupt normal neurotransmitter chemistry in the brain.

Think about it. When you connect the dots, if the brain is malnourished and shrinking, then it's not working correctly. The chemicals are "off." Imbalanced chemicals in the brain can express themselves in symptoms that run the gamut from moodiness to brain fog, difficulty concentrating, to depression, rage, and, yes . . . insanity! Brain fog alone makes the normal course of going to school virtually impossible for some. Our children have been exposed to chemicals and toxins from birth and the negative effects are coming to their logical conclusion.

Children's brains are not fully formed until their mid to late twenties. Taking this precious unformed resource and making it *tox*-sick with dangerous chemicals is not only stealing their brains but disturbing the delicate balance of the GI tract and the overall health of everybody. The youngest among us are taking the hardest hit.

As you now know, sugar, in all its forms, and toxins have destroyed the lining of our GI tracts by eating little holes in the epithelium, allowing for leaks into the bloodstream. As these toxins roam through the bloodstream looking for a new home, they search out the fattiest organs. Our livers are already groaning from the toxic overload, so the toxins start looking around to choose their new homes. Perhaps it is the largest organ, the skin (causing eczema), or the pancreas (triggering diabetes), or the lungs (cancer), or the sex glands (halted hormones). But what they really are after is the fattiest organ of all . . . the brain.

The brain is like a sexy beach house for the chemical microbes.

The brain is composed of approximately 65 percent fat!

Understand this: Bad pathogens love to live in fats (especially fatty organs), but don't like to "eat" them (Suzanne-speak, not science-talk). They instead thrive on sugar. That's why flooding our GI tracts with fat essentially "starves them out" while also sealing up the barrier wall of the GI tract. Bad pathogens crave and live to eat sugar. They drown in fats and die of starvation. Real fats are essential to life and are satisfying comfort foods. Real fats make us feel good and complete. Why? The body has wisdom, and most of the time our body knows what it needs. It's time to listen to the good sense inside all of us. When we used to eat butter and real fats, we didn't crave all the crap that returns us to the fast-food restaurants or that pantry filled with bags and boxes of preservative-filled, processed, chemically laden foods.

A diet of low-fat and processed foods is making us sick.

The brain cannot live or thrive without fats. Cholesterol is crucial for brain health. This is the dirty little secret big business doesn't want you to know. In the next chapter you will find out that statins are big business, and it is in the best interests of those who are making money off them to keep as many people as possible thinking they must have these dangerous drugs. As Dr. Stephen Sinatra will explain, statins are only beneficial for those who have high Lp(a) (small dense razor-sharp particles). So if your doctor suggests you take these drugs, you are going to have the knowledge to ask the proper questions. Drugs can be lifesavers if they are absolutely necessary, but if there is a natural nonharmful protocol, why wouldn't you try that first?

As I said, bad pathogens in the gut *must* eat sugar to thrive but like to *live* in fat. Fats are the elixir of the brain. The brain has to have fat (cholesterol) to be healthy. It craves fats. Toxins love to take up residence in fat. With the low-fat craze, the brain is not being given its most important ingredient so it *shrinks*, giving toxins lots of room to hang out in the brain and grow and make trouble. If you consume a lot, or in some cases (like mine) a little bit, of sugar, the "bad guys" have a plentiful supply of happy food from the sugar you take in through your gut. Follow the pathway of all this dysfunction and you realize it all originates in the gut from these leaks and your food choices, and now they are causing brain fog and brain disorders.

> In 2011, a study conducted by Harris Interactive for MetLife Foundation showed that 31 percent of people fear dementia more than death or cancer.

It's a cascade. In addition to this destruction from toxic exposure, our hormones become disrupted because the hormone "executive" (order giver), the hypothalamus, resides in the brain, but due to toxicity and a liver unable to handle the toxic assault, it is not being stimulated to do its job because toxic chemicals and pesticides are running interference with the natural processes. Now this poor unsuspecting person has a hormone disaster, with disrupted signals. At this point the liver is so overloaded with toxins, it throws all the hormones back into the bloodstream, causing a hormone overdose and all the uncomfortable symptoms that accompany hormone imbalance. With brain dysfunction there are no neuronal signals telling the other hormones what to do. It's like a symphony without a conductor.

An unclear brain caused by a digestive tract that is in constant distress equals a full-body disaster! These two major organs are inextricably intertwined. No fat in your diet causes actual brain shrinkage, and then the toxins move in and with all this extra "room" they multiply until the brain loses its ability to operate at optimum. This is the beginning of brain fog, which leads to other and worse conditions or diseases.

> The fate of your brain is not in your genes. It's not inevitable. And if you're someone who suffers from another type of brain disorder, such as chronic headaches, depression, epilepsy, or extreme moodiness, the culprit MAY NOT be encoded in your DNA. It's in the food you eat.
>
> —Dr. David Perlmutter, *Grain Brain*

The brain cannot tolerate housing toxic foods and chemicals. Period. So let's learn how to clean house.

ENVIRON*MENTAL* ILLNESS: AN INTERVIEW WITH SHERRY ROGERS, M.D.

Dr. Sherry Rogers is an environmental doctor who has been in the trenches for more than forty years, long before most doctors realized there was an environmental assault on the human body. She was one of the first doctors in the United States who realized the limitations of orthodox medicine relative to the changed planet. She has a deep understanding of the scope of chemical pollution, and her protocols for preventing disease and treating chemical overload have saved the lives of thousands of patients. People come to her from all over the world at the end of their ropes, desperate after having been to numerous doctors to find an answer, to find relief. She has been a leading environmental medicine authority for more than twenty years and has authored books for both health professionals and the general public that have contributed significantly to the "changing of the guard" in medicine. Her book Detoxify or Die *is a tour de force that demonstrates the importance of understanding the role toxins, both from the outside world and produced inside our bodies, have on the origin of illnesses.*

SS: What an honor to speak to you, Dr. Rogers. Your work with toxicity and environmental issues is renowned. I am eager for my readers to hear your take on the effects and dangers of environmental toxins and how you are able to clear them from the body. I read your incredible book *Detoxify or Die*. Is it really that dire?

SR: Absolutely. And, in fact, I think you'll agree a thousandfold after we're done today. We are the most toxic humans to ever inhabit the planet Earth.

SS: How did you become this person? How did this become your specialty? Is this part of the medical school curriculum?

SR: No, it isn't. I'm no smarter than any other doctor. I was just sicker. That was what forced me over the last forty-five years to learn the molecular biochemistry of how the body heals, instead of just bludgeoning every symptom with the latest drug.

SS: First of all, you and I are of similar ages. When I was a girl, women didn't become doctors. How did you pull that off?

SR: I'm the oldest of eight children from a then poor family and nobody had ever graduated from high school, and when I told my family I was going to be a doctor they said, "Oh, that's nice, but you don't understand, that takes a lot of money. You have to go to college and then you go to medical school, and by the way, they don't take women in medical school" (that was in the '50s). So I went to the guidance counselor and asked, what can I do? He said, if you study like crazy and you are an "A" student, you could win a scholarship. So that's what I did . . . I won scholarships and worked all the way through college and medical school. One day in medical school, I asked a question of a dentist, who had just lectured to us, and he took one look at me and said, "Oh my gosh, you poor starving medical student. I see you have a mouthful of mercury amalgams that have probably been in your mouth since you were about seven years old, let me give you a discount and repair your teeth." I thought, *Well, this is good*, so he took out all the mercury and put in brand-new mercury.

So I'm one of the few living people who has had such enormous levels of mercury in their body for decades. That was toxin number one, and then there were many other things; I used to strip furniture, antiques and things, with my bare hands with toluene and xylene and benzene, et cetera, and multiple other things requiring chemicals. We later had a farm. I drove the tractor. We sprayed herbicides and other pesticides on the cornfields, you name it. But that wasn't all. For example, my first office was in the early '70s when we thought formaldehyde was the great thing: the UFFI, urea-formaldehyde insulation. It was the latest and greatest way to insulate a building—you just blew it into the wall cavity—so we did and I got severe formaldehyde poisoning.

And then, of course, that produces mold. I eventually ended up having my own mycology lab so that I could study mold and actually grow the molds from people's homes all over the world, because we were seeing such a deluge of people who were mold-sensitive as well. And it snowballed into the whole scenario of multiple chemical sensitivities [MCS] where people would come to my office who had become wildly sensitive to foods, chemicals, molds, and much more.

Like me, these folks were sensitive to environmental pollutants that most people aren't even aware exist.

As it turned out I realized we unsuspecting chemically sensitive people are the canaries. Sadly, we're the ones who show you how disease works. In fact, now we know there are only two causes for most disease: the nutrient levels go down and the toxicity levels go up. So that's what we do; we assay and find out what we have to do to correct deficiencies and toxicities to bring the body back into balance, and that is known as "healing."

SS: So the answer to this toxic dilemma is good nutrition and detoxification? And yet it's not quite as simple as that, right?

SR: Yes, absolutely.

SS: How did you know that you had formaldehyde poisoning?

SR: It began with being exposed to the high levels of formaldehyde in the autopsy room in medical school. Years later (I wasn't tuned in), I would walk into my office [with UFFI] and my eyes would burn, or I would get a migraine headache. In fact, I had such serious migraine headaches, I thought I had a brain tumor, because I thought there's no way migraines could be this painful.

I had so many incidents that didn't add up; I couldn't think straight, I had no energy, I had blinding migraines, asthma, eczema, sinus headaches. I broke my back six times. I wore a body cast. I blew out a shoulder, knee, elbow. Those were just the orthopedic issues. I've been through a lot. When I was thirty-five, they told me my bones looked like I was seventy-eight.

I was allergic to most toxins and nightshades but didn't know it then and the allergy attacked my soleus muscle in my back and mimicked a ruptured disc.

SS: Was your nightshade consumption potatoes?

SR: No, the hidden stuff. Things you wouldn't think were allergens: Who would think a paralyzed leg mimicking a ruptured disc could be from ingredients like spices, paprika, starch? My book *Pain Free in 6 Weeks* describes it all.

SS: So your pain and dysfunction led you to environmental medicine?

SR: Yes. No one was addressing it, like it didn't exist . . . I went through the practice guidelines for major cardiology, internal medicine, emergency room guidelines for physicians and how they should practice their recipes for what they do day to day, and there was practically nothing on cause and cure.

Today my focus is to find the cause and the cure of every symptom; the label is irrelevant, whether it's chemical sensitivity, brain fog. Why are we having this epidemic of people with brain diseases, starting with the young right on into Alzheimer's? We now know exactly how it all started and how to fix it, and that's the beauty of this. By the way, everything I say today is backed by the full scientific references, the evidence somewhere in my seventeen books and twenty-five years of newsletters. I have to admit, I am a medical doctor who's a reference junkie. I have to have the biochemical backup for everything that I say because that's just the way I operate.

SS: What was your impetus? What made you want to learn everything?

SR: It's been a forty-five-year quest, the luckiest thing that has ever happened to me because now we get tearstained letters from people so grateful for their healing. For example, one might say, "I had multiple chemical sensitivities and I cleared it," or "I had rheumatoid arthritis," or "My child had juvenile drug-resistant diabetes or hypertension and now it's gone," or "I have atrial fibrillation resistant to ablation."

SS: That's rewarding work. These conditions are supposed to have no known cause, no known treatment, yet your readers are healing?

SR: Yes. That's how we ended up writing *The Cholesterol Hoax; The High Blood Pressure Hoax; Wellness Against All Odds; Pain Free in 6 Weeks; Depression Cured at Last;* et cetera. Because I learned that there was a plethora of decades of research by all these brilliant people to substantiate how we should be looking for the cause and the cure in medicine as opposed to just drugging everything. I realized I had to get the message out. So, yes, it's been very rewarding in many ways and a quest that still continues.

SS: You said in your great book *Detoxify or Die* that we are all afraid of cancer. But no one understands that the damage produced by pesticides is more pervasive and that it has the opportunity to affect so many different areas, organs, and glands in the body, right?

SR: Oh, absolutely. There are volumes of research on this. In fact, a lot of times, for example, one of the nastiest brain diseases is Parkinson's disease. Do you know how they create it in the lab to get five hundred rats with PD, so they can study some new drug? They give them an *organic* pesticide. And guess what, they can create PD. So you could imagine what a nonorganic pesticide would do. That's partly why there's this catastrophic explosion of insidious brain deterioration and mental disease in the United States.

Brain disease, as the *Wall Street Journal* recently showed us, is affecting more than one in twelve children and they are now on mind-altering drugs, whether it's Ritalin or Adderall for ADD, ADHD, OCD, autism, depression, learning difficulties. Altering a young mind like this makes it possible to morph into violence and crimes, all because of multiple chemical sensitivities. For some it morphs into schizophrenia. We have record suicides in teenagers now, and in adults, we have bipolar disorder, schizophrenia, OCD (obsessive-compulsive disorder), depression. Then it can morph into MCI, which is a misnomer because they call it mild cognitive impairment. There's no such thing; this is like being a little bit pregnant! MCS is the precursor to dementia, Parkinson's disease, and the dreaded Alzheimer's.

But the good news is we know how to fix all this, and it's been known for decades. In fact, what most people don't know is that by putting back the best nutrients for rejuvenating the brain, you can return to levels of better health than you ever had before.

SS: Where do multiple chemical sensitivities start?

SR: They start in the gut. In fact, the gut is called the "second brain" by many researchers. There are many things that damage the gut.

One of the first things is all the antibiotics that kids are given right away as soon as they have their first ear infection and so forth. This can change the ecosystem and can cause overgrowth of one of the many fungi in the human gut called *Candida albicans*. There are other species: *C. krusei, C. parapsilosis, C. glabrata,* et cetera. The antibiotic does not just go to fix a sore throat; it goes to the gut and kills off multiple bacteria, creating an imbalance. When this happens (we're just using this yeast as one teeny, tiny example of bugs or organisms that can change the function of the body's second brain), the imbalance creates inflammation in the gut lining, which goes on to cause a leaky gut and autoimmune disorders like multiple sclerosis and rheumatoid arthritis. More important, it causes the body to make antibodies against the person's own thyroid gland. In other words, as the food and bacterial antigens leak across this inflamed gut, the body sees these new antigens as foreign invaders (bugs that the body never recognized before) like candida, et cetera, and it says oh, we should attack. The inherent wisdom in the body is to protect the body. In doing so, some of the antigenic sites on the thyroid are similar to the ones in intestinal bugs that have leaked through along with certain foods. That's one of the many reasons why we have an epidemic of thyroiditis in the United States.

SS: So you are saying antibiotic intake at an early age sets the stage for problems down the road, throughout life, including thyroid problems?

SR: Yes, and another reason is the PBDEs: polybrominated diphenyl ethers. These are one of the nastiest chemicals we have introduced in the United States. Back in the '70s PBDEs were required for circuit boards as flame retardants. Then they were legislated by law to be in mattresses, couches, cushions, airplane seats, car seats, beds, you name it. The high level of bromine from PBDEs actually kicks the iodine out of the T3 thyroid hormone. As a result, the tests for thyroid function can look normal, but the thyroid doesn't function normally in the human body.

So now we have a person who's tired, brain fogged, depressed, and gaining weight and has high cholesterol, metabolic syndrome X, and high triglyciderides. And they can't figure out what's wrong with them, and their doctor says their thyroid tests are normal. It's even worse if a pregnant woman is low in thyroid; that child is born with an IQ at least ten points lower than he or she normally would have had. Then the candida causes food allergies, and we have epidemic food allergies now, such as the gluten enteropathies, brain fog, inability to concentrate, depression, bipolar disorder, and so on, which go to the brain. For a lot of people, the brain is the target organ. There are opioid receptors in the human brain that actually cause addiction to wheat and milk products, which are the number one and two most common food allergens.

But as we wrote in *Pain Free in 6 Weeks*, plus I published a medical paper as well to substantiate it, three out of four people who have any type of arthritis—one joint, two joints, many joints, fibromyalgia, juvenile rheumatoid arthritis—have been totally cured. Cured. We don't use that word in medicine. Cured if they just don't eat the Solanaceae family; this was my problem, allergies to the nightshades—potatoes, tomatoes, peppers, cayenne, chili, paprika, modified food starch, modified food protein, starch—which are hidden in so many foods as the term *MFP* or the generic word *spices*.

SS: Natural flavor. Very deceptive.

SR: Yes, it is, and so many people get hurt unnecessarily. Because of this lack of understanding, starting with antibiotics, there's a whole epidemic of joint replacements, and in progressively younger people. Furthermore, the gut houses half the immune system and half the detoxification system for the whole body. So if the gut isn't healthy, you can't make the brain healthy, and then you can't clear multiple chemical sensitivity, arthritis, coronary artery disease, and IBS. You can't clear up anything. The gut is the starting place.

SS: But people are stumped about their gut. I see on the Internet people sharing advice and no one knows what to do. The antifungals aren't working, and the antibiotics are making it worse.

SR: Well, the first thing people need to do is look at what's growing in the gut and test to see if it's in abnormal amounts, and what it's sensitive to. A lot of people have a gut full of yeast. We can see this by an elevated arabintol on a urine test, and we can also see it by culture on the comprehensive stool. So the first line of defense is to heal the gut. On the flip side, when you look at their chemistry, if you see that they're low in many crucial nutrients, maybe the first thing that you have to do is correct some of those deficiencies. You can't heal unless you are playing with a full deck of nutrients.

SS: What nutrients are you talking about?

SR: As just one example, many people have low magnesium levels; some so low it is like they should have had a heart attack a year ago and died. They're just making do. They're pulling magnesium out of the bones and other storage places to make do in the body because they're magnesium depleted. This deficiency is literally epidemic and rarely diagnosed.

SS: And when magnesium levels are seriously low, are these people experiencing bone weakness?

SR: Yes, you get osteoporosis from it. And taking calcium makes it worse, if it is not balanced with magnesium. This lack of balance hardens arteries in the heart, brain, and extremities and is a major cause of death.

SS: Yeah, but let me be the devil's advocate for a minute. So then you just take a little Fosamax, right?

SR: Oh, we've done a lot of articles on that; sure, if you want jaw rot and to have all your teeth fall out. When I consult with readers and I see their records from the last three years, the people who are on Fosamax are depleted in D_3 or K_2, but physicians rarely look at that. You can't heal a bone without K_2 and D_3 for starters.

SS: Does a newborn child inherit the gut flora of the mother?

SR: Yes, there's evidence that not only do children inherit the gut flora of their mothers, but they inherit the nutrient deficiencies of the mothers. These studies have gone on for three generations. If the mother is low in zinc, then the child does not make enough hydrochloric acid (HCL) from the enzyme carbonic anhydrase, which is a zinc-dependent enzyme in the stomach. If you don't make enough HCL in the stomach, then you can't absorb your minerals well. So you get deficiencies from that, which lead to brain problems and MCS. It doesn't matter what you call the disease. What matters is, what is the cause and what is the cure? So without sufficient HCL, acid bubbles up from fermented food. The esophagus is not made for any acid whatsoever. So even the littlest bit that's there causes acid reflux and the person thinks he or she needs something like Prilosec or Nexium, which is the worst thing in the world because this lowers B_{12} and magnesium. It actually promotes Alzheimer's and many different types of nerve and brain degenerative problems. Clearly, stifling a symptom with a drug eventually snowballs into an avalanche of many seemingly unrelated symptoms and diseases. Low magnesium leads to high blood pressure, angina, atrial fibrillation, depression, back pain, and more.

That's why we wrote *No More Heartburn*. These drugs also lower your magnesium levels, so now the person has back spasms, like I had. Then he's off to the orthopedist. We actually have documented back spasms so serious that they mimicked a ruptured disc and the person should have had disc surgery, and it was just due to the nightshades. But it can also be due to magnesium deficiency, which, of course, is a major cause of sudden cardiac arrest. Then there's another organic acid that's put out by candida called tricarballylate, and it actually chelates out your magnesium. So in spite of taking it, you don't get better.

Clearly, there is no substitute for an in-depth analysis of all your bio-chemistry at once. How else will you know where to start?

SS: And this is why people are on so many drugs requiring more drugs because they are not really treating the problem but actually exacerbating it?

SR: Correct. Magnesium deficiencies cause depression and fatigue, atrial fibrillation, and so forth. And nobody knows why you're not ab-sorbing your magnesium, because first of all, they rarely measure it, and generally if they do, they measure the wrong one; they measure (serum) magnesium. You never want a doctor to measure just your serum magnesium as that represents only 1 percent of the body mag-nesium. You want the RBC, red blood cell, intracellular magnesium; that's where about 95 percent of it is, and if that is low, you are set up for sudden cardiac arrest: the new epidemic for people in their thirties and forties, who suddenly die.

SS: All from magnesium deficiencies, caused by yeast and other toxins?

SR: Yes, and everybody says, "But they were so healthy." There are many other things that this yeast does, but this is just one example of one organism out of over five hundred in the gut that can cause seri-ous problems in every organ in the body.

SS: So the kid starts out behind the eight ball because of the toxic burden he's born with, coupled with the poor diet of most Americans and the inherited bad ecosystem and nutritional deficiencies of the mother. Now it's becoming clear why we are here with this unbeliev-able epidemic of children with "mystery illnesses."

SR: It gets worse. There's a lot of research showing that the moth-er's diet clearly influences the child's brain when he's in utero. For example, if she does not have enough DHA, docosahexaenoic acid, the number one fatty acid in the human brain, the child has a big problem, for not only is DHA (in cod liver oil) essential for the mem-brane surrounding every nerve and every other type of cell, we need it for the mitochondrial membrane because that is where we make energy. If the mother doesn't have enough, then the child will most likely be born with a low IQ. He will have more need for glasses, and other problems, because this is fundamental chemistry in the human body. And if, heaven forbid, she should have yeast from antibiotics beforehand as we were just discussing, then the child will have accelerated health problems.

Another thing the yeast makes is acetaldehyde, which causes brain fog, body aches, chemical sensitivity, and depression symptoms that nobody can figure out. Unfortunately, most doctors are working totally blind. They do not measure vitamins, minerals, fatty acids, amino acids, and organic acids. But that's the only way you can find the cause and the cure. Another major cause of brain deterioration through the gut is the prescription drugs that people take. The statin drugs, as we showed in *The Cholesterol Hoax*, actually starve the brain of its daily repair of cholesterol that it needs. You eventually rob the brain of the cholesterol it needs to make new memories and happy moods.

SS: Yes, Dr. Sinatra goes into that in detail in his interview for this book. It's terrible so many are taking that awful drug.

SR: Yes, and statins also lower the eight crucial forms of vitamin E. Four of the eight forms of vitamin E are called tocotrienols and they're HMG-CoA reductase inhibitors. In other words, they work in the same way by lowering cholesterol, but they don't damage the genes and bring on cancers, Alzheimer's, and sudden amnesia as do statin drugs. Statins also promote diabetes, as evidence recently stated in the *Wall Street Journal*. So those people who are on Lipitor or Crestor, et cetera, are literally starving their brain every day from the crucial repair needed via cholesterol.

But rather than show people what is wrong with medicine, I'd rather show them how to get themselves well. In an October 15, 2014, article in the *Journal of the American Medical Association*, the authors described a telling example of how misguided medicine can be. The title of the article was "Effect of High Dose Vitamin D_3 on Hospital Length of Stay in Critically Ill Patients with Vitamin D Deficiency." The researchers used the wrong cutoff (30 ng/dl) to diagnose the deficiencies, and then they grossly undertreated. There were many false statements in the paper that we documented.

SS: What did they consider a high dose of vitamin D_3?

SR: Well, first of all, they only used 300 milligrams, which is less than the RDA. With most people we find they need 10,000 units of vitamin D_3 a day. You cannot cure diabetes, high blood pressure, depression, a poor immune system, or recurrent infections without enough

D$_3$. And there are numerous scientific reports documenting that most people need anywhere from 4,000 to 10,000 IUs a day.

Anyway, besides the statins are drugs like Zetia or a statin combination called Vytorin, which is a statin plus a cholesterol absorption inhibitor. So now, you not only have a statin, which brings on diabetes, Alzheimer's, cancers, and so on, and sudden amnesia, but you are robbing the body of essential cholesterol. Many of the freak accidents we have where planes and subway trains suddenly crash are often attributed to the drugs the operators are taking . . . but the investigators and reporters rarely ask what the people are on and most pilots are on Lipitor.

Zetia, as a cholesterol-absorbing inhibitor, also inhibits the absorption of fat-soluble vitamins: A, D, E, K, CoQ10; the fatty acids. Everything you need to heal. And it gets worse; a real common drug is a calcium channel blocker (like Norvasc) for arrhythmias and high blood pressure. These are proven to shrink the brain in less than five years, yet these are prescribed forever. Then Motrin and Aleve and the nonsteroidal, anti-inflammatory drugs can actually potentiate arthritis and mysterious pain in the joints because their chemistry deteriorates the chemistry of cartilage repair.

So now we have this epidemic of people with knee replacements. Well, most of them ate a lot of nightshades (N-shades) for years before this happened, plus they can cause leaky gut just like candida. Prilosec, Nexium, and the proton pump inhibitors, decrease your magnesium, decrease your B$_{12}$, which leads to heart attacks, depression, muscle spasms, high blood pressure. In fact, recent papers have shown that individuals who are put on drugs like Prilosec or Nexium while they're in the hospital increase their chance of getting pneumonia by 30 percent. It begs the question: Why has the FDA decided they are safe enough to no longer require a prescription?

And then we have people who are on Coumadin and Warfarin because they've had pulmonary embolus or a heart attack or stroke, and they need to thin their blood. But that poisons vitamin K, which is crucial for the sphingomyelin synthesis needed for brain repair. So, just so much, and we have only touched a few categories of drugs. Clearly, once you stifle a symptom with a drug, you create an avalanche of new symptoms.

> The sick get sicker quicker with drugs!

Food toxins also damage every part of the body; they can bring on every disease from MCS to heart and vascular disease to diabetes. There are a number of toxins that are not talked about that much but are extremely potent.

> Phthalates (known as plastics) are the number one toxin in the human body. Phthalates are so potent that if a mother is drinking out of plastic water bottles while she's pregnant, she can be programming her unborn child for adult diabetes, poor brain and nerve function, breast cancer, prostate cancer, and much more.
> —Environmental Health Perspectives

SS: Is this the obesity crisis?

SR: Oh, absolutely. Yes. Phthalates are unavoidably ubiquitous twenty-first-century toxins that damage our body chemistry in multiple pathways. That is why they are able to literally create any disease.

SS: All our little overweight children and they never had a chance.

SR: Yes, and don't forget that all our little fat children, as the *Journal of the American Medical Association* documented in 2014, have morphed into an epidemic and a 30 percent increase in children in the United States with diabetes in just the last eight years.

SS: Why aren't the mothers being warned?

SR: It's stupid; orthodox doctors are unread. The word *phthalates* did not even appear once in the journal articles. I see this over and over in many scientific articles in the conventional medical literature; the word *phthalate* never appears. All these researchers from twenty different hospitals and high-profile medical centers thought that childhood diabetes was caused by the obesity epidemic.

SS: Rather than the other way around.

SR: Worse! That's like saying auto accidents are caused by car salesmen.

Anyway, back on the phthalates, we cannot escape them because they're everywhere—in our air, food, and water. Ketchup and mustard used to be in glass, now they're in plastic, baby bottles are plastic, and then there are the construction materials in our homes; carpeting, furniture, everything is plastic, even the electric wires and plastic coatings that outgas phthalates. That's why they are the number one pollutants in the human body and damage brains, because they poison many fundamental areas of human chemistry needed for healing and normal functioning.

For example, plastics damage beta-oxidation; what does that mean? It means that you can take the best cod liver oil in the world, for example, to fix your cell membranes. But you can't do it because you don't have enough of the chemistry in your body for it to work because it's been poisoned by the phthalates. And for any readers who don't believe (because there are many naysayers) this stuff about plastics and BPA, which is a cousin of phthalates, who believe it is not all-pervasive in the world, think about this: the Arctic polar bears, who have the cleanest air, food, and water on the planet, now have human diseases—osteoporosis, hypothyroidism. This shouldn't be. Our pollutants have literally reached the most remote corners of the planet.

SS: Because the chemical phthalates are in the air?

SR: Air and water. They're everywhere. You cannot escape them. In fact, Yale researchers were studying breast cancer cells in plastic petri dishes, but before they added the carcinogen, the breast cancer cells were growing like crazy as though the carcinogen had been added.

SS: From the plastic of the petri dishes?

SR: Yes, that's how they discovered that plastics are huge carcinogens and that they were creating the rapid growth of breast cancer cells. Most environmental chemicals—pesticides, heavy metals, phthalates, and others that we'll mention—are what we call "EEDs," environmental endocrine disruptors. They can destroy any gland and they can do it silently, because, for example, the PBDEs, which are the brominated flame retardants that are in most of our furniture—cushions, foam, mattresses—kick out the body's iodine and substitute, instead, bromine in the T3 or T4 molecule. So, now, when you have a blood test for thyroid, the doctor says "you have enough thyroid, I just measured it."

Next, when the thyroid hormone attaches to the cell, it doesn't work right because the body recognizes it doesn't have the right number of iodine molecules. They have been substituted with bromine.

And worse, once the thyroid hormone hooks onto the cell receptor for thyroid—the place where the thyroid hormone hooks in to turn on the energy process in the cell—the cell membrane doesn't have the right fatty acids in it to make the thyroid work. Phthalates have destroyed the beta-oxidation. Unfortunately we don't have sufficient physicians interested in this type of chemistry, which is hugely evidenced. Endocrinology records that I review from readers show the very fundamentals were ignored by these "specialists." They never ever checked the iodine or the membrane thyroid receptors for adequate fatty acids, phosphatidyl choline, tocopherols, and so on.

SS: Is it too soon to ask you how we clear phthalates from the body?

SR: First it's about diet. *Brassica* vegetables: cabbage, cauliflower and Brussels sprouts, broccoli, kale and mizuna, collard greens, et cetera. There are many more of them, including radishes and turnips, rutabaga. The *Brassica* vegetables are also called "cruciferous." They rev up glucuronidation (a phase II detoxification pathway occurring in the liver in which glucuronic acid is conjugated with toxins), which is the main way that we detoxify phthalates.

There are other things we put in the body that damage the gut and then damage the brain right away; one big offender is high-fructose corn syrup. It's an FDA-approved sweetener that's in most processed foods and used to create diabetic rats for research. I thought to myself, how could corn syrup be that potent to create diabetes? I mean, it's only a different form of sugar. So I looked up how it's made and, lo and behold, I found the answer that we evidenced in the *Total Wellness 2014* report. The process of making high-fructose corn syrup or corn syrup, cornstarch, or corn sugar is a mercury chlor-alkali process. It loads the victim with one of the most toxic heavy metals, mercury. This alone can mimic a litany of common and mysterious disease states.

SS: What does that do?

SR: HFCS actually gives the person who has an average amount of corn syrup a day—average, not the people who go overboard—equivalent mercury to having one tooth in their mouth filled with mercury every day for the rest of their lives!

And I know many people whose mercury amalgam healed with the removal of just one tooth. Once they got that mercury filling out, their high blood pressure, their shoulder pain of a year, their MS, their leukemia, all sorts of conditions disappeared.

In my book *Pain Free in 6 Weeks*, we have the dental map of the organs showing which different teeth are connected to which organs or areas of the body through acupuncture meridians. If you have a root canal or a mercury amalgam in those teeth that are connected to certain organs that are a problem for you, that may be the answer.

Anyway, back on the PBDEs, people might say, "I never heard of that," "I don't like these chemical names, how can that be so bad?" Well, that's probably the number two most toxic environmental pollutant in the human body. Yet the United States legislated it into mattresses, couches, and chairs so some smoking drunk wouldn't burn himself up at night.

As a result, the U.S. populace has 40 to 100 percent higher levels of PBDEs in their blood than do the Europeans, and our levels are doubling every two to four years because PBDEs are one of those environmental pollutants that are called POPs: persistent organic pollutants. They never leave. There's no way to metabolize them. They are even imprinted in circuit boards and electronics. For that reason a lot of people need to take the iodinated compound nonprescription Lugol's; depending on iodine and other levels, four to eight drops a day is the usual starting dose for nonprescription 2% Lugol's solution.

SS: Iodine or iodide?

SR: It's both. Four drops of 2% Lugol's contains 5 milligrams of iodine and 7.5 milligrams of iodide. It tastes terrible, but it's a wonderful way for people to decrease ADD, chronic fatigue, schizophrenia, breast cancers. Also there are so many other brain destroyers like fake sugars, MSG, trans fats, and there's the canola con.

> We had good evidence before that aspartame most likely
> produced cancer and now we know it does for sure.
> —Dr. Russell Blaylock, neuroscientist

Promoters convinced regulators that canola oil, which is genetically modified, was better than the trans fats. Well, canola has trans fats in it, but they are deceptively not listed on the label. This damages the membrane chemistry until you do an "oil change." And then, of course, we have genetically modified foods. Most babies are brought up on soy, and that's genetically modified. Eighty percent of soy is GMO. The body knows when it is not getting the real McCoy, plus soy is an EED (damages glands).

SS: What is the effect of GMOs on the human body? Where is this going?

SR: It's huge. The body cannot be fooled. It knows when it's getting something fake. And we wrote a lot about that in this year's newsletter *Total Wellness 2014*. Some of the things GMOs can bring on are food allergies and gluten enteropathy, which, of course, can have brain manifestations as well as joint and muscle manifestations. It's probably the reason for the epidemic of people who say, "I'm gluten sensitive," now; and by the way, a lot of people are told by their gastroenterologist that once you're sensitive, you'll always be sensitive. Not true. For many people, if they get their body healthy enough, they don't have sensitivities anymore. The healed gut can stop making antibodies that attack itself, as we have seen with many autoimmune diseases.

SS: That's uplifting.

SR: That's the uplifting part about all of this. I would not be spending my semiretirement years (I closed my office after forty wonderful years of practice) writing books and newsletters and talking on radio shows if we didn't get all the wonderful letters. That's what motivates me.

SS: I run into so many people who say, "I just can't be bothered, we're all going to die sometime." But you're saying no, we can live this long life and we can heal by taking the proper steps, right?

SR: Right. But it's dependent on the whole package that individuals bring to the table and then how they decide to empower themselves to modify their health regimen. It's your heredity, your environment, but mainly it's your knowledge and your ability to want to do the right things. None of us is perfect. Do I have plastic wrap in my kitchen? Of course I do. Do I have some plastic containers? Of course I do. We can't be perfect. But we can know enough.

And my motto is always: "Let's make people too smart to fail in their quest for wellness."

SS: Are there tests that would indicate brain deterioration? And what are those tests?

SR: There are scores of tests to indicate silent, early reversible brain deterioration, One test we wrote about in the 2013 newsletter tested for high levels of quinolinate. It shows brain deterioration years before it appears. It's usually due to the person not having enough zinc. So they cannot convert B_6 to its active form P5P, pyridoxal 5 phosphate. Once they do that with enough zinc or they take P5P, the quinolinate goes down.

SS: If the liver of a person is groaning from toxicity and can't handle it anymore, is zinc going to do any good?

SR: For a "groaning" sick liver, zinc will not do any good until you identify the following: (1) the deficiencies that need correcting; (2) the toxins that need to be depurated (to make or become free from impurities); and (3) in which order these steps need to proceed in accomplishing the task for this individual.

We have composed a twelve-page assay, and we tell people how to order their own assays in *How to Cure Diabetes*. Not only does the assay look at levels of vitamins, minerals, fatty acids, amino acids, but it looks at organic acids. What does that mean? It means if, for example, you draw somebody's B_6 level and it looks normal, then your doctor says there's no problem here, that can't be the cause of your brain deterioration or your brain fog or your chemical sensitivity or your ADD. Then he's not looking at how much *you* as an individual need. That is just looking at the level. A functional assay shows if you need more than the "normal"" amount to make your chemistry of healing soar.

SS: It works the same way with hormone replacement. The amounts I need are different from the next person.

SR: Right; if you then go and look at other examples of where B_6 is not being utilized, you'll see further evidence of your particular need. For example, is your B_6 being converted to its active form? We know that even though you may have a "normal" zinc level, it may not be normal for you. That's the beauty of organic acids. It tells you the functional assay or whether or not you have enough for your chemistry. Even if your zinc level is great, if your beta-carotene is high and your vitamin A is low, you're not converting the beta-carotene into two molecules of vitamin A, because that's a zinc-dependent enzyme. We went into a lot of those zinc-dependent enzymes in this year's newsletter just as a review for folks, because we're always trying to get them smarter and smarter. I try not to snow them with chemistry, but keep it pragmatic.

So back to your original question, which, of course, was so good: How do we fix the brain? Many ways. In fact, the chemistry that we use to fix the brain is the same chemistry that you use to fix everything. First of all, Suzanne, I hate to say it, but we are fatheads. We have more fat in the brain than anywhere else because the cell membranes around the nerves are made up of fats.

SS: What are we, about 65 percent fat?

SR: Yes, 40 percent to 65 percent, depending on which areas of the brain you're looking at. When you start healing brain fats, you also heal the fats around every cell in the body—the heart cells, the liver cells, the kidney cells—and you start healing the nerves as well. It's so important for people to understand that the cell membrane is like the computer keyboard; that's where all the messages from the cell come out and say okay, put out the cytokine that kills cancer or put out this protein that regulates the heart rate, and so on. We analyze the fatty acids in people's cell membranes (and I go over their molecular biochemistry with them on the phone in two dozen countries), and we find that for most people, their cell membranes and their brains are literally starving. In fact, their brain and mitochondrial and cell membranes are not only starved for the right fatty acids but are simultaneously choked with the wrong fatty acids. They can never heal whatever their goal is without correcting this. They are stranded.

SS: Is the antidote as simple as essential fatty acids, phosphatidylcholine, and eight forms of vitamin E? Is this the "recipe" for body repair?

SR: I wish it were that simple. When I consult with folks on the phone, I have them send their last three years of medical records from everywhere. So I get to see Johns Hopkins, Cleveland Clinic, Mayo Clinic, Harvard. I get to see the crème de la crème. Shockingly to me, these institutions are still not even assaying all this wonderful chemistry that has been known for decades. They're working blindly. They just prescribe drugs and then procedures like ablation. In order to bring about wellness, you need to see as much of the chemistry at once as possible. You need to see the grand inclusive picture of what is wrong. To have only a "snippet" like fatty acids is not enough.

Last year, I consulted on a ten-year-old child who had SVT, supra-ventricular tachycardia, a cardiac arrhythmia that goes about 250 times a minute and drops him to the floor unconscious. He had been to all the best cardiologists for three years. I saw all the records. I did the twelve-page assay to look at his chemistry and found that he was low, desperately low, in selenium, magnesium, phosphatidylcholine, and on and on. So often the solution can be incredibly quick and simple.

Once we corrected these, in one month, his three years of arrhythmia—totally gone. Cured. And yet the cardiologist had wanted to do ablation, where they slip a catheter up into the heart from the groin and turn on the juice and ablate or permanently elec-trocute and destroy parts of the nerve and muscle of the heart. This is not a cure. The cure is to find out what's wrong, what's missing, and how the person can fix it: not destroy forever parts of a child's heart!

When we started out, I said I'd talk about other nutrients that the brain definitely needs. Bruce Ames, a very famous M.D. researcher, did some great studies that showed how merely two nutrients can make brains revert to more youthful levels. So just imagine what hap-pens when you look at the whole package!

Acetyl-L-carnitine and lipoic acid are crucial for moving the fatty acids into the brain and restoring brain function. Well, guess what phthalates do? They destroy ALC, acetyl-L-carnitine, and lipoate!

Connect the dots . . . And that's why it brings us back to what peo-ple are putting in their guts. They can make intelligent choices about what they're putting in their mouths. Once they understand that if they have a choice between glass and plastic, if they have a choice between making this food or buying a processed food with fourteen ingredients on the label that they don't even know how to explain, then they can start to change the chemistry of their bodies.

For example, researchers selected five families in California and taught them how to *not* eat phthalates, how to reduce the amount of plastic and how to rev up the brassicas. All of them dropped the phthalate levels in their blood within a few months by 96 percent! That's powerful. And then, of course, there's R-lipoic acid. It should be criminal not to prescribe R-lipoic acid for diabetics because it is proven to decrease the side effects that diabetics get: early heart attacks, early Alzheimer's, early cataracts, early phlebitis, gangrene, and amputations.

In fact, R-lipoic acid is extremely potent against mold; when there is no other cure for Amanita poisoning, R-lipoic is the remedy. Amanita poisoning comes from when people have been on a picnic and picked poisonous mushrooms they thought were good and ate them. Most of them die because medicine does not have a remedy for it. R-lipoic as a remedy is not taught in the schools where guys are getting their degree as emergency room physicians, because we don't look for the cause and the cure.

Also, you have to have R-lipoic acid to get rid of candida, same to get rid of poisonous mushrooms, to rejuvenate and bring the brain back to youthful levels.

SS: In your book, you talk about your detox cocktail of glutathione, ascorbic acid (which is powdered vitamin C), and R-lipoic. Is it always important to take your lipoic acid with the vitamin C?

SR: No, the order doesn't matter. You can take those components—glutathione, R-lipoic, ascorbate—anytime. They can be separate. It's just that we tried to make them into a cocktail because we showed people that you have Phase I of detox and then you have Phase II. You also want to recycle some nutrients like C and E, so that you can get more mileage out of them, and that's what R-lipoic acid does. Also phosphatidylcholine is very crucial, and then of course, more zinc and magnesium. There are numerous studies (which we've referenced) showing groups of children six years of age, who are not from poor families, but from well-to-do wealthy families, and 40 percent of them were low in vitamin E and were low in D_3. No wonder they are prescribed antibiotics that start gut deterioration when pediatricians are identifying and correcting these epidemic deficiencies.

SS: And why are children having record deficiencies in the land of plenty?

SR: Because of the way we eat today. Foods are the vehicles for toxins like the phthalates and the PBDEs and the genetically modified foods and the trans fatty acids often hidden in canola oil and mercury-laden corn syrup.

SS: Well, the market on canola oil has been tremendous. They have convinced most people that this is a healthy choice. I'm in agreement with you that the healthy oils are so important. What are the oils that you recommend?

SR: Well, first of all, it's a balance; the most important oils are the omega-3s, like cod liver oil.

SS: What brand do you recommend?

SR: We use Carlson's lemon-flavored cod liver oil, because when it comes to oil-soluble nutrients, I want a company that is ironclad about ethics, transparency.

SS: The common complaints today (and I have this in my own family) are Lyme disease, mold, chemical sensitivities, food allergies, gluten, and people pretty much allergic to almost all foods.

SR: Which is what I was; I had eighty-five foods I could not eat and only six foods that I could tolerate for ten years. Now I eat everything but the nightshades and junk food. But every disease has a cause and a cure. It just depends on how damaged the person is and how much about the chemistry of healing their physician knows.

SS: Is the recipe essentially the same for people who are loaded up and toxically burdened?

SR: Yes. You have to fix the chemistry. Lyme disease; I consult on so many of those people. They have never had an assay of the nutrients needed to fight infection! They've had some scattered nutrients; they've got all sorts of other assays they send me, genetic testing and different virus titers in the body, and so on. But they're not playing with a full deck; when you see what's missing, then you know why they're sick. For example, if their doctor did a vitamin D_3 level and believed that the cutoff that the commercial labs all use (30 nanograms per deciliter) was normal and they were 32, then he would tell them you've got enough "D," so no problem with that. Well, you can't fight off Lyme disease, mold, chemical sensitivity, food allergies, without a "D" over at least 80 nanograms per deciliter. It's really tragic if they haven't studied enough to know the commercial lab cutoff is over fifteen years behind; what do you think they know about the rest of the total load needed to cure?

SS: Many people with Lyme disease go to their doctor for IV antibiotic treatments two and three times a day. How do you feel about that?

SR: By fostering candida and not identifying the nutrient deficiencies, many orthodox doctors push these folks deeper into sickness.

They create thyroiditis, brain fog, and body pain. These people have rampant candida, which progresses into worsening symptoms. Candida makes an enzyme that destroys vitamin B_1, thiaminase, so no matter how much you take, you can't get it in the body. Candida makes an organic acid, tricarballylate, that chelates out magnesium. So people think, I'm taking all these wonderful nutrients, but they're not helping, all because the practice guidelines (recipe for doctors' practices) focus on drugs. This leaves this type of doctor practicing blindly; he has no idea of how to find the cause and cure.

SS: And you measure by a test?

SR: The best starting test is by Metametrix, which has been bought by Genova Labs. But you have to be sure that you get the original cardio/ion Metametrix test. It's twelve pages of molecular biochemistry. Very few doctors are trained in interpreting it. And that's why in the newsletter, we actually put tests, little surreptitious tests where you can innocently ask a question of the doctor. He won't even know he's being tested. But that will show you if he's competent to analyze your twelve pages of molecular biochemistry or not.

Back on the farm when I was forty-four and driving the tractor spraying atrazine on the cornfields, I had my last period and never had another period because atrazine kills your ovaries.

SS: Some people can walk in the same room that's loaded with chemicals and not be affected by it, but the next person is affected; why is that?

SR: I was once that person. People with MCS are not detoxifying as fast nor as much as the others. But the chemical can still affect the "unaffected" person. They may be adapting and stuffing the volatile hydrocarbons (like benzene from carpet) into a particular organ, which eventually will bring problems like leukemia.

SS: I guess you mean the toxins will eventually accumulate and one day come to haunt you. So the toxins build up in the body, the toxins find organs and glands of opportunity via the bloodstream, but the person may not know there's a ticking time bomb in him until it explodes and one day he awakens with a symptom?

SR: Correct. Many toxins take ten to twenty years to create levels high enough to create a cancer of organ malfunction. We all have them right now.

SS: Everybody? You? Me?

SR: Yes, NHANES, the National Health Assessment, shows that all Americans have phthalates. We can't get away from it now, because nobody's going to go back to a less sophisticated lifestyle. We can't live without our modern interiors, factories, and computers, so we have to learn how to compensate for the need for more detoxification.

SS: You and I are close in age, but we had one advantage when we were children and that was if you collected bottles from everybody in the neighborhood, you could put them in your wagon and take them to the grocery store and turn them in for money. We didn't have plastic bottles when you and I were kids.

SR: That's right and one reason why a child born today has, by age six, levels of toxins that used to take us until our forties to accumulate. That's why kids now have adult-onset diabetes and more cancers. These are normally diseases of adults.

SS: I think the switchover to glass bottles would go a long way in changing the health of America, especially when I go to our market and I see the pallets of water bottles in the parking lot sitting in the hot sun.

It's like a minefield to go into a restaurant these days trying to get a clean glass of water from a bottle, and just trying to eat some food that's not going to kill you.

We both have to go to restaurants because of our work. I'd like to control my food, but it's very difficult when you are not at home. When you come home from a restaurant, what do you do to offset the restaurant food?

SR: Start with your detox cocktail.

SS: One teaspoon powdered vitamin C and three capsules of R-lipoic acid and 800 mg of Recancostat, the only form of glutathione proven to be orally absorbed. (Or a LifeWave Glutathione Patch; click on LifeWave on SuzanneSomers.com.)

SR: There's so much more to take; for example, one more nutrient proven to make brains twelve years younger in three months is phosphatidylserine. It's crucial in the sphingomyelin (a particular type of lipid that makes up the majority of the fat content of cell membranes) chemistry of the brain nerve sheaths (the lining around the nerves in the brain and everywhere in the body).

SS: How often is Parkinson's misdiagnosed when it's really symptomatic of toxic burden?

SR: Well, often the first thing that Parkinson's starts with is a tremor. And that's classic for heavy metal toxicity. Most people with Parkinson's have serious heavy metal and/or pesticides or both. In fact, we can use one dose of an "organic," "safe," pesticide to create PD in rats during experiments.

SS: How frightening. I think of all the people I know who live on golf courses and what they are breathing in twenty-four hours a day: pesticide city. Is chelation an antidote?

SR: It depends. You want to check people's levels. In the book *The High Blood Pressure Hoax*, we show how to do the tests to see if you need chelation because everybody has a different load or toxic burden. We don't all have heavy metals as the primary toxicant.

SS: When one has tremors, what's the cocktail?

SR: As I said, tremors are usually pesticides or heavy metals. You can start with a provocation urine test. The best test for this one is RBC Minerals and Toxic Elements by Doctors Data, Inc. (see doctors data.com). But first one must assay your detoxification capability, or chelation can make you worse.

SS: You're about the solutions. What do you think is going to be the long-term effect of all these children who are on amphetamines?

SR: I think we're going to have a nation of kids who are less intelligent, less motivated, and on more drugs than ever before. Right now we have more kids on drugs than ever before in the history of the world. As the drug industry executives will tell you, they concentrate on drugs that people have to take for a lifetime. They don't really care about drugs that you take as a quick fix. Their new focus is on drugs for kids.

SS: Tragic . . . and now college kids are using these amphetamines to make their brains sharper for finals the next day and also for recreational use.

SR: I know, but that chemistry also leads to depression and then later in adult life, brain deterioration. You don't get something for nothing. You don't rev up unnecessarily and expect it to just go back to normal. And drugs use up nutrients in the work of detoxifying them, nutrients that kids are not smart enough to put back in their brains like cod liver oil or phosphatidyl choline, or phosphatidyl serine, or tocotrienols. How many kids in college have a bottle of cod liver oil in their refrigerator?

SS: One antidote to detoxification lies in far infrared saunas. If you can't afford a sauna, what could you do?

SR: You can get a church, a synagogue, a club, whatever interested in it, and then multiple people could use it and take benefit.

SS: And what if they could just exercise till they sweat, or will they not have the energy to exercise till they sweat?

SR: They often don't have the energy if they are toxic, plus it's a different kind of sweating. The far infrared wavelength molecules actually create a little dance under the skin and drag out some of the drugs with infrared saunas.

SS: You mentioned in your book that as you are sweating in a far infrared sauna to keep wiping down so you don't reabsorb, right?

SR: Yes, correct. Otherwise you can merely reabsorb the toxins you just mobilized into the sweat.

SS: What are the most important supplements that you take every day?

SR: It varies. It depends on what I'm doing and where I'm going and what's happening in my life. That's why we advocate that people get themselves smart enough to make these decisions for themselves. I do more minerals if I've had a far infrared sauna or a vigorous tennis match.

SS: So once you know your deficiencies, you take more minerals like magnesium after an infrared sauna?

SR: Yes.

SS: How do individuals read their own body "language"?

SR: Well, for instance, if you suddenly have a muscle twitch in your eye. You know, whoops, I'm low in magnesium. I better take some. Or it could be potassium or calcium or some other nutrient too, but most likely it's mag.

SS: I got a letter yesterday from a woman about a ringing in the ear. I guess that's tinnitus. What's that deficiency?

SR: It can be anything. In fact, we just did some articles in an upcoming newsletter on tinnitus. And that article was on DHA. The number one most important fatty acid that's in the brain, and it's in cod liver oil. But it also could be a mineral. It could be zinc.

SS: So, on this damaged and polluted and changed planet, which all pretty much has happened in the last fifty years, you remain, it seems to me, hopeful and excited at the possibilities of true health if people understand what to do?

SR: I'm happy with my work because my mission is to make people too smart to fail, too smart to fail in their quest for wellness. The key for every person is to take responsibility for his or her health. They must read and learn because medicine is focused on drugs, devices, and surgery.

SS: If someone wanted to set up a phone appointment, can they? And of course there's a fee, right?

SR: Yes, that's correct. They go to PrestigePublishing.com in the States; and in Canada they call 1-800-846-6687.

But I highly recommend that people read three or four of my books and three or four years of newsletters (at least from 2010 forward) before they talk with me.

SS: You don't want to deal with the equivalent of a kindergartner?

SR: Yes. It's a time waster. Once they educate themselves, we can go to higher levels of wellness.

Personal responsibility is the important thing. They have got to be that interested in order to get well. It's a partnership. They work *with* me. Abdication of personal responsibility first began with Original Sin. When God turned and said to Adam, "What is this you have done?" He said, "It was that woman, she made me do it." Adam denied his responsibility for his action. Then to make matters worse Adam blamed the only other person in his universe and said: "And you gave her to me"!

SS: That's funny!

SR: The point is, the diagnostic label you have been given is meaningless; labels are just words that describe your symptoms. What you need is to find the cause and then find the cure. I've seen people heal conditions that I, as a double-board-certified physician, would never have thought was possible. What I offer is anyone who has a cancer just has to go to the website or call the number and for free they will get a cancer issue. I've had readers who were given two or three weeks to live and had exhausted everything that traditional medicine could offer and then get well through detox. So many of these people have been gracious enough to give me all their records from their oncologists—X-rays, blood tests, everything showing exactly where they were. Afterward I got to meet them; now it's twenty years later and they are totally well. Some of them I still see on a regular basis. As it says in First Corinthians, "Has God not made foolish the wisdom of this world."

When everything medicine has to offer fails, go on a diet. Just eat good food.

SS: Thank you, Dr. Rogers. I do deeply appreciate your time and wisdom.

GO FROM *TOX*-SICK TO NOT SICK

1. Our environment is toxic.

   REMEDY: Dr. Rogers's Daily Detox Cocktail—1 teaspoon ascorbic acid (powdered vitamin C) and 3 capsules R-lipoic acid, 1 or 2 times daily. R-lipoic acid heals candida and rejuvenates and brings the brain back to normal levels. Also take 800 mg Recancostat glutathione capsules.

2. To see what is growing in your gut: test for elevated arabintol for abnormal amounts of candida and sensitivities.

   REMEDY: Have your doctor order Metametrix testing for blood and stool for candida, looking for tricarballylate.

3. Fosamax depletes D_3 and K_2. You can't heal a bone without K_2 and D_3. Most people need 4,000 to 10,000 IU of vitamin D_3 a day. You cannot cure diabetes, high blood pressure, depression, poor immune system, or recurrent infections without enough D_3. You can't fight Lyme disease, mold, chemical sensitivity, food allergies without a "D" over at least 80 nanograms per deciliter.

   REMEDY: Vitamin D_3 and vitamin K_2 supplementation daily.

4. If a birth mother is low in zinc, her child will not make enough hydrochloric acid (HCL). If you don't make enough HCL in the stomach, then you can't absorb minerals. These deficiencies lead to brain problems and MCS (multiple chemical sensitivities). Without sufficient HCL, acid bubbles up.

   REMEDY: HCL (hydrochloric acid) supplementation with every meal.

5. Magnesium deficiencies lead to back spasms sometimes so serious they can mimic a ruptured disc. Not having enough magnesium is also a major cause of sudden cardiac arrest. It's necessary to measure RBC (red blood cell), intercellular magnesium. If this reading is low, sudden cardiac arrest can occur.

REMEDY: Daily magnesium supplementation.

6. DHA (docosahexaenoic acid) is the number one fatty acid in the human brain, feeding the mitochondrial membrane, which is where we make energy essential for the cell membrane of every cell. (If a newborn doesn't have enough, the child is likely to be born with a low IQ.) Cod liver oil, phosphatidylcholine, and vitamin E heal brain fats and fats around every cell in the body.

REMEDY: Essential fatty acid supplementation daily (fish oil), phosphatidylcholine, vitamin E daily.

7. Phthalates destroy ALC.

REMEDY: Supplement with acetyl-L-carnitine (ALC) and lipoic acid to move fatty acids into the brain and restore brain function. To clear phthalates from the body, avoid drinking from plastic bottles. Consume brassica (cruciferous) vegetables: cabbage, cauliflower and Brussels sprouts, broccoli, kale and mizuna, collard greens, radishes, turnips.

8. High-fructose corn syrup damages the brain and the gut.

REMEDY: Avoid foods with HFCS forever.

9. POP, persistent organic pollutants, never leave the body.

REMEDY: To neutralize them, take 5 percent of the iodinated compound Lugol's, one or two drops every day.

10. There is a test to scan for brain deterioration: it's called quinolinate, and it shows brain deterioration years before it appears. With enough zinc in the body, the quinolinate goes down.

REMEDY: Zinc supplementation daily.

CHAPTER 5

THE HEART

It's okay to be fat. So you're fat. Just be fat and shut up about it.

—ROSEANNE BARR

THE ACCEPTANCE OF OBESITY IS QUITE TROUBLING. IT'S NOT about the outward consequences; fat bodies are just as beautiful as thin ones. It's the health consequences that are worrisome. In this section I am going to explain how we get fat. It's not what you think. It's about your toxic burden. You will learn that the higher the amount of toxins in your body, the more fat you need to store them. This puts a different spin on being fat. Now it's not about body shape, but more about what the toxins are doing to your health and especially your heart.

Conventional thinking has been that *fats are bad*.

Now you know the truth . . .

The *bad* unhealthy fats are

- Processed fats
- Trans fats
- Hydrogenated fats and cooking vegetable oils

Bad oils cause atherosclerosis, heart disease, and cancer. This has been proven by real science. Yet it's a travesty that so-called healthy fats such as vegetable oils (canola, sunflower, safflower, and others) were touted as heart healthy. What a crock. We bought into it and we got *tox*-sick as a result! Millions of dollars were spent by agriculture and food manufacturers to convince us of this lie.

As Dr. Sinatra eloquently says in the interview that follows:

Contrary to popular propaganda, research is now showing that animal fats have nothing to do with heart disease, atherosclerosis, and cancer. Our human physiology needs these fats and they are important for us to eat daily. We also now know that saturated fats are heart protective; they lower Lp(a) in the blood. Lp(a) is a very harmful substance that initiates atherosclerosis in blood vessels.

To truly understand, let's take a look at the breakdown of the fats nature has provided for us to thrive, grow, and be healthy.

We can all agree that breast milk, the first nutrition nature has provided to help us thrive, grow, and be healthy, is loaded with fats.

Look at this breakdown and be amazed!

Breast Milk
33% monounsaturated fat
16% polyunsaturated fat
48% saturated fat

Now let's look at the foods we have been warned to avoid:

Butter
30% monounsaturated fat
4% polyunsaturated fat
52% saturated fat

How about . . . ?

Beef
47% monounsaturated fat
4% polyunsaturated fat
49% saturated fat

Pork
45% monounsaturated fat
11% polyunsaturated fat
44% saturated fat

Lamb
38% monounsaturated fat
2% polyunsaturated fat
58% saturated fat

As you can see, the fat composition of breast milk, butter, beef, lamb, and pork are all virtually the same!

Discovering this blew my mind. . . . Are you connecting the dots? Our babies thrive beautifully on this composition of fats in breast milk, and the largest part of it is *saturated*. We need all the natural fats in natural foods, and saturated and monounsaturated fats actually need to be the largest part of our fat intake. If our mother's breast milk started our life with healthy fats and lots of it, then doesn't it make sense that nature intended that we continue on in life with healthy animal fats like those listed above?

Recently I saw on the news a new government plan to wean Americans off meat because of the amount of land it takes to feed animals and the methane gas they emit. (Think of all the *gas* bloating humans emit!) The government is now urging us to eat a plant-based diet. To most people this makes sense. Something worth striving for, and anyway, it's no big deal because we have all been scared off meat of any kind anyway due to the lies we've been told. Remember, *meat is bad*?

Did nature screw up?

I think not.

We screwed up!

Again, when we look at the composition of breast milk compared with butter, red meat, lamb, and pork, we see that it's virtually the same composition. Our bodies use every bit of the fat content, including the saturated part. If this is the grand design, then no wonder we have all gotten so far off track by switching from healthy fats and vegetables to processed foods, sugar, high-fructose corn syrup, and chemical/pesticide-laden foods.

How could that possibly work?

It doesn't!

That's why fats are necessary (and delicious) to achieve true health!

Yet over and over again, we are told by our doctors and on TV in "special reports" to avoid saturated fats! Give up butter and steak. How sad. Some of the smartest people I know are unconvincible regarding cholesterol and their statin drugs. They have been brainwashed into believing this is what is keeping them alive.

The human body has one stomach, and that stomach was designed to digest animal proteins. Ingested animal fats form the gut wall barrier (immune system) to provide the protection from dangerous pathogens. A cow has several stomachs, perfect for digesting grass (the only food a cow should be fed). They are perfectly capable of digesting a plant-based diet.

This box will be surprising to you:

Vegetables should and need to be a big part of a healthy diet, but if the gut wall barrier is damaged, then high-fiber vegetables are "grabbed" by the dangerous pathogens on the gut wall (bad guys) because there is not enough good flora (probiotics) available to extract the nutrients and benefits of the vegetable. Instead the dangerous pathogens "grab" the vegetables and turn them toxic, releasing them into the bloodstream, allowing them to look for a new home (again, their favorite hang-out place is the brain).

THE PROBLEM YOU REALLY NEED TO WORRY ABOUT IS INFLAMMATION

My dear friend and nationally recognized, board-certified neurosurgeon Dr. Russell Blaylock says, "It has long been established that as we age our bodies, including our blood vessels, become progressively more *inflamed*. Along with *inflammation*, we produce considerably more free radicals and lipid peroxidation products, as well as a lot more advanced glycation end products (AGEs), which are nasty little bits of damaged proteins, fats, and carbohydrates."

Sadly, we have created an inflamed society by eating inflamed plants, inflamed animals, and inflamed fish. We eat inflamed food and become inflamed ourselves.

The medical community has finally begun to realize that inflammation is an underlying cause of or contributor to most chronic diseases, especially coronary artery disease. Diabetes is an inflammatory disease, smoking cigarettes is inflammatory: the results of both are linked to heart attack risk. Inflammation can get turned on systemically: in all your tissues, in your blood, and in your organs. Whatever system is weakest in you will break down first with chronic inflammation.

With age, toxic substances begin to accumulate in tissues and organs, kicking off the process of atherosclerosis. Special structures within cells remove damaged or abnormal proteins and other cellular debris in a process called "autophagy." However, we are starting to learn that as people age, this process becomes defective.

In addition, the energy-producing parts of cells called mitochondria start to wear out, which greatly increases production of "free radicals."

Lowering your *inflammation* levels is your responsibility. Toxins create higher levels. You know they are out there; we are all being bombarded by them every moment of every day. So taking the proper supplements and thinking carefully about your dietary choices is imperative. In today's world we have to eat as though our lives depend on it. Healthy foods—fruits and vegetables along with quality fats and protein—all are *anti-inflammatory* and will help you to lower your inflammation levels.

Now you know: Ever since the *low-fat* movement, the digestive tracts of Americans from toddlers to seniors have become seriously damaged. Contrary to popular belief and long-held theories that are now being proved wrong, it is clear: The human stomach, brain, HEART, and entire body were designed to operate at optimum on healthy fats and animal protein. We now know (going back forty years or more), that fat has been misidentified as the culprit behind heart disease, when all along it's been sugar.

Sugar and processed foods cause inflammation. You want to have a very low level of inflammation.

A high-sugar diet raises your risk for heart disease by promoting metabolic syndrome—a cluster of health conditions that includes high blood pressure, insulin and leptin resistance, high triglycerides, liver dysfunction, and visceral fat accumulation. Insulin and leptin resistance is caused by factors inherent in our modern lifestyle, including diets heavy in processed carbohydrates, sugars/fructose, refined flours, and industrial seed oils. Making matters worse, the average American gets inadequate exercise, suffers from chronic stress and sleep deprivation, is exposed to environmental toxins, and has poor gut health (dysbiosis). This is the perfect storm for chronic disease.

Mad yet?

Feel screwed over?

Now you realize you are able to eat real food and healthy fats. You *CAN* have butter again! Healthy dietary fats will not make you fat or sick. Toxins make you fat and toxins cause inflammation. But right now, let's dive in and find out what else you can do to protect this most precious and vital organ, your heart, as Dr. Sinatra sheds some much needed light.

THE FAT LIES HURTING YOU:
AN INTERVIEW WITH STEPHEN SINATRA, M.D., PH.D.

Dr. Stephen Sinatra, author of The Great Cholesterol Myth *and many other important books listed in the bibliography, will validate what you have been hearing me say about cholesterol and the necessity of healthy fats. He is a friend and my go-to doctor for all things involving the heart. He is the leading integrative cardiologist (and also a psychologist; he deals with the mind and the heart) in this country. He will further explain and validate the need for healthy fats not only for the GI tract but also as a means for keeping the HEART healthy and strong.*

SS: Hello, Stephen, thank you once again for your time. You are, to say the least, a very interesting combo . . . integrative cardiologist/psychotherapist, plus you don't believe in the low-fat movement. The low-fat movement (diet/heart hypothesis) has been called the greatest deception of this century. How did the low-fat movement originally take hold?

SINATRA: Nice to talk to you again, Suzanne. It dates back to over fifty-five years ago when President Eisenhower had a heart attack. It was known that he loved his bacon, eggs, butter, and toast, and the public and politicians were concerned about his health. Around that time, Ansel Keys conducted his Seven Countries Study and found that people in countries that consumed the smallest amount of fats had the least incidence of heart disease. The problem was, Ansel Keys cherry-picked his data to prove this hypothesis.

Also, around that time George McGovern was secretary of health, education, and welfare, and the thinking was just beginning to take hold that fat in a diet was likely the cause of heart disease or heart attacks. Educating people to that fact, he thought, would be doing a good thing for the country.

SS: And the public was encouraged (for instance) to switch from butter to margarine as the healthier choice, right?

SINATRA: Right! Margarine and other new fake chemical foods were advertised as a better choice and a means of lowering the risk of heart disease. So once the low-fat health movement was in full swing, the food manufacturers came up with more choices; they rolled in so-called heart-healthy oils: corn oil like Mazola and others. And this low-fat myth got further propagated when the Framingham study came out, showing a linear relationship between higher cholesterol and more cardiovascular events. So it appeared reasonable to the medical community that cholesterol was a risk factor in heart disease.

SS: Is this when the drug companies got into the act?

SINATRA: Yes, because now cholesterol was considered a major problem. They wanted to create a drug that could reverse or neutralize it. They created statins in the late '80s, and cholesterol levels started going down, so doctors believed cholesterol was clearly the cause of heart disease and statins were the answer. I was one of the choirboys as well; I believed it, and I was chief of cardiology at my institution at the time. Not only that, I lectured for Merck and Pfizer and I was paid very well. I did it because I truly believed in the cholesterol theory of heart disease. In fact, for a few years, I literally taught doctors about the dangers of cholesterol and heart disease as I lectured extensively throughout the Northeast, USA.

SS: What turned you around?

SINATRA: Well, after a few years, we were realizing that something was wrong; we made all these changes in our diets, yet the incidence of heart disease was skyrocketing.

SS: Why?

SINATRA: Because of the food. Corn oil, margarine, and all the other new foods that were trans fats; we had not realized that these fake foods and poor-quality oils were dangerous. What an irony; we gave up butter and steaks and got sicker and fatter!

Then I had an epiphany relative to statins; I realized I was barking up the wrong tree. It was 1993 when I read an article showing that statin drugs diminished CoQ10, which is a vital nutrient made in every cell in the body and is a major nutrient for the production of cellular energy. Also CoQ10 is critically important for the strong pumping action of the heart.

I had started using CoQ10 with my patients a decade before, in the early '80s, and was very impressed; I was able to avert a heart transplant with a patient I put on CoQ10. So I had to ask myself this question: How can a statin drug that's supposed to be so good for the heart deplete it of CoQ10, the most vital nutrient for the heart to survive? It didn't make sense!

Then I discovered that Merck Pharmaceuticals had a patent on CoQ10 in the same pill called Lovastatin or Mevacor, meaning they knew that statins would deplete the heart of CoQ10 but kept it hidden from the public. So I had to wonder, If Merck knows about this situation, why don't they exercise the patent?

SS: Yes, why?

SINATRA: Probably because the drugs were selling so well, and the doctors had been convinced to believe they were so safe.

SS: But if you were Merck Pharmaceuticals, and realized that statins depleted CoQ10, and you had the patent, why wouldn't you put out the new superdrug?

SINATRA: Why alert people to a problem when the drug is the darling of the industry?

SS: They had to know at some point they were going to get found out.

SINATRA: Yes, but think of all the money they would make before that happened. Statin drugs are some of the top-selling drugs in the world.

SS: Doesn't CoQ10 activate the energy center of the cell?

SINATRA: Correct. CoQ10 is the spark plug that ignites the energy process; the mitochondria produce energy and the dietary fats are the fuel source.

Did you know: Heart cells require mostly fat to produce energy?

Did you know that? 60 percent to 70 percent of all the energy of
the heart comes from the burning of FAT.

SS: That must be why so many men my husband's age have no
energy. They get lost in a haze of Lipitor and low-fat diets, all because
they are terrified that fats will give them a heart attack. It sucks the
energy out of them, like they are out of gas. Women are also terrified
of fats. When you go out with most any woman, she will just order
a salad. If she orders soup, she always asks for no cream. People on
no- or low-fat diets get dried out and lifeless. Also, I think of men we
know—cool guys, creative cool guys—who now, courtesy of orthodox medicine, are slumped over with no vitality or energy. Why has
this "recipe" of orthodox heart treatment continued?

SINATRA: Because the diet/heart hypothesis made us all believers,
especially the doctors. Yes, these men and women may be out of gas
on Lipitor, but it's even worse; some of them are going to develop
congestive heart failure and heart disease from CoQ10 depletion and
the lack of healthy fats. There's an entity called "statin cardiomyopathy": over time when CoQ10 levels drop, the heart suffers. We call it
diastolic dysfunction of the heart, and it can lead to congestive heart
failure.

SS: Interesting . . . CoQ10 and healthy fats are intricate to making
the body run! Most people would think that information is crazy.

SINATRA: The low-fat movement is ingrained in most people's
minds. Because of lower healthy fats in the diet and diminished
CoQ10 from statins, we are seeing more statin cardiomyopathy nowa-
days even though the incidence of coronary disease is going down.
So these guys or friends that you know may not have a heart attack,
but they may develop heart failure or develop premature Alzheimer's.
They may get sexual dysfunction. They may lose the bounce in their
step or become weak and fatigued. They may get muscle pain and
more quality-of-life issues, which can be troublesome.

SS: As in, no "juice"?

SINATRA: No juice. These people are running on fumes, and
when some really run out of gas, we hope they don't experience heart
failure.

You see, once the diet heart hypothesis took hold, the public was
convinced that two things were going on: Cholesterol was demonized
and saturated fat was named the enemy. And worse, carbohydrates

were now touted as heart healthy, so everyone started eating pasta. That's when insulin resistance, diabetes, and heart disease soared. There are studies pointing to an association between increased saturated fat intake and cardiovascular risk, but there are a few things to know about those studies; in many of these studies, the major risk examined was cholesterol. But then, as scientists looked more carefully at the association between saturated fat in the diet and levels of cholesterol in the blood, they concluded: saturated fat raises overall cholesterol levels. But here's the important factor: its effect is more *positive* than *negative* because it causes the HDL to go up more and it shifts small LDL to a less invasive, larger LDL particle.

SS: We know HDL is the "good" cholesterol, but can you explain to my readers that there are two levels of LDL, each very different from the other? Most doctors only measure the total LDL. Why is this an incorrect way to measure?

SINATRA: The particle size of the cholesterol molecule and the number of particles are more important than the total cholesterol and LDL numbers; the smaller the particle, the more inflammation.

Saturated fat has a positive effect on particle sizes of both LDLs. It makes more of the less invasive LDL (big fluffy particles), LDL pattern A, and less of the small particles (small, dense inflammatory particles), LDL pattern B.

SS: Are small, dense inflammatory LDL particles what is referred to as arterial plaque?

SINATRA: Well, yes, to an extent. If these small inflammatory LDL particles become oxidized and angry, they can create the beginnings of an inflammatory response. In a nutshell, specialized blood cells called "monocytes" can become agitated, forming foam cells, leading to more inflammation. Adhesion particles are created, and if the local environment has other endothelial unfriendly constituents, like heavy metals, trans fats, cigarette smoke, chemicals, excessive insulin, and so on, a perfect storm can result in a major inflammatory response, setting the stage for endothelial dysfunction and then later plaque infiltration. Remember, if the plaque ruptures and occludes a strategic vessel, a heart attack or a stroke may occur.

SS: Does the inflammation of the small dense LDL result from the fact that small particle LDL are (for lack of a better description) like sharp razor blades on the sides of the arteries?

SINATRA: Yes, to a degree. If the small particle LDL becomes oxi-dized and angry, it can set the stages of inflammation as I mentioned before. The worst kind is Lp(a); these are very, very small particles of cholesterol. They cause enormous inflammation in the blood vessels and blood clotting at the same time. To me, it's the number one risk factor in the cholesterol theory of heart disease and is the real truth regarding an association of cholesterol and heart disease.

SS: So saturated fat is not the problem, and there is no real reason to be concerned about high cholesterol if this very small particle Lp(a) count is not high?

SINATRA: Right. Lp(a) is most often a genetic trait and it's a vari-ant small particle cholesterol, so actually statins can make it worse in some cases. But the drug companies won't tell you that. The way to neutralize Lp(a) is with natural nondrug supplements, either lumbro-kinase or nattokinase, which thins the blood.

Sometimes understanding the heart is not black-and-white or simple. I asked Dr. Sinatra to go in depth for the sake of any cardiologists who are reading.

SS: Stephen, I'm confused about this Lp(a) notation as well as the LDL subtypes. Can you take a moment to explain it in more detail?

SINATRA: Okay, this is the complex answer. When it comes to LDL, the most important thing is fractionization of the particles. The prototype of LDL cholesterol can be particle B, particle A, or a combi-nation AB. The particle B size is very small and it is the most inflam-matory. If your pattern is more AB, it is inflammatory but to a lesser degree.

If you are pure A, the particles are fluffier, but they too can cre-ate inflammation if they become oxidized. However, it is far better to have the particle A pattern as this is the least invasive of the three.

Now Lp(a) is the worst pattern to have as this is the smallest cho-lesterol particle that is clearly the most inflammatory and most in-vasive. It is very important to measure this pattern in anyone with a malignant family history of early heart attack or sudden cardiac death as this trait can be transferred genetically.

So what would be the worst cholesterol picture to have? If the patient had large calculations of Lp(a), or if they had high LDL cholesterol that was pattern B with a high number of particles, that is, greater than 1,000, with a low HDL, that is a very, very inflammatory pattern. If some of these people have high triglycerides, then we have to consider the possibility of metabolic syndrome, which has inflammatory cholesterol patterns.

SS: Okay, that was way over my head, but I get that the worst scenario is Lp(a) and very few people have this condition. Therefore it seems to me that a lot of people are on statins when they are unnecessary. That is the takeaway from this. As a layperson I believe knowing that the dangerous reading of Lp(a) is the most important thing to know. It's also nice to know that a natural supplement can do the job of blood thinning better than a drug. So many adults are on Coumadin (a drug blood thinner) and there are significant bad side effects. How do the natural supplements work?

SINATRA: Unfortunately, many patients do need to stay on traditional blood thinners like Coumadin, especially in the setting of metallic or plastic cardiac valves or in situations of atrial fibrillation associated with a large left atrium and a leaking mitral valve. However, in some cases, natural supplements can be utilized instead of Coumadin such as in the situation of "lone" atrial fibrillation in which the patient has a normal-size left atrium where blood clotting is minimized. In these situations, I've used supplements like garlic, omega-3 essential fatty acids, nattokinase. When I'm dealing with Lp(a), lumbrokinase can actually target and lower the very bad Lp(a), and it also helps dissolve fibrin, which is involved in the clotting process. There are other important supplements like omega-3 essential fatty acids as well as fast-acting niacin, which helps to neutralize the toxic effects of Lp(a), the blood clotting and inflammation.

SS: Time-released niacin?

SINATRA: No. Not the time release. People can have terrible side effects with high doses (2 to 3 grams a day). In my experience, it has not been very effective. Just over-the-counter niacin, from 250 up to 500 mg three times a day is more effective. But it can produce flushing and itching, which is frequently not tolerated very well.

SS: Will this thin your blood and keep blood pressure down?

SINATRA: Yes, it does both while helping to reverse inflammation at the same time.

SS: Great information, simple natural nondrug options to protect from catastrophic heart disease. And clearly the low-fat movement was wrong.

SINATRA: Here's the real scientific truth backed up by research:

Saturated fat predicts absolutely nothing about a person's risk for cardiovascular disease.

SS: How great! Bring on the organic butter!

SINATRA: And olive oil! Yes, I encourage my patients to eat healthy fats and cut down on sugar and carbs. In one meta-analysis, in the researchers' own words, after examining 21 studies and 350,000 people, the authors concluded: "There is no significant evidence for concluding that dietary saturated fat is associated with an increased risk of coronary heart disease or cardiovascular disease." Even when the researchers factored in age, sex, and study quality, it didn't change the results. Saturated fat did nothing wrong! In fact, it showed the opposite in another major study; that is, less stroke and heart disease. I'm referring to the famous Primary Prevention of Cardiovascular Disease with the Mediterranean Diet as reported in the *New England Journal of Medicine* in 2013. I had the pleasure of moderating the Saturated Fat, Cholesterol, and Statin Controversy panel with one of the lead authors of the PREDIMED study, Dr. Miguel A. Martinez-Gonzalez, at the American College of Nutrition Conference in San Diego this past November. After the conference, he even shared some more recent studies demonstrating exciting data regarding olive oil and fat in the prevention of diabetes as well.

Saturated fat: found in butter, cheese, eggs, meat, coconut oil, palm oil

Monounsaturated fat: found in olive oil, macadamia nuts, avocado

Polyunsaturated fats:
- Alpha linoleic acid (ALA): found in walnuts, flaxseed
- Docosahexaenoic acid (DHA): found in fish, grass-fed meat
- Eicosapentanoic acid (EPA): found in fish, grass-fed meat

Everything we learned in the past was wrong! Most people shudder in horror because they have bought into the idea that saturated fat is the worst thing ever. It's hard to convince people of the idea that butter with its high content of saturated fat could be a better choice than those inflammatory omega-6 vegetable oils that are continually pushed on us. It is in direct opposition to fat theology: the deeply held belief that saturated fat and cholesterol are the root of all heart disease. That notion has been the prevailing dogma about saturated fat, cholesterol, and heart disease for decades but there's one problem . . . IT ISN'T TRUE!

The information on saturated fat has been a misguided public policy on diet and heart disease for most every major government and mainstream health organization, including the American Heart Association.

SS: And have they changed their position on this theory?

SINATRA: Yes, it's happening. Today health professionals have re-examined the case against saturated fat and are finding that it was based on very little evidence. Although saturated fat, when taken in the diet, converts to cholesterol, remember it supports HDL levels, and saturated fat is the least prone to oxidation when compared to the pro-inflammatory canola, corn, cottonseed, and vegetable oils.

SS: So what you were reading in the literature and what you believed as a younger cardiologist, you weren't seeing clinically?

SINATRA: No. So now I had a second question: If cholesterol is so bad, why am I seeing people with heart disease with low cholesterols and people with high cholesterols with the absence of heart disease? It didn't make any sense. For instance, in my own personal practice, I'd be doing an angiogram on a patient with cholesterol of 320 expecting to find this person riddled with coronary disease, but instead I found normal coronaries in so many of these people. Conversely, I would do an angiogram with somebody with cholesterol levels of 150, 160, 170, and they would be loaded with coronary disease.

In 1993, I wrote an editorial for a medical journal questioning the cholesterol dogma. Once my beliefs changed, I immediately reversed course and I canceled all my lectures for the drug companies. I told them I couldn't do it anymore because I no longer believed in the cholesterol theory of heart disease, as I had believed in the '80s and early '90s. I had been the choirboy for cholesterol because I believed it with all my heart. I had no choice but to discontinue lecturing because of this reversal in thinking based on research studies and my clinical practice.

SS: Where would you be today if you were still delivering that message?

SINATRA: Oh my God. I would be [laughs] reaping the rewards: golfing trips, all the meals, all the lectures; they paid me very handsomely. I'm embarrassed to tell you what they paid me.

Once I knew the truth, I stopped immediately. You could have paid me millions and I would not have given that information out to doctors and people, because I now knew it was questionable and in some cases dangerous information.

Remember, in medical school, I took the oath: do no harm! In the early '90s, I was seeing the side effect of statins, and yet the literature was saying the side effects of statins were minimal. But my patients were complaining of fatigue, impotence, memory problems, muscle pain, joint pain, even inability to focus the eyes, flulike symptoms, weakness. One of my patients said, "Geez, I played doubles tennis, I'm a great tennis player, and I couldn't get out of bed the next day, my muscles were so sore."

SS: What is that called?

SINATRA: Muscle pain is referred to as myalgia, and when it becomes severe with muscle tissue breakdown, rhabdomyolysis (renal [kidney] failure from statins) may occur. And that's what happened with the Baycol disaster, to which around 60 deaths were attributed years ago. That was a major disaster. Baycol was a very powerful statin that caused such muscle breakdown it would cause renal (kidney) failure and people died. The FDA fortunately removed it from the market quickly.

> Take the cholesterol drug Baycol, which was removed from the market after killing 100 people. Baycol is a statin (cholesterol-lowering) drug similar to Mevacor, Zocor, Lipitor, Pravachol. Was there a need for tens of millions of dollars to be spent developing another statin drug? Drug companies think so because the FDA readily recognizes statin drugs so they are easy to get approved.
> —*The FDA Versus the American Consumer*

So I began putting together my own data about the side effects and realized the side effects were grossly underreported because doctors were asking the wrong questions.

I began to question what was going on. For example, I was at the National American College of Cardiology Meeting with thousands of cardiologists in the audience, listening to lectures on the fabulous benefits of statins and reporting the reduction in cardiovascular events. Guys would be running out of the room, calling their brokers to buy stock. I mean it was idiotic. It was sickening.

SS: It sounds almost as good as being a congressperson allowed to participate in insider trading.

SINATRA: Ha ha! Yeah. The pay phones were jammed. They didn't have cell phones twenty years ago.

I began to try and ruffle the feathers about the importance of CoQ10, saying, look, we have to use caution. But nobody was buying the CoQ10 situation, despite the fact that a few years before it was reported that CoQ10 was diminished in people taking statins.

I do peer review analysis for medical journals, which means that when a doctor or a group submits research, sometimes it's referred to me to review, and I'll suggest to either rewrite the article (or suggest making a minor revision, perhaps a major revision) or reject the article.

One author wrote an article on cholesterol for the *Southern Medical Journal* and the editors asked me to review it. It was a party-line article, Suzanne, meaning the usual wrong information: high cholesterol risk, high saturated fat causes cholesterol to soar, cholesterol causes heart disease, and you have to treat it with statins. There was no balance to the article. It was like grandstanding for the cholesterol theory of heart disease, vilifying saturated fats, and using statins. I told the editors I thought the article was well written, but it was way out of balance. The information was not 100 percent accurate. The editors came back to me and said, would you write an editorial? I thought about it and said okay.

I literally spent dozens of hours researching and writing the editorial for the *Southern Medical Journal*, and it was placed in the same journal where the original article was written. I believed I was right, and this new information was absolutely incredible, and I needed to get this word out to doctors.

That's when I realized statins have a light side and a dark side. The drug companies wanted us to believe that cholesterol causes heart disease. I knew some forms of cholesterol were markers like oxidized small dense LDL and Lp(a), which causes inflammation, but I was like a salmon pushing upstream, believing that native nonoxidized cholesterol is harmless and vital for the body.

I realized, when I did the research, that cholesterol is found at the scene of the crime, but it's not the perpetrator. In other words, cholesterol plays a very small part in the genesis of inflammation, which is the root cause of heart disease.

Statins had positive effects in some populations, especially in high-risk smoking males, because one important effect of statins is blood thinning. I read the WOSCOPS Study in Scotland and, if you used a statin drug, particularly in smoking males with low HDL, these males had a significant benefit with statins.

And the researchers recognized that the cholesterol lowering was not the reason these men did better on statins; it was because statins were thinning the blood. In other words, they improved blood viscosity.

SS: Wouldn't there be a less damaging way to thin the blood than to take statins, like the nattokinase supplements?

SINATRA: Of course, but high-smoking males, with low HDLs, are a ticket for heart disease. So if your blood is like red ketchup, you need something to thin it, and if you have a physician that only believes in drug medicine, then choosing statins would thin their blood, which is a good thing. Also, statins are anti-inflammatory and antioxidants as well, but drug companies can't sell that. So statins can do good things especially for male patients who have thick blood or who smoke and for those with documented coronary artery disease. In fact, this is the bright side of statins; with any male under the age of seventy-five with a history of heart attack, bypass surgery, stent, or angioplasty, I will use statins regardless of the cholesterol level. Statins and coenzyme Q10, 100 to 200 mg, in males with coronary disease, is good medicine as the benefits outweigh the risks.

I rarely use statins in women, as they have many more side effects, and almost never in children.

SS: Considering the terrible side effects of statins, and knowing there is a natural supplement to thin blood and that we need cholesterol for life, it's shocking that because of business interests we are still trying to make fats the enemy and eradicate essential cholesterol when the real problem is inflammation!

I have many friends that, even with a crowbar, you couldn't get animal fats like butter or cream into their mouths. These are smart people indoctrinated by their orthodox doctors. Beliefs are virtually impossible to change until the information is so smack-dab in your face as it was for you.

SINATRA: Healthy fat is essential for your body.

Statins diminish fat in the brain, and that's the ticket for cognition problems. The brain needs fat. Low-fat is one of the major reasons we have an epidemic of Alzheimer's disease in this country and there's also another important issue: we are eating too much sugar and not enough fats.

Sugar causes the brain to age quicker, and healthy fats are not only a great fuel for brain cells, but they also offer protection at the same time. Statins diminish the phospholipids in the brain, and that's why people are having memory problems. We need cholesterol for the whole body. We need it for hormones; we need to lubricate the skin; and we need it to make vitamin D. When the sun hits our skin, the cholesterol in our skin activates the vitamin D pathway. We need cholesterol for neurotransmission in the brain. We need cholesterol to block infections.

The higher your cholesterol, the better you are protected against GI infections and respiratory infections. When people have HIV that turns to AIDS, and the cholesterol drops below 90, their health goes downhill because HDL forms of cholesterol support the immune system and protect us from infectious disease.

The early data from the Framingham study that initially showed that higher cholesterol was unfavorable is now obsolete. After forty years of research, higher cholesterol levels now predict a longer life.

The most recent data shows that people with the highest cholesterol live the longest.

This same data has also been replicated in an Italian study as well, showing that the higher cholesterol, the better the longevity.

SS: I remember discussing with Larry King (on the air) what he missed in his new "heart healthy" diet since his heart attack; he said he missed lamb chops and that he wanted to be able to eat all the crispy fat. He talked about them (fats) like he was recalling an old lover.

SINATRA: Right. He should have eaten them!

SS: It seems to me if nature started us out on the breast with a high-fat diet, then that's what nature wanted us to continue in our life. I avoid sugar and carbs but load up on healthy protein, animal fats, butter on my vegetables, olive oil. I have four teaspoons of coconut oil daily. I feel great and energized. I'm thin, weight is not an issue, and my system and brain are working great; no lost thoughts like so many of my peers.

SINATRA: I completely agree with you. That's why the Paleo diet, which is a modified Mediterranean diet (without pizzas and pastas and bread), is great. It's not going to elicit a significant insulin response, and we know insulin is the primary cause of endothelial cell dysfunction and inflammation in the blood vessels.

The problem is that we're a sugar society. The average person takes in about 154 pounds of sugar yearly. Sodas, high-fructose corn syrup, sweets, breads, bagels, pastas, potatoes, white rice—all these high-glycemic foods elicit an insulin response, then throw in wine and other alcohol. If you are going to have a cocktail, at least wash it down with a couple handfuls of nuts. The fats and the protein in those nuts will help balance the sugar in the wine, so you will get a slower insulin response, thus protecting your blood vessels.

SS: What about vegan diets? No fat, no animal protein?

SINATRA: If a patient can do it and stick to it, there are benefits from the high-fiber, high-nitrate vegan diet. Personally, I believe in some animal protein as a way to consume protein as well as essential fats. However, as a cardiologist, when you have patients under threat of death from a heart attack, who don't believe in animal protein or high fat to protect their health, if they are motivated to go on an all-vegan diet and stick to it religiously (because they'd rather survive than die), I will support them. If this is what they feel they need to do, whatever the motivation, I don't want to destroy that. As a doctor, I strive to empower the patient in taking more responsibility in getting well. So if a person wants to do the opposite and not eat animal protein and go on a high-fiber, no oil, vegan or vegetarian diet with lots of vegetables and no inflammatory omega-6 oils, I will absolutely support it. I would coach them on adding omega-3 essential fatty acids, coenzyme Q10, alpha-lipoic acid, as well as B vitamin support, since many of the pure vegan/vegetarians are compromised on these vital nutrients because they are frequently found much more in the animal domain.

SS: But if the truth on dietary fats in the diet were to be made available to the mainstream, things would change. The public is fed only what the manufacturers want them to hear. I agreed with you in your book *The Great Cholesterol Myth* when you said you can avoid heart disease and enjoy food by understanding that your enemies are sugar and high-carb diets. I have written several books making the same claim. I now feel that grains are just another form of sugar. *Grain Brain* was a very enlightening book for me. Since I gave up grains as well as sugar, my young body has returned. That's motivating, and then to think that my heart, brain, and GI tract are protected . . . it's a win/win, right?

SINATRA: Exactly. Sugar, in addition to any of its forms like grains and flours, is the number one enemy of heart health. People who are on a low-fat diet and eating lots of carbs and grains like wheat and rice may be putting themselves in harm's way compared to people consuming olive oil and healthy fats. Eating the fats, including a couple handfuls of nuts a day (which also have a lot of healthy omega-3 fats), is giving the body what it wants. Seventh Day Adventists are a true testimony to this theory. They eat a lot of nuts, and they have a very low incidence of heart disease.

SS: I have "stores within stores" at an organic healthy food chain called Clarks in Palm Desert, California, where I sell my toxic-free organic skin care and makeup products. One of the stores is in Loma Linda, which is called a "Blue Zone," one of the spots on the planet where the people live long lives without disease. These people have healthy diets and don't drink or smoke; these are superhealthy people.

SINATRA: Yes, and it is known they consume a lot of nuts— macadamia nuts, walnuts, almonds, pistachios—which are fat and protein. These foods don't elicit a significant insulin response. Healthy fats are a key component for health. In the PREDIMED Study reported in the 2013 *New England Journal of Medicine,* more than 7,800 patients over a study time of 4.8 years who consumed healthy fats—like four tablespoons of olive oil a day or two handfuls of nuts per day—had less diabetes and heart disease and fewer strokes as compared to their counterparts eating a lower-fat and higher-carbohydrate diet.

SS: Yes, and I bet if President Clinton (a vegan) knew the real truth, he would love to have a grass-fed juicy steak with a pat of butter melting on top of it!

SINATRA: I love organic butter, but I prefer olive oil since I grew up on it. My father is Italian and he used a lot of it.

SS: Let's clear it up right now. You are no relation to the other famous Sinatra?

SINATRA: You know, Suzanne, I really don't know. My grandfather and Frank's father grew up in the same town in Sicily, but the library burned down in 1896 and all the records were lost. Maybe they were brothers, cousins, or just friends.

My grandfather, like my father, loved olive oil. When I was a kid, I remember him dousing everything with it—vegetables, salads, even meat, so I grew up with olive oil being served at every meal. He also passed at age ninety-nine. When I became a doctor and a cardiologist, I read a lot about the benefits of olive oil, and the research showed that it raised HDL, and made small particle LDL fluffier, supported endothelial cell function, plus lowered blood pressure. I realized I had an advantage by being Italian as olive oil is in my blood. Olive oil is good for the skin, it improves depression, and it protects against Alzheimer's disease. The "secret sauce" of the Mediterranean diet is olive oil. In addition to all the great cardiovascular benefits, it down-regulates pro-inflammatory genes!

SS: That means it protects against inflammation?

SINATRA: Yes, and that's significant, because we live in a toxic environment. Healthy fats such as olive oil help certain people do better with inflammation as opposed to others because epigenetics play into this.

Some people are just more sensitive because of their genetics, and the environment selects those among us who are genetically predisposed or more vulnerable. We call that "epigenetics." When you liberally consume olive oil that can suppress pro-inflammatory genes, you're attenuating inflammation. I personally believe it may support longevity as well.

SS: Dietary fats like olive oil taste so great, it's nice to know the enormous benefits of consuming lots of it.

SINATRA: Olive oil protects against inflammation and when you have less inflammation, the body thrives. Unfortunately, I have also discovered that all olive oils are not pure, so you have to be careful. A lot of olive oils out there are cut with canola, corn, or vegetable oil. If the olive oil is cut with canola, with 75 percent olive oil and 25 percent canola, it is still legally classified as 100 percent extra-virgin olive oil.

SS: That's disturbing and upsetting. Canola is usually genetically modified, so canola in olive oil undoes all the good. Readers, beware and ask questions of your grocer!

SINATRA: The organic growers in California have a certification program, and it's a truthful program on 100 percent olive oil. It's the purest form of olive oil; it's 100 percent organic, and it's 100 percent clean.

SS: What olive oil do you use?

SINATRA: The manufacturer is B. R. Cohn. They sell wine in Sonoma, California. The olive trees aren't sprayed, no insecticides or pesticides, and they only use 100 percent pure extra-virgin olive oil. I also love their Picholine variety, which is not certified organic, but the owners have told me no sprays are used.

SS: Okay, changing gears. Where do you feel testosterone comes into play for our health?

SINATRA: Testosterone is important for both men and women. Remember, our sex hormones are derived from the biochemical base of cholesterol. So again, when you are taking out cholesterol with statins, you could be adversely affecting your sex hormone production at the same time.

SS: It's all connected.

SINATRA: Yes, it is. . . .

SS: What do you eat?

SINATRA: Good question. I love fresh seafood. I won't eat the farm-raised salmon that's confined. But if I can get tidal water organic salmon, I'll eat it. I love sardines packed in olive oil from Vital Choice; they have the highest amounts of CoQ10 and omega-3, especially DHA, which is also in salmon, pasture-raised beef and buffalo, and calamari. I use Calamarine oil in my omega products because it is higher in DHA. As a cardiologist, I know that DHA is taken up by the heart, retina, and brain. So I like supporting these organs and tissues while having some protection against inflammation at the same time. I eat a lot of fresh vegetables, fresh fruits, organic as much as I can. I love the taste of buffalo, especially the tenderloin. I slice it up and eat it on the rare side because I want the enzymes. I cover it with a sprinkle of sea salt, lots of pepper, and my extra-virgin olive oil. You'd think you died and went to heaven. Like you, I don't eat a lot of carbs. I love salads and nuts and again a lot of olive oil on my steamed vegetables. I'm a cooking cardiologist. You gotta see me on my website, HeartMDinstitute.com. I have these videos of me cooking.

SS: I love your website.

SINATRA: And my videos show lamb—rack of lamb is one of my favorites—is very healthy for you, as is avocado. I love coconut. I love dark chocolate, but in moderation.

SS: You are an eater! Ha ha! Do you have a cocktail with dinner?

SINATRA: I'll occasionally have a Ketel One or a Tito vodka martini. I cut back on wine big time. But I drink my son's Freespirit Wine because it's organic; there are no insecticides or fungicides, which can be especially toxic to people.

SS: Last question. What do you think about salt?

SINATRA: Salt's fine. I mean, here's the deal. Salt has a bright side and a dark side as well as a sweet spot, as too little or too much can be harmful.

It's not the salt you sprinkle on your food, but it's the hidden salt in a lot of these foods, like dehydrated soups, dill pickles, processed chickens, potato chips, French fries, et cetera. You can get two grams of salt in one sitting. People need to read labels. If the sodium is higher than the potassium, I tell them to consider avoiding it. Potassium is the most important mineral you take in the diet and I believe taking in generous amounts of potassium will not only help to prevent major illnesses like stroke and heart attack but cancer as well, as it affects the acid base balance of the body. I take 500 mg of powdered potassium every day as part of a vitamin and mineral electrolyte drink. If you can take in more than 3 grams of potassium a day, that's a good thing.

SS: What about sprinkling sea salt on your food?

SINATRA: I like Celtic salt and Himalayan salt because they have some minerals. Salt is crucial, and too little salt in your diet is not good.

SS: Is salt okay if you have high blood pressure?

SINATRA: Sure. Just sprinkle a little on your food to taste and just remember to avoid the hidden salts in boxes and cans. I usually allow my patients up to 2.5 grams of salt per day. But some people may be more salt sensitive than others. It is important to remember that too little salt can raise blood pressure via excessive hormonal responses in the kidney. So salt has a sweet spot. Too little is especially undesirable, particularly in patients with heart failure, as it can create undesirable vasoconstriction in the kidney; and too much can be harmful as it can create volume expansion leading to higher blood pressure. Generally I don't like more than 3.8 grams for anyone, but for most people, including those with high blood pressure, 2 to 2.5 grams is reasonable.

SS: Essentially, for heart health you are touting the benefits of saturated healthy fats and that cholesterol is not the problem, that the human body needs fats, and there are benefits from sea salt for the heart! They must love you at cardiology conferences! And then . . . on top of all of this, you are also a psychotherapist.

SINATRA: Well, I did years of training in bioenergetic psychotherapy. Early in my cardiac career I learned that cardiology is frequently an illness from the neck up. I can't tell you how many times I resuscitated people in sudden death situations that were precipitated by stressful and emotional situations. Everybody knows that every physical illness also has an emotional component. Just think of a time when you were ill with the flu; frequently depression and sadness and feelings of despair come in. Positive intention is vitally important. Healers must support this. Positive thinking in any illness is so important as it empowers the patient, helps to alleviate fear, and in my experience patients do remarkably well if they focus on the positive and not the negative "what ifs." It also allows me to ask my patients emotional questions, like, what are the most important emotional issues in your life?

SS: That kind of interaction with your cardiologist must diminish stress, which can only be good for a heart patient.

SINATRA: The most important thing a physician, or a cardiologist like me, does is understand when the patient is suffering emotionally. When the patient knows that you "see" them in their struggle and you understand their suffering, it reduces their stress remarkably.

Any time you can decrease or eliminate stress in a patient is huge. I will tell you that right now. Being in touch with your feelings is crucial. For example, so many people have so much anger and are in total denial. Others have sadness and totally suppress it. One of the reasons I wrote my book *Heartbreak and Heart Disease* is that I had a deep understanding that suppressed emotions and emotional toxicity are frequently at the heart of illness. It became very clear to me that forgiveness is the key, and loving one's self and others is healing. Anger, rage, and emotional hostility are definitely toxic to the heart.

SS: Can't get well when you are toxic (physically or emotionally). You are very special. Thank you for this great information. And coming from you, it's going to open many eyes and be very validating.

I'm going to the kitchen now to grill my artichokes with olive oil and fresh lemon, sea salt, and put butter on my asparagus. And I feel great about it!

Give me your website again.

SINATRA: For additional information, please see HeartMDInstitute .com, and for specific nutraceutical solutions, then it's DrSinatra.com.

SS: What a pleasure! Thanks. You are changing the paradigm. I'm proud to be your messenger.

Clearly, cardiologists like Dr. Sinatra have rethought the prescribing of statins and have confined their dispersal to only a very small percentage of people who would benefit. Yet, still today, they are the biggest-selling drugs in the world. Could it be that using pharmaceutical-sponsored research as the basis for making decisions could be compromising us? Are we the losers in this one? Have we become *tox*-sick as a result? That is how deep the low-fat, no-fat, "cholesterol is bad" myth has become embedded.

When you factor into your health equation that healthy fats will now be a regular part of your diet, you will find that you will be satiated. If I am craving something (anything), where I once would have gone for sugar or carbs, I now get myself a piece of cheese, or I have a slice of my fabulous toasted seed bread slathered with organic sweet butter. Once a major sugar addict, I find that being able to eat healthy fats has taken away my cravings; fats are delicious, they satiate my cravings for sugar and carbs, and as a result, I am at the best weight of my life.

GO FROM *TOX*-SICK TO NOT SICK

1. Cholesterol is not the enemy; it is inflammation we need to worry about.

   REMEDY: Measure inflammation with a highly sensitive CRP blood test to test C-reactive protein levels.

2. Dietary fats like coconut oil, avocados, extra-virgin olive oil, and the omega-3 essential fats found in sardines and squid are crucial to health for the heart, brain, and the GI tract. When fat levels drop in the body, the heart suffers.

   REMEDY: Enjoy and use healthy fats freely.

3. When measuring cholesterol, the so-called bad LDL should have two readings: one measure for large fluffy particles of LDL, and another measure for small-particle LDL.

   REMEDY: If your small particles levels of LDL are high (>1,000), you need to make some changes in your diet. Eliminate all sugar and all carbs and consume healthy dietary fats, grass-fed, organic proteins, and organic vegetables.

4. Small particle LDL is the dangerous reading, especially for people whose genetics predispose them to Lp(a).

   REMEDY: You must avoid trans fats and consider lumbrokinase or nattokinase supplementation to thin your blood, plus over-the-counter, non-time-release niacin, and definitely omega-3s. (By the way, bioidentical estrogen for women and testosterone for men have also been shown to have a positive impact on lowering Lp(a), especially when there is hormonal deficiency.)

5. CoQ10 is a vital nutrient for the heart and the body.

   REMEDY: Supplement with this key nutrient, particularly if you're on a statin.

CHAPTER 6

THE EFFECTS OF TOXINS ON YOUR THYROID AND OTHER HORMONES

JUST WHEN WE THOUGHT WE HAD THE HORMONE REPLACEMENT puzzle figured out, just when we were starting to feel "right" again, we hit a wall. Sadly, the intercept is toxicity. Toxins blunt hormone production, and toxins overload our livers so the individualized, pre-scribed, as-per-lab-work hormone creams that have revived quality of life and health for so many are now getting "kicked out" of the liver due to toxicity, leaving these hormones to roam around in the blood-stream. The effect is a hormone "overdose." If you are symptomatic again—gaining weight, itching, sweating, and more—a toxic liver is most likely your issue.

The young are affected also. My granddaughter Violet experi-enced the effect of her toxicity when it threw her hormone system completely into chaos, creating uncontrollable moods, depression, sadness, and acne. As described earlier, she was only fourteen years old when this invisible enemy attacked her quality of life. Up until that point, hormones were something she had never thought about relative to herself; at her age the hormone-making machinery does it all automatically . . . except when toxins interfere. Sadly and sud-denly, her hormone pathway was intercepted by her toxic overload from an HPA axis (hypothalamus/pituitary/adrenal) that stopped getting the correct signals due to toxins residing in the brain. The toxic attack knows no age or gender. People from their teens through their twenties, thirties, forties, and on are now subject to severe hor-monal "storms" from toxic exposure.

For those who are in actual hormonal decline due to age, the remedy is not to stop taking your hormones. The answer, and the only answer, is to detox your liver so your body can clean out and go back to normal.

Environmental plasticizers or phthalates can damage thyroid glands (major hormone) and make them hyper- or hypoactive. Environmental chemicals can sit in every cell membrane hormone receptor, blocking the activity of hormones. The body may be able to make sufficient hormones on its own were it not affected so negatively by chemical toxins. This explains why younger and younger women experience severe hormonal decline. Children and teens are now tragically experiencing imbalanced hormones due to chemical exposure, and their doctors are stymied as to what to do.

This hormonal roller coaster causes emotional problems, from rage to depression, brain fog, premature menses, and breasts and bodies these children are not ready to handle. Chemicals are causing a complete interruption in nature and no one seems to be very concerned.

It's difficult enough as a woman when we first experience hormonal decline in midage, so try to fathom what it must be like for a little girl or boy.

Connect the dots from ingested chemicals to the damage they cause to the protective barrier of the GI tract, which causes leaks. These leaks result from toxins eating their way through the GI lining that then lead to toxic travel up to the fatty brain. Now these toxins disrupt the hypothalamus (that lives in the brain) and disables it. This is consequential because the hypothalamus is the hormone "director," whose job it is to tell the rest of the hormones what to do (and in particular, the thyroid). As a result of the toxic damage, now the hormones operate inefficiently, discordantly, or not at all. The result is a "crazy" feeling. You're feeling out of control, like having PMS every day twenty-four hours a day, and now not only is your GI tract damaged, but your immune system is also weakened, and your brain is not operating at optimum. All from toxins!

There's more. Breasts can stockpile plastic, and prostates can stockpile cadmium. Men who experience heart attacks often have low testosterone levels that have been stunted by toxins in the body.

Toxins affect your entire body, but the hormone system takes a major hit, and the effects are uncomfortable and difficult to explain. You go to a doctor who is not up on environmental illness and you will be treated for everything with allopathic medicine, meaning, here's the pill to fix it. If, in fact, it did "fix" it, you could rationalize the use of these chemicals, but it doesn't fix or cure. In many if not most cases the doctors' allopathic arsenal aggravates the condition. Hypothyroidism, Graves' disease, Hashimoto's thyroiditis, infertility, prostatic hypertrophy, endometriosis, cancers of the prostate or breast, polycystic ovaries, and abnormal Pap smears are all linked to or rooted in today's toxicity.

In this section I am going to concentrate quite a bit on the thyroid, one of our major hormones. I have written extensively on how all the hormones work in my other books, all of which are listed at the back of this book. (Or, if you are anxious to find a qualified bioidentical or environmental doctor right away, please go to ForeverHealth.com, a free service that will connect you to the right doctor nearest you.)

If a major hormone like the thyroid is low or missing chronically and continues this way, you won't live very long. That's why a well-working thyroid is so crucial. But the thyroid is under attack from toxicity, and doctors once again are for the most part guessing at how to handle the problem. So many people are walking around with false diagnoses of MS, fibromyalgia, or lupus when in fact their problem is a dysfunctional GI tract, leaking toxins into their bloodstream that then find their way to the thyroid or the hypothalamus in the brain. Here's why that is important to connect. The hypothalamus is located in the brain along with the pituitary gland. I like to call them the president and the vice president. They are "command central" for all the other hormones. In other words, they are responsible for telling all the hormones what to do.

They have an "executive assistant" who does the day-to-day work, and that is the thyroid. The hypothalamus speaks directly to the thyroid, and the thyroid obediently goes into action and directs the minor hormones: estrogen, progesterone, testosterone, DHEA, and pregnenolone. There are other minor hormones, but these are the key ones. When they are low or missing, you feel awful, and not in control of your body; weight gain appears, and/or hot flashes, night sweats, flushing, itching, or moodiness can all occur. You might find that you are unable to sleep or you might experience body pain and joint aches, headaches, and a loss of interest in sex. All because the thyroid has gone awry.

When the thyroid is "off" in a child or a teenager, these children don't grow properly. Very short people usually have thyroid or other hormonal deficiencies like human growth hormone (HGH). What does the thyroid gland do? Just a few key things, like these:

- Controls and maintains your body temperature, which is why when the thyroid hormone is low, your hands and feet are always cold.
- Helps get rid of cellular waste; if the thyroid isn't working correctly, you get puffy skin on the face, arms, and thighs.
- Provides critical immune function; when low or too high, you get chronic colds and flus.
- Stimulates increased blood flow, but if the hormone is low, you get brain fog and cognitive impairment because low thyroid slows blood flow to the brain.
- Stimulates oxygen consumption in the heart, liver, skeletal muscles, and kidneys.
- Helps with sleep and mood; if your thyroid levels are too high (hyperthyroid), you can't sleep and feel agitated and slightly "crazed" all the time. If your thyroid levels are too low or too high, you fatigue easily and feel very tired.

That's a thumbnail of why the thyroid is so important. People with chronic low or high thyroid hormones have a very poor quality of life. And here we are under this massive toxic assault; these toxins get into the bloodstream via the leaky gut, and the thyroid is often assaulted by them. It's the same pathway taken by all the toxins. Any organ or gland that the toxins decide to attack will result in severe changes in health and quality of life.

Let's not accept this. It's time for a change.

WHY YOUR BHRT MAY NOT BE WORKING:
AN INTERVIEW WITH GARRY GORDON, M.D.

Dr. Garry Gordon is an internationally recognized expert on chelation ther-apy and antiaging medicine. He is also a consultant for various supplement companies and the coauthor of The Chelation Answer, *plus he lectures extensively on the topic of health, hormones, and toxicity. He is on the Board of the Homeopathic Medical Examiners for Arizona, is cofounder of ACAM (the American College for Advancement in Medicine), and is a board member of the International Oxidative Medicine Association. He does telephone consultations for patients from around the world, offering second opinions on any type of health issue, from his offices in Arizona.*

SS: Thank you, Dr. Gordon. You are one of the pioneers in func-tional medicine. People flock to your seminars and lectures. What's the big complaint today? What are people asking you?

GG: I hear over and over that people feel like they are going crazy! Brains under attack.

SS: Sad but true. You know so much about lead poisoning and che-lation, and so many other topics, a lot of which you and I discussed in my book *Bombshell*. But today I specifically want to talk to you about hormones, especially the thyroid. Let's explore the effects of toxins on the thyroid; what can we do about it?

GG: Well, we know that it's about the chemicals and now the chemical assault on the human body is even affecting babies in the womb; unfortunately, the exposure never stops. In 2005, the Environ-mental Working Group released a hallmark study using cord blood to assess the chemical exposure of neonates in utero. The placenta has long been thought to shield the developing baby from pollutants in the environment. The study's alarming results dispelled this as a wishful myth. It concluded that, "The dangers of pre- or post-natal ex-posure to this complex mixture of carcinogens, developmental toxins, and neurotoxins have never been studied."

SS: I guess it's never been studied because it opens a can of worms they most likely want to keep closed. But any thinking person can re-alize that the human body was never meant to process this chemical assault. So let's start with the child; how does this affect a newborn?

GG: It's disastrous for the developing immune system and the health of the GI tract. Within hours of emerging from the womb, a newborn is given a dollop of antibiotics in the eyes, injected with the hepatitis B vaccine, with known neurotoxic properties, and jabbed with a vitamin K shot, which contains 9 mg of benzyl alcohol. In 1992, Golding published concerns that vitamin K injections could be associated with a doubled risk of malignant disease in children, particularly leukemia. While there have been considerable doubts about whether the association is coincidental or causal, the controversy has never been completely resolved.

SS: So now that the child has been bombarded with toxic molecules, what can we do?

GG: Detoxification must be done daily by everyone today, children and adults. It is now essential that detoxification is a part of everyone's everyday life in order to live long and healthy. Preventing illness and feeling your absolute best is predominantly done through living a healthy, responsible lifestyle. But to achieve lasting wellness in today's toxic world, there are steps that must be taken. Detoxification must be a daily, lifelong pursuit.

SS: We know that environmental pollution and the natural aging process produce damaging free radicals. Please explain what free-radical accumulation over time contributes to hormonal disruptions.

GG: Free-radical damage confuses the body. This damage not only is responsible for brain and gut issues, but also is a key component associated with thyroid and hormone imbalances. Detoxification and hormonal restoration are key elements of my F.I.G.H.T. health program, along with protocols designed to cleanse and heal the body every day, all year long, for life.

What we do to provide ourselves with the optimal environment of necessary nutrients for energy production, repair and function, elimination of toxins and wastes, and proper positive mental outlook is absolutely crucial to health, happiness, and longevity.

SS: If the thyroid is severely affected by toxins, explain the trouble caused when the thyroid isn't working correctly.

GG: A thyroid that is malfunctioning creates lots of challenges. Patients complain of symptoms that are overt hypothyroidism; their fingernails aren't growing, hair's not growing, they're cold all the time.

But thyroid testing is grossly inadequate; individuals can have every conceivable picture of hypothyroid, but they often fail the thyroid tests.

SS: So many readers tell me that. They go to the doctor and complain of symptoms that are clearly thyroid related, but the test comes back saying normal. Why are they missing it?

GG: In the Dark Ages, we used to use a simple test like underarm temperature and that was very telling. But we have such a sick population today. Normally if your under-tongue temperature is 98.6, the underarms should be 97.6, but almost nobody is achieving the right numbers these days due to toxicity. We can determine by symptoms and if the patient complains of fatigue and no energy that thyroid supplementation is often the answer. It gives the patient that extra burst of energy for more activity, and then they also lose weight. Contrary to most thinking, the thyroid function can restore itself as the body heals and detoxifies. The good news is you haven't turned off a switch.

Top doctors feel the American public is not being informed of the many reasons the thyroid gland isn't happy; bromides in bread and chlorine that's in so many different things all challenge our body's ability to get the iodine. The thyroid is dependent on sufficient iodine.

SS: So iodine supplementation is important. What are other thyroid functions? What does the thyroid do?

GG: It controls the rate of repair of your body; it controls metabolism. In other words, when you have slow metabolism, nothing works correctly. Alarmingly, I'm finding early signs of thyroid cancer in virtually every thyroid I check. It's that bad and that misunderstood.

SS: What are doctors and the labs that conduct this testing doing wrong?

GG: Most doctors don't know how to interpret the labs. Of the four thyroid hormones, blood levels of T4 are the highest, approximately four times higher than levels of T3. However, T3 is far more potent and biologically active than the others. The body makes a lot of T4 and converts to T3 as needed. T2 hasn't been well understood until recently when research clarified that it stimulates enzymes critical to producing T3.

T2 has also been shown to increase metabolism in the liver, heart,

Hypothyroidism occurs when the thyroid gland does not produce enough "energy-generating" thyroid hormones. Weight
gain is a classic symptom of this dysfunction. In such cases,
levels of thyroid-stimulating hormone may rise in an attempt
to spur more production and secretion of thyroid hormones
from the thyroid gland.

Some Signs of Low Thyroid (Hypothyroidism)

Weight gain

Chronic constipation

Fatigue

Feeling cold when others
  are hot

Brittle hair, hair loss, or
  nails that break easily
  and split

Longer, heavier, and
  more frequent periods

Dry, scaly skin

Bruising easily

Depression

Mental confusion

Trouble sleeping

Low libido

Sensitivity to light

Recurrent infections

Headaches or migraines

Some Signs of High Thyroid (Hyperthyroidism)

Anxiety

Racing heart

Difficulty sleeping

Diarrhea

Shortness of breath

Sweaty hands and feet

Thickening of the skin
  around eyes and neck

Signs of a Sick Thyroid

Selenium deficiency: Selenium is a mineral necessary for the
  conversion of T4 to T3.

Estrogen dominance: Estrogen suppresses thyroid function.

Mercury toxicity: Mercury is a toxic metal that can contaminate the thyroid gland.

muscle tissue, and fat tissue. T2 breaks down fat without breaking
down muscle tissue.

SS: That's complicated information, but suffice it to say that a doctor reading thyroid lab tests needs proper education. No wonder these
tests are so often misinterpreted. So toxins interfere with all this important signaling. A toxic body manifests a malfunctioning thyroid,

resulting in underactive thyroid (hypothyroidism) or overactive (hyperthyroid). When toxins interfere and the T3 and T4 drop too low, what happens?

GG: The pituitary responds by making more thyroid-stimulating hormone (TSH), which stimulates your thyroid to produce more T3 and T4; but increased TSH means your thyroid hormone levels are dropping and now your body starts reacting with all the signs and symptoms of low or high thyroid, and quality of life suffers.

SS: When do women tend to develop hypertension?

GG: At the time of menopause, and that ties in to bone breakdown that is accelerated by toxicity. It's all connected. But now we can clearly see that bones are breaking down faster because of lead accumulation. Now you have hypertension, which is part of the end result of lead. Dr. Dorothy Merritt, a Houston internist, has discovered that bone lead turns out to not have any correlation with blood lead. *Blood* lead is useful. *Bone* lead is an old chronic problem.

SS: Why aren't orthodox doctors concerned about lead levels in a human body?

GG: Lack of information . . . when you decline in hormones, you become inactive because your energy is zapped without hormones (including thyroid) and if you are not replacing hormones with bio-identicals, you are going to break down bone faster plus you will have more lead being released. Then your doctor is going to tell you your blood pressure's going up and he or she is going to give you a drug for it. But in fact, all you needed to do is thyroid replacement and learn about oral chelation to get the lead out, which has been available to every doctor working with lead workers.

On my website, to make it easy for doctors who do not understand this, they can go to Gordonresearch.com and they can put in the Search area "507 EDTA articles." It links to the published papers written about workers in a lead battery factory. This is such a dangerous occupation that if one of those patients came to me, I couldn't let them continue to work at the plant. But if I give them oral EDTA, it mixes with blood lead, and then they get so much better that I can let them return to work and earn their living.

EDTA protects organs from getting rancid in your body because of its antioxidant effects. It also protects against liver cirrhosis. EDTA taken by mouth is generally recognized as safe. I'll say it again: people need to understand that we all need some form of detoxification every day of our life because of the tremendous toxic assault in today's world. I am an expert on the measurement of lead, mercury, cadmium, arsenic, and zinc, and we know for sure that these heavy metals are very bad for us.

SS: Is the oral chelation something a person would drink every day?

GG: EDTA is available in powder and tablets. EDTA is also sold as a rectal suppository and, yes, it's taken every day.

SS: This is a book about the effects of toxins on our health. Recently a woman I know who's very beautiful and thin and gorgeous put on thirty pounds in an alarmingly short period of time, for no apparent reason. I'm sure it had something to do with hormones, but she said she couldn't handle natural bioidentical hormones, that she'd take them and feel worse. Her face was puffy, her eyes were puffy, her eyes were yellow, her stomach was distended, she was constipated, and she was in chronic pain.

As I was thinking about her, I ran into another friend of mine and he was experiencing exactly the same thing. And then I heard about another. It seems to be happening to women more than men, but it just could be that I interact with women more than men. What's going on? It doesn't appear to be about a recent increase in calories (none of them had changed their eating habits), so is it toxic thyroids? I mean, why are people who are young and should be healthy, suddenly having their bodies and faces blowing up and their stomachs distended? Why have their systems stopped working correctly?

GG: The microbiome has been changed in people's bodies by the ingestion of the chemicals that enter our systems every day, including the antibiotics we inject into our food. Most people are suffering with failing health as a result. It's like a Sherlock Holmes mystery waiting to be solved. Harvard studies conclude that everybody correctly tested is going to have cytomegalic viruses living in the plaque of their arteries. If they don't have that, they'll have chlamydia or coccidiomycosis or Lyme. The poisonous, pesticide-ridden food we ingest, infections, genetics, heavy metals, hormones injected into GMO corn-fed protein, and toxins are all trying to bring us down. My program called F.I.G.H.T. is an acronym trying to help people solve their problems. Some people just need to get gluten out of their diets. Some people

need hormone replacement, but if their house has formaldehyde leaking out of the plywood that's holding the kitchen cabinets together,
or if the stove is leaking and that gas is permeating throughout the
house, you are going to have health problems and that takes the kind
of doctors who understand the environmental assault.

SS: Feels daunting.

GG: Yes, but remember this . . . the body is self-adjusting, although
getting well requires several steps to rid the body of toxicity. Taking
out the lead in your body through chelation is only part of the picture;
diet has to be looked at and understood as well as hormone replacement.

SS: What else is interfering with our hormones and health?

GG: David Ewing Duncan, a professor at University of California,
San Francisco, was stunned to find that he was loaded with polybrominated diphenyl ether (flame retardant). Turns out he flies a lot.

SS: Because the thinking is that if an airplane crashes the seats
have been made fire retardant and the person has a better chance of
surviving?

GG: Yes, regulations have insisted that every seat be fire retardant.
The problem is that flame retardants are dangerous chemicals not fit
for the human body; so all the fire-retardant seats do is expose passengers to harmful chemicals for long periods of time, and THEY are
also ineffective.

SS: We are at present having a lot of wildfires in California. I
watch the news with airplanes dropping this red, smoky-looking wet
stuff over the fires.

GG: Yes. That stuff is essentially like dropping poisons on the fire,
and all those in their path get infected. We had fires in Arizona this
year and the water of our nearby lake became filthy with it as a result.

SS: If we don't take steps to detoxify in today's world, how long
can we expect to not only live but live healthy?

GG: Before we decided to poison our earth, living to 120 years
wasn't really that rare.

SS: But I believe you can outsmart the assault and keep your own
body clean and healthy. It just takes focus, determination, and consistency.

GG: I agree, and I believe by taking the steps that I do on a daily basis to detoxify will help me achieve long life. I am healthier than I've been my entire life and I am seventy-nine.

SS: I will vouch for that. Whenever I see you there's a spring in your step that most forty-year-olds would like to have. Your eyes are clear, and I truly believe clear eyes are a window into health.

GG: I've been on daily detoxification for thirty years. I designed a program for me and my patients called *Beyond Chelation Improved*. Why? Well, know that each day of your life you're going to take in a little lead, mercury, cadmium, and arsenic from the food you eat, the water you drink, and the air you breathe. But most people are not aware that they will also be a little bit more poisoned on a daily basis as the old bone makes new bone and the old bone releases lead.

SS: So chelation, and EDTA, releases lead, mercury, cadmium, and arsenic heavy metals. What about the degraded food, GMO food, food from convenience stores, and food that really isn't food?

GG: It is sad because the long-term outcomes of poor-quality food, and the amphetamines that are prescribed so readily to people of all ages who have toxic brains, are nothing but negative for brain function and addiction. The literature is out there, including from the AMA, which has a special journal for internists showing that all causes of morbidity and mortality are tied to how long you are carrying lead in your body, affecting your brain and reflexes. Why do old people drive into storefronts? Their reflexes are off. Think about the amount of lead they have stored up in their bones. By the time you reach your seventies and eighties, you will have a thousand times too much lead in your bone, and that lead changes the neurotransmitter function in your brain; in other words, that is why everybody is having trouble reaching that 120 years of lifespan.

SS: Where are we getting the lead exposure?

GG: When we started mining and disturbing the earth's surface, the lead material went up in the air; and what goes up has to come down. It's all the same, whether you talk lead, mercury, cadmium, or is it the coal that we burn? There is no easy solution. The solution that works for me and the lucky people who believe in my protocol is to take chelation; they clean out their bodies, and they can feel as good as I do.

SS: What about mercury exposure?

GG: Folks, we're all mercury poisoned. I don't care whether we talk lead, mercury, or cadmium, which is tied to so many illnesses. The FDA and EPA do not even agree on what's a safe level of mercury in your body.

SS: What fish are safe? Any fish absent of mercury?

GG: You really can't find anything on the face of the earth that has mercury absent. Selenium tends to neutralize the adverse effect of mercury, though.

SS: What are the effects of mercury on the human body?

GG: You can be depressed or tired or have chronic fatigue as a result of a mercury diagnosis. The big problem is that most doctors are not environmental doctors. It takes a lot to learn all of this.

What's the one nutrient you can't live more than two minutes without? Oxygen, right?

Once you understand the importance of oxygen, then you have to understand "Redox Signaling Molecules." What does that mean? That within your cell, the mitochondria has to know what the nucleus wants done in the life zone. Every part of the cell has to talk to the other part and guess what does that? Signaling molecules. Now when you are young your signaling molecules are so high, it's wonderful, boundless energy.

Unless you're near dead, you still have about 98 percent oxygen. But when I measure the oxygen in your plasma (blood), it's another story.

Linus Pauling pointed out as long as your PO2 (the oxygen blood level in your body) is over 60, you don't get cancer. It's when it drops under that you set the stage. Cancer grows in an anaerobic (no oxygen) field. ASEA gel (go to GordonResearch.com to find out more about it) will increase your oxygen, making your energy increase while protecting you from cancer and other diseases (providing you are watching your diet).

SS: Now consider the brain conditions of today: ADD, ADHD, OCD, autism, bipolar disorder, schizophrenia, asthma, dyslexia, dyspraxia, and so on. Are these all things that could benefit from ASEA?

GG: Yes. Oxygen is always on the top of the pile, yet it's been the most neglected component. That's the basis of Linus Pauling's work.

It takes effort to be well today and there are a lot of complexities to getting everybody well, but oxygen is going to help you burn all the toxins you are carrying in your body. No matter how you avoid it coming in, you haven't started to get it out of the tissues and that's where ASEA is a great advantage.

SS: You speak of the supplement "Pueraria mirificia." Why?

GG: Pueraria mirificia is neuroprotective more than any substance we have ever found. It is a great protector of the brain and goes a long way in protecting from dementia.

SS: And my understanding is that I would also take this if my libido was off?

GG: Dr. Christiane Northrop claims she has women who couldn't be sexually active for fifteen years, who are now chasing their man up and down the hall.

SS: Are you still hot on colloidal silver?

GG: I believe in silver. It works and is extremely beneficial for the GI tract and the gut/brain connection.

SS: What are the benefits of Epsom salts? What do you think of them?

GG: Epsom salts are essentially you bathing in magnesium. Your skin soaks it in, which has a calming effect, makes you sleep great, and is excellent for detox. Magnesium changed my health. So, yes, regular Epsom salt baths will assist in fighting the environment and keeping you healthy.

SS: Why do you do this? Why do you keep on keeping on? I'm watching people my age, your age, my husband's age degrade on this present form of allopathic medicine. The fact that you're keeping yourself alive and healthy and your continuing interest in new technologies is remarkable. You could give it up. You've done so much; you've been fighting the fight. Do you think the fight will become less intense as time goes by?

GG: If we motivate people, that will cause them to stay on our kind of health-promoting programs. Their feeling of well-being will be the motivator.

And for me, I'm turned on by helping people and doing no harm.

SS: It's worth going after this new health. Life is so enjoyable if you are healthy and you have a good working brain and strong bones. I'm so enjoying aging as a result of all the things that I do. You know, people say to me, "It's so much work . . . you have to take all these supplements and follow so many protocols." I always say, "It's a lot more work to be sick."

Thank you, Dr. Gordon, for your wisdom and enthusiasm. You make me a believer.

> For more information on Dr. Gordon's F.I.G.H.T. program and personalized health consultations, go to the Gordon Research Institute website at GordonResearch.com.

GO FROM *TOX*-SICK TO NOT SICK

1. Iodine supplementation is necessary if you have low thyroid.

   REMEDY: To test for thyroid-stimulating hormone (TSH) contact Life Extension Foundation or ForeverHealth.com to obtain blood work and an interpretation of your tests, so your doctor can prescribe as needed.

2. Know your numbers.

   REMEDY: Go to either website and obtain:
   • A chemistry panel and complete blood count: this will give your doctor a quick snapshot of your overall health. It will provide a broad range of diagnostic information to assess your vascular, liver, kidney, and blood cell status
   • Fibrinogen levels: increased fibrinogen levels can indicate a heart attack risk and inflammatory disorders, such as rheumatoid arthritis
   • Hemoglobin AC: to measure blood sugar
   • DHEA levels: frequently referred to as your antiaging hormone
   • Homocysteine levels: high homocysteine is associated with increased risk of heart attack, bone fracture, and foggy brain
   • C-reactive protein (C-RP) levels: to test for inflammation
   • Estradiol levels: a minor hormone that needs to be optimal for best quality of life
   • Testosterone levels: both men and women have testosterone, and these levels need to be optimal for best quality of life

3. Detoxification is essential for regaining hormonal balance. Like the doctor says, detox first, then replace hormones. My other books lay out anything you need to know about hormone replacement, but start first with Dr. Gordon's Detox Program, as another of the many ways to regain balance in the body. His protocol can be ordered from his website and/ or by a phone consultation.

CHAPTER 7

THE REST OF YOU

One of the biggest deterrents of the exposure of mold-related illnesses is because mold illness is acquired from flaws in the indoor environment. If there is a flaw, then someone caused the flaw and that means liability. With liability, someone might have to pay to correct the flaw and the illness. Given the number of people in buildings with too much moisture, there is a staggering number of dollars potentially involved.

—DR. RITCHIE SHOEMAKER

WE ARE FINALLY BEGINNING TO REALIZE THE HARMFUL EFFECTS of mold. It is common in so many of today's homes and is highly underrated as a dangerous toxin to the brain and body. Left unchecked, it can silently eat its way through our intestines, causing massive stomach and brain damage. My husband took you through his encounter with mold, a condition that made his life very difficult. It was a saga to detoxify this mold out of not only his but both of our bodies. But the real danger was that we were unknowingly already toxic from the environment, and the mold put us both over the top. That's what happens to so many; you never know what will be your tipping point. It might be the car fumes at the gas station or the "new car smell."

As I've spoken to more and more people with mold disease, no one—no landlord, no building—can be held responsible. It's a can of worms no one wants to open. Yet we personally have spent thousands of dollars out of our own pockets, as have so many, because insurance does not recognize this as a viable condition. If it is diagnosed as Parkinson's, or fibromyalgia, or MS, or brain dysfunction, you have a shot at getting insurance to pay, but it's likely you will also be given a myriad of unnecessary drugs when detoxification is the answer.

Most patients are written off as hypochondriacs, yet mold illness is real and it is debilitating. For those who carry the HLA gene, the body becomes extremely sensitive to mold and other toxic substances. From my experience and that of my husband and granddaughters I can say firsthand, mold is not in your head. It's real, and unless aggressively treated, it can bring down a person's health and quality of life.

Below is a typical mold story. It will give you some idea of the devastating effects of this illness. Some people have had to leave not only their houses but their furnishings, and almost all their possessions, if their exposure is drastic. Some people's reactions are less extreme than others', but when you read the story of this family you will recognize this: mold is no joke.

I was experiencing a burning in my chest for a few months; then I noticed a musty smell in my house and air conditioner. I had it cleaned twice. They told me the air conditioner was probably drawing something from the environment. I was convinced it was not my clean house that was the problem and made inquiries about getting a new air conditioner. I was advised by the saleslady that she had had the same problem at home, and replacing the air conditioner did not help. We proceeded to clean mold that we found around the back door and the windowsills. The air became musty and hard to breathe so I ran out onto the back veranda and told my husband I was going to my mother's until it settled. I returned a week later and my glands and lymph nodes began to swell up again and the burning in my lungs returned. So I left and told my husband I could not go back there. The next day my tongue swelled on one side and I got ulcers, so I went to the doctor, who gave me antibiotics. We had the carpets cleaned and the outside of the house cleaned, but the house still smelled musty and I still could not enter into that environment. Finally, we had to move. My husband is working eighteen hours a day to afford a mortgage and rent. I am at home with my baby and she suffers with a rash and silent reflux. But we have gotten better since we moved. I have never been so stressed in all my life. I just want to enjoy our baby daughter and not have to go through all this upheaval. If this happens at your house, if it smells musty or if you notice mold, just get out and stay somewhere and have a mold professional come in to deal with it. Do not clean it yourself. I am grateful we got out alive.

Dr. Ritchie Shoemaker (www.chronicneurotoxins.com) is one of the foremost authorities on mold in this country. I asked him to lay out the pathway for us. It is daunting, but try to follow so you can see how pervasive this insidious disease can be and how it takes hold of your body and doesn't want to let go.

MOLD AND HOW IT MAY BE HARMING YOUR HEALTH: AN INTERVIEW WITH RITCHIE SHOEMAKER, M.D.

Dr. Ritchie Shoemaker knows all about mold. Hailing from Pocomoke, Maryland, he wanted to be a rural doctor, but his aspirations were waylaid by patients with mystery illnesses who were showing up at his office, a few at first, then in droves. As a result, he switched focus and became known as the foremost authority on mold in America.

If you think mold may be your issue, devour this information. Read it and then reread it. Mold is so incredibly complex that it will take that kind of concentration. But within these next pages you might just find the missing piece to your health puzzle. This is cutting-edge science and medicine from the controversial world of toxic mold.

SS: Dr. Ritchie Shoemaker, it's so nice to speak with you. I was thinking this morning that mold has been around forever—it's even mentioned in the Bible—but up until recently the mold-fear we are now experiencing was nonexistent. I remember as a child we had mold in our bathroom, always in the cracks in the tile, and my mother would get some Clorox and get it out; we never thought about it. Is mold different today, or are our bodies just so toxic that we can no longer tolerate it in a way we were once able to handle?

RS: Thank you, Suzanne. Well, that's a series of questions. The Leviticus discussion about indoor mold is one that people always will talk about, but we know that there were some rather dramatic changes in fungi (mold) beginning early in the '70s. The Pittsburgh Paint Company started adding a fungicide to paint so that it was easier to clean and therefore easier to maintain. The particular compound created mutations in fungi, and just about all the players that make people ill indoors now come out of this mutated line. The toxic compounds made by these mutated fungi I worry about have a different shape compared to the same compounds made by earlier generations of fungi. Our immune systems recognize this compound as foreign and create a much greater immune response to them than they did in the unmutated form.

So the simplest answer is no, the fungi we had then are not the same as they are now.

SS: Is mold simply a tipping point, the final straw of an accumulation of toxins: car fumes, exhaust fumes, pesticides, mercury, PCBs in the fish, then you throw in mold and the person's health is now over the top?

RS: Bill Moyers did a piece on environmental chemicals that were found in the cord blood of newborns and there were hundreds of different toxic compounds. What's fascinating to me about mold is that we are born with particular chromosomes and there is a group of genes called the immune response genes; the acronym that we give to it (I know how much you like acronyms) is HLA, or histocompatibility locus A.

SS: You do have a tendency to speak in initials, ha ha, but fortunately I happen to know of the HLA gene as I carry it. My understanding is that it is particular to (but not exclusive to) the English, Irish, French, British, Welsh, German, Spanish. But then again my husband is Eastern European and he and his family are carriers.

RS: Hey, all right. Now, there are 6 of at least 54 different haplotypes of those who carry the HLA gene that make up over 95 percent of our proven mold cases. Those with HLA have more relative risk, which is something you're born with, so when does this illness get started? Using your terms, when do you go past the tipping point? Well, there's no one chronological time. I've had two-year-old toddlers becoming ill for the first time and eighty-five-year-old men getting ill for the first time. It has a lot to do with inflammation, creating an event I call "priming."

SS: Priming? Meaning if you are an HLA gene type and then you get exposed to mold, you are more likely to get sick?

RS: Yes. A classic example is this wonderful artist living on the

Front Range outside Denver who had a basement that basically had a forest of mold blooming away like crazy that never made her sick, until she had a temperature of 104 for a week or so, from pneumonia, then darn near died. When she came home she became sickened by the fungi and all the other organisms in her basement, which didn't bother her before she got sick.

SS: Did you start out being the mold/Lyme doctor expert?

RS: No, I think fate finds people for a reason. I always wanted to be a rural family practice physician. That idea is a little old-fashioned these days, but I always thought there should be one doctor who would be out in the boondocks, who would take direct personal responsibility for a group of patients as they traverse through the health-care system.

It's personalized so I know if you come to see me and something's wrong, I am familiar with your history and will recognize something present in you that I haven't seen before. If you need a cardiologist, I'll send you to the cardiologist who takes care of the problem, and then he or she sends you back to my care.

SS: A lovely thought. I grew up like that, with a family doctor.

RS: Well, that was the ideal I wanted.

SS: What happened?

RS: I lived in the flatlands of Maryland and was very happy to be taking care of rural people in my rural way until *Pfiesteria*, a little critter called a dinoflagellate that lives in estuaries, started growing because of man-made chemicals.

SS: Was this mold?

RS: Well, it's a toxic microorganism. Fungicides, namely copper and dithiocarbamates, killed the things that ate *Pfiesteria*, which then changed its eating habits.

SS: So why was this a problem?

RS: This was 1996, and I was a physician for people who worked around the water; people who caught crabs and "orsters," as we call 'em, and fish, suddenly started being affected by the waters that were previously safe.

Pfiesteria poisoning was the first of the biotoxin illnesses, but no one knew the mechanism by which it made people ill. In 1998, two years after working on *Pfiesteria*, I had my first mold case. What we saw is that these particular toxins that are made by a dinoflagellate, a blue-green algae, or a cyanobacteria around Lake Erie and Toledo were now in the water and the city said it was okay to take a shower, but the water was not safe to drink.

SS: That doesn't make sense.

RS: Of course it doesn't. You can get ill by breathing in bio-aerosols of this stuff, especially in the bath or shower.

SS: Meaning you are taking it in through the lungs and skin?

RS: Yes. Mostly through the lungs.

SS: So your patients all of a sudden were coming in with weird illnesses that you hadn't been aware of before?

RS: Multisystem illnesses, cognitive problems, fatigue, weakness, aching, muscle cramps, cognitive issues, difficulty with recent memory, difficulty with concentration, difficulty with word finding, confusion, disorientation. But then there was the cough, and shortness of breath and diarrhea, abdominal pain, and funny neurologic problems of numbness and tingling and weaknesses that would come and go. Now we know that the cognitive problems were coming from the central nervous system. But back then, psychiatrists were telling patients, "I think your fatigue and cognitive issues are all in your head." I was able to show that in fact "it is in your head," but not in the way the psychiatrists implied, and that we could verify it with NeuroQuant, a software program that's done on an MRI.

SS: On an MRI you could look inside the brain at the central nervous system where the patient might be having tics or spasms or Parkinson's-like syndrome?

RS: Yes, and for that I would want a NeuroQuant, which takes ten minutes to do on the brain. The company is in San Diego, and it costs eighty-nine dollars to do the test and give you results.

It's interesting that you picked tics and spasms and Parkinson-like things; those are all representations of a part of the brain called the caudate nucleus. When I first read about it, I had not done any neuroanatomy for years and the caudate is near the hypothalamus.

SS: The bottom part of the brain?

RS: Right, and incredibly important in integrating pathways that run from the front part of the brain to the back part of the brain.

SS: Why is the caudate significant?

RS: The caudate is full of dopamine, but with mold you get disruption of dopamine-functioning nerves because you start losing caudate. Forty-five percent of my patients have a Parkinson-like tremor, but it's not Parkinson's. It's fascinating that over the years, people have talked about classic Parkinson's disease but they've also talked about Parkinson's syndrome, which is different and is related to toxins.

SS: So it's the mold toxin that causes the tics and spasms?

RS: Well, certainly what you find in a water-damaged building includes mold and mold toxins, but more important than mold toxins are bacterial toxins found inside water-damaged buildings. Also, the breakdown products of mold fungus and other things create the same inflammation response that toxins do, setting off inflammatory responses from the immune system. It's the innate immune response that causes the damage.

SS: When someone comes in with one, ten, or twenty of these symptoms, do you have a protocol, a template?

RS: Sure do; there are 37 symptoms of mold exposure I have recorded in every one of my patients. Fatigue is about 95 to 98 percent, cognitive issues 90 to 95 percent, and 30 percent of my patients have things like unusual sensitivity as well, such as to light touching of the skin. I have a complete list of symptoms in my book and the *Surviving Mold* website.

SS: So what do you do about it?

RS: Antibiotics and fungal killers will not take care of inflammation. If you have a sinus infection from a fungus, you're going to need an antifungal; if you have a fungus ball on your lung, you're going to need an antifungal.

But what has developed over the last twenty years in my world is a protocol that has twelve steps, and each one of these steps allows us to check and see what to do and when. It's been a process of trial and error.

First we want to remove people from exposure from the interior environment of a water-damaged building, then they need an inflammagen binder and there are two: cholestyramine and Welchol. Cholestyramine removes bile acids from the body by forming insoluble complexes with bile acids in the intestine, which are then excreted in the feces. When bile acids are excreted, plasma cholesterol is converted to bile acid to normalize bile acid levels. This conversion of cholesterol into bile acids lowers plasma cholesterol concentrations. Welchol lowers LDL, the bad cholesterol.

SS: So are these two substances the remedy?

RS: They are one of the first steps. Cholestyramine and Welchol are orally administered medicines. I don't use IVs. I see no need for them.

In the world of Lyme disease, so many people get antibiotics for months and months; and then when the veins give out, doctors have a port inserted into your body just like you get from chemotherapy to make access easier. But peripheral IV treatments are asking for trouble, because the compounds, even if they're done perfectly, are not welcomed by veins.

SS: I'm trying to get a history. So these people started coming in with these symptoms and at first you are realizing that your usual arsenal is not working. Did you come up with your protocols yourself, because very few doctors understand mold and Lyme?

RS: Yes, my protocol is mine. Everything I use is my own use of established medications. I participated in the creation of use of a compound called VIP, or vasoactive intestinal polypeptide, but it's not my invention.

SS: How do you administer VIP?

RS: It is made into a solution that's sprayed into your nose, which is a wonderful mucous membrane resource. In fact, we can get medications across the nose into the brain within twenty seconds.

SS: Interesting. So . . . your first step is removing all the mold from the environment you are living with? How drastic is that? Do you have to throw out all your furniture and your clothes and everything to be effective?

RS: You know, I use the term "hair pulling" to describe what people have to go through. We can say that nonporous items like wood and glass and plastic and metal can be cleaned and they can. But, unfortunately, porous items are the bulk of what we have, and you start saying, my goodness, I've got to throw out my books and my carpets? Yes, you do. And then they ask, how about my photos? Well, those can be reprinted or copied. How about the nice fabric frame with the photo from my tenth anniversary? Well, that frame is trash. And you say, Grandma's sofa? Okay, take off the upholstered material, and take out the filling, and you've got the frame you can clean.

As far as clothes go, they can be washed. But the truth of the matter is, the fabrics that people wear can be cleaned and those are not the same fabrics that you put on your sofas and your floors.

SS: So if you are diagnosed with mold, if you really want to get well, you must adhere to step one: get rid of anything that could be harboring the spores.

RS: There is difficulty in giving you a simple yes, which is what I'm tempted to do, but HLA has six variants that increase susceptibility, and two of those are way worse than the others. So those two (if you'd like the identifying numbers; the 4-3-53, and then the 11-3-52b) are the worst ones, and the level of cleaning that you are going to need to do with those is more intensive.

It's stunning to see that what is good for one guy who doesn't get sick from mold won't do for the other guy who has one or more of these susceptible types, and that's the person who has got to discard all his porous materials.

SS: But now you have the air you breathe to deal with. What do we do?

RS: If you just take an air filter and you put it in the middle of the room, it will clear particulates out of two thousand square feet, assuming eight-foot ceilings. And you say, well, that will just take me a day or so to clear out my whole house, but those things work to create a cone or a vortex of air that's pulled through the filter. And every time you have a particle caught by the filter, the filter gets more clogged than what it was two seconds before, so you need to be changing filters.

Here's where it gets tricky; the rest of the air in the room kind of laughs and says, *I'm not moving.* This is called boundary layers; if you use a filter, you need to move it from spot to spot around the room on a day-to-day basis; one day you have it six feet up in the air, and the other day it's six inches up in the air, then another it's north, east, south, west, and this will work.

This is why the idea of whole-house filtration just doesn't work, because most of the air that goes into the filter will return, then that air gets filtered and pumped into the rest of your air, and now your home ends up being recycled with harmful particles.

SS: When a building is sick, and you have the entire building remediated, do you ever really kill the mold spores?

RS: Moving is the easiest thing to do at first glance, but the National Institute of Occupational Safety and Health now says that 50 percent of our buildings are wet; whether you're in L.A. or in Bangor, Maine, all have moisture problems. When we did testing of fungal DNA from the EPA, we found once a person is identified as having mold illness, the chance of this person finding a house or an apartment or a living situation that's safe is about one in seven. It's just incredible.

So moving doesn't make a whole lot of sense. And if you are not able to move to a tent in Arizona because you can't leave your work, then how do you clean your house? It used to be that we would say there's not too much you can do, but now we have learned so much about the size of the particles that make people sick.

You have to stop all water intrusion so the building envelopes are cleared and watertight. Then you have to get rid of porous materials and clean the nonporous, and usually get rid of the carpets. You must install a HEPA filter and then and only then can you start using particular fogging solutions provided by the manufacturer. The good ones that work have Borax in them, and that's about it. You can actually take a home that was unfixable and now make it clean.

SS: I'm feeling relief. For a moment there I thought it was sounding hopeless. So that's a big step unless you are one of the unfortunate ones with the HLA gene with all the numbers behind it?

RS: Yes.

SS: What lab do you use to test for your gene type, to see if you're maybe HLA?

RS: Labcore, ARUP, and Quest do these tests called HLA-DR by PCR.

SS: What's next in this process?

RS: I'll do monthly modules with my patients, one thing at a time. And then we want to analyze where we are with labs at each step of the way.

SS: To be clear, anyone can be susceptible to mold, but HLA heightens the prospect of being infected?

RS: Yes. Now we're going to go over your labs. If you have genetic susceptibility, you could have a lack of regulation of regular inflammation. Then there's the other inflammation of what I call the innate immune system inflammation.

SS: No wonder this is such a difficult thing to unravel.

RS: The language gets to be terrible. In a way, it's like trying to tell somebody how to drive from Chicago to L.A. without using route numbers.

SS: Okay then, why should I care if I'm pro- or anti-inflammatory?

RS: One type of inflammation is melanocyte-stimulating hormone, or MSH.

It primarily is made in the hypothalamus, but it circulates through the blood and will affect skin membranes and mucous membranes; it affects blood, it affects tissue, and it especially affects the *gut*. I know the GI tract is one of your passions and it's important you factor MSH into some of your analyses. MSH is a big-time player especially when we look at *gut inflammation*.

SS: It seems that the gut is always affected by toxins of every kind. Your job as a mold doctor is much like being a detective.

RS: Exactly, and the focus of my therapy is to bring people back to what is not in excess either way. But it's complicated; it turns out that MSH manufacture in the hypothalamus is incredibly hard to measure and detect. You can't see these areas where there is interaction between the pituitary and hypothalamus on an MRI. You've heard of the portal system that affects the liver, affecting blood going to the gut as well as blood coming from arteries; well, the hypothalamus and the pituitary also have a portal system.

And that portal system can be disrupted when MSH production starts to fail, but there are some people who never get MSH back again.

SS: Why does MSH matter?

RS: A life without MSH is being chronically tired, chronically in pain, and having problems with leptin (the hormone that helps burn fatty acids). If leptin isn't working right, then you get insulin resistance.

These people get leptin resistance and that is manifested by weight that won't go away by eating less and exercising more. We talk about the explosion of weight problems in the U.S.; 35 percent of people are now called obese and this is a national epidemic. But if we look at those people with leptin resistance, at least 50 percent are mold patients.

SS: This is a big piece of the puzzle. I hear this all the time: "I'm working out more, I'm eating nothing, and I'm gaining weight."

RS: Yes. When you look at the mechanisms for that syndrome, there is a fascinating interaction between a compound called "adiponectin" and leptin; it's called high leptin, low adiponectin. If you want to induce adiponectin, the workout protocol I've published works very nicely but it's a lot of work.

Adiponectin is literally the hormone that tells your body to burn fat for fuel. It's like your body's "fat-burning torch." The research is clear that low levels of adiponectin are associated with a higher incidence of obesity. The more fat you have, the lower your levels of adiponectin, making fat loss difficult.

SS: What is hard about your adiponectin workout protocol?

RS: It's forty-five minutes daily, and it's boring because it's repetitive. I never let patients go beyond their ability to use oxygen for aerobic metabolism. If they go beyond their anaerobic threshold, they're not delivering oxygen properly in capillary beds.

The mitochondria (energy center of the cell) is where 95 percent of our glucose is metabolized from glycogen, and that's where our ATP (adenosine triphosphate, which transports energy in cells) energy comes from. But you don't get that energy if you have reduced delivery of oxygen in capillary beds, so we make sure patients don't go beyond their ability to deliver oxygen to the capillary beds.

SS: Why?

RS: If you don't deliver oxygen to the capillary bed and then on to the muscle cell, it's not going to do anything to help you. Mold is an illness that chokes down on blood flow. We can measure that flow using an MRI with a special chemical detector that these magnets can create. It's called "magnetic resonance spectroscopy" (MRS), which allows us to look at the chemical makeup of people's brains. We can see the amount of lactate they have. Remember if you don't have oxygen being delivered to a muscle that's exercising, the glucose can be converted to lactic acid; the higher the lactate, the worse the blood flow.

SS: When I envision the hypothalamus, I see it as the hormone CEO up there in the brain, telling everybody what to do. Is that why so many people with mold issues also have severe hormonal issues?

RS: If you'll permit, the CEO (hypothalamus) needs to be called a regulator; if there is mold in the brain, it will knock out regulation of ACTH. *ACTH is a hormone that stimulates the adrenal glands.*

Over 60 percent of patients will have a lack of MSH or a lack of

ACTH, and about half of them have both. If patients have an inability to control their salt and water, or difficulty controlling testosterone and estrogen levels, and if they cannot regulate inflammation with ACTH (which controls the cortisol from the adrenals), then the hypothalamus is the one little guy who is controlling the whole mess.

SS: What are the symptoms of a hypothalamus gone awry?

RS: Rapid mood swings—sad or mad. Appetite swings. Some days hungry, some days not at all. Sweats, especially night sweats. It's MSH, but most doctors write it off to menopause.

SS: So it's simple. You give your patients MSH and then everything is okay?

RS: Not so fast . . . problem is, the FDA won't allow it. It's illegal. If it were legal, the sweats would go away in a day. When you give people VIP, which is legal, the sweats go away in a couple days. And then the last symptom is difficulty in controlling body temperature; always hot and always cold. With missing MSH, people also lose normal circadian rhythms, so they can't get to sleep at nighttime; they toss and turn, and they're exhausted during the day.

SS: That sounds like the thyroid is not getting the right signaling?

RS: The thyroid is fascinating. But thyroid disease and TSH is not regulated by MSH.

SS: I'm under the impression the hypothalamus has a regular conversation going with the thyroid.

RS: It does, but the assumption that thyroid disease is a big player or that bioidentical hormones are the way to go might be right if MSH didn't have a role. But with mold patients, MSH has everything to do with it.

SS: Relative to hormone replacement, you are saying if mold is your issue, you've big problems to deal with before you even get around to replacing hormones with BHRT?

RS: A lot of medical practitioners don't recognize the role of the hypothalamus as the regulator. So they respond with an antidepressant or some sort of mood-stabilizing drug. Or they say, you've got adrenal fatigue, let's give you cortisol; how many times have you heard that?

SS: Often, but in the absence of mold, natural cortisone replacement can be the missing link to hormone balance.

RS: But with mold patients, as soon as you give cortisol, predni-

sone, Cortef, you will disrupt what little bit is left of the ACTH/corti-
sol interaction.

SS: So then you would be dependent upon that replacement for life
because you had killed your own ability to rev up?

RS: There are other issues involved; cortisol compounds are directly important in making the adverse effects of TGF beta-1 get
worse. People on long-term replacement with steroids get a lot of different illnesses that are unusual, called "immune suppression."

TGF beta-1 is a compound that is genomically active, but if it is
suppressed, it changes and results in many different characteristics
and is a huge player in these different illnesses. So if I'm communicat-
ing properly with you, you're starting to see . . . that this is a multi-
headed beast. Genetics are involved, regulation of neural peptides is
involved, and then we have inflammation levels to deal with.

SS: This is exhausting information. No wonder everyone's going
from doctor to doctor, because what you're talking about is incredibly
complex. It is my understanding that this is not what med students are
presently learning.

RS: I think your understanding is correct. When I was in med
school at Duke, we had ten minutes on toxins and we only talked
about botulinum toxin. I always thought the professor was kidding
when he said botulinum toxin was going to be therapeutic at some
time; I thought you'd put it in somebody's toothpaste if you wanted
to kill the guy.

SS: And now people are injecting it to be beautiful.

I've never met a *country doctor* who understands this language you
are speaking; it's very complex to take all the steps it takes to become
well when you have mold. Let me ask you, can mold patients become
well?

RS: Yes. Now that we have the knowledge about genomics, gene
activation, and gene suppression, we know that, fundamentally, while
people may recognize symptoms and doctors are trained to look at
blood test results, deep down it all comes from differential gene activation. We are able to show that out of 22,000 genes, about 350 are
of critical importance in mold patients, which is different from those
in Lyme patients, and different from *Pfiesteria* patients. Today, we can
actually use a computer to create a fingerprint for these different illnesses.

When we start to use therapies that are genomically active, we can reverse the very basis of this illness.

Until I saw genomics in action, I would never permit anybody to use the word *cure*. We could control and help people return to function and to work and to family interactions, but not cure. But now we're using a different term, because we can recognize that the different gene activation is fundamental.

SS: How do you apply this to a patient?

RS: The fascinating results are coming from our work with brain injury. We found that by using NeuroQuant there was a discrete fingerprint for (brain) atrophy.

NeuroQuant® is a breakthrough medical device that can make quantitative MRI measurement a routine part of clinical practice. It brings sophisticated, accurate, and fully automated MRI post-processing capabilities to the physician's desktop. This software provides neurologists, radiologists, and clinical researchers with a convenient and cost-effective means to quantify the volume of the hippocampus and other structures.

Atrophy is a condition in which cells in the brain are lost, or the connections between them are damaged, not just in gray matter areas but in individual areas like the caudate.

NeuroQuant is a marker for what happens in the brain with mold. Then we finish with VIP (vasoactive intestinal polypeptide) and the nucleus (the cell nucleus contains the majority of the cell's genetic material) regrows.

SS: In English, please . . .

RS: It boils down to regrowth of individual brain nuclei with an externally or orally administered medication.

SS: Thanks! But orthodox medicine is responding with drugs, an abnormal use of amphetamines to replace the brain chemicals they say are missing in mold and Lyme patients. Do you use these drugs as part of your protocol?

RS: Yes, if I have to, but my treatment is looking at the whole idea of reestablishing brain connections.

GFAP (glial fibrillary acidic protein) is released when you're inside your mother's womb, which controls the development of the size of your brain to the size it's supposed to be, as in, not to be too big. GFAP is important because it shuts down brain regrowth.

In traumatic brain *injury* you turn *on* GFAP, so you won't heal. With mold I want to turn *off* GFAP, because what stimulates GFAP is TGF beta-1; so if I am able to lower TGF beta-1 (which controls cell growth), and if I can knock out GFAP, the brain heals.

SS: In serious mold cases, there's so much missed: time at school or days, hours, months, years at work; serious mold can devastate a family financially.

The other problem with drugs as an antidote is how those toxins migrate from the liver to the portal vein to the GI tract, then to all different parts of the body and in particular the fatty organs. The brain is the fattiest so here's the connection of mold to stomach issues. When the person is already toxic from environmental exposures, then you throw in mold, then you add to the cocktail amphetamines, it seems to me that long term you are asking for big troubles. I keep hearing that docs feel amphetamines are necessary because the patient is not making sufficient dopamine and these drugs can stimulate dopamine production. What's the effect of people taking Adderall, Vyvanse, Concerta, Ritalin, and what's the long-term effect? Is it effective for the work that you're doing?

RS: I wish I had the answer for you. In my work there are some people who are undisputedly functioning better because of drugs like Vyvanse. I ask my patients how many days a week they can take a holiday from it. If they say, I need it four days a week, then I'll say okay, that's fine, every other day. But when someone needs it every day, I don't see that person having the same ability to recover from inflammatory issues that come down the road. When those patients relapse, they relapse worse. Why that is, actually I don't know. How that is, I sure don't know.

NeuroQuant imaging allows me to look into the brain. Caudate (brain) issues are incredibly important in attention deficit (ADD) and hyperactivity (ADHD). We know in PTSD (post-traumatic stress disorder) patients that the hippocampus is abnormally small; we know in mold patients, for example, that the hippocampus is abnormally large. Does that small hippocampus have something to do with behavioral disturbances? Because those folks with PTSD end up not only being on amphetamines, but as many narcotics and pain relievers as they can.

SS: A friend who was at my house yesterday is taking Vyvanse and I noticed her hands shaking. Is that a manifestation of that drug?

RS: Well, it sure is. We used to call them "speeders" back in college; all the speeder drugs will give people tremors.

SS: Is that the body talking, like, whoa, hold it? Enough of this?

RS: Well, you mentioned dopamine, and I told you this, 40-plus percent of my patients with this illness have a Parkinson-like tremor. So the fact that she's got a tremor, I can tell you is an amphetamine at baseline, but if she has tachycardia and a tremor, and is on Vyvanse or something similar, the question has got to be, is this hyperstimulation from this drug a good idea?

> Tachycardia is caused by a disruption in the electrical signals from the brain to the heart. It can happen from high blood pressure, smoking, or heart disease.

SS: There is an epidemic of Parkinson's at present; how often do you think it's misdiagnosed and instead toxic related or mold or Lyme disease?

RS: I wish I had statistics on that. When I saw MSH being used in treatment (when there is MSH deficiency), combined with use of erythropoietin, because it is neuroprotective, the Parkinson's compounds drop and then the Parkinson's patients improve like crazy.

> Erythropoietin (EPO) is a hormone produced by the kidneys that stimulates red blood cell formation and controls the rate of the formation through negative feedback.

My work is trying to reestablish dopamine emerging pathways in the brain that are disruptive.

SS: Many people, particularly older men, have red watery eyes these days; but now younger people are getting red eyes. Is that because of mold in old buildings and a lack of understanding from strictly allopathic approaches to healing?

RS: Tearing and tears are under control of the cranial nerve system, which is very frequently injured in about 60 percent of these biotoxin illnesses. All cranial nerve nuclei are hooked up in the back part of the brainstem.

SS: Makes sense; they are all living right next door to one another up there.

RS : When people have vertigo, and the room is spinning and they are so disabled they can't stand up or go to the bathroom, my job as doctor is to watch their eyes move. If they have nystagmus, then it could be posterior brain problems (the brainstem issue), or the vestibular neuron, and not a cranial nerve problem in the inner ear.

> Nystagmus is a condition of involuntary eye movement, acquired in infancy or later in life, that may result in reduced or limited vision.

These people will often have difficulty with facial muscles. They can also have cranial nerve and vagus nerve problems, which brings nausea and vomiting. Sometimes they won't be able to walk normally; these things are interlinked.

SS: VIP is part of your protocol; can the patient administer it themselves because it's oral?

RS: Everyone who gets VIP needs to pass certain criteria, so we do a test dose in the office to make sure that you tolerate the drug. If so, we then send you on your way after twenty minutes; that's the minimum time we need to observe you. Then people can give the drug to themselves without any need for physician supervision. They'll start off spraying a total of one spray, to either the left or right side of the nose, doesn't make any difference, four times a day. People can take more if they need it; if they need to have twenty-eight sprays a day, it's not a problem; the only problem with that dose is paying for it.

SS: I keep thinking about the people in New Jersey with that flooding last year where their basements were filled with water. I'm not aware that mold education is being stressed explaining the serious effects of mold on the human body; are whole areas like that going to get sick?

RS: Of course. At present 24 percent of them are already suffering the effects. In New Jersey there's an outbreak of post-traumatic stress disorder, an outbreak of asthma, an outbreak of depression, and an outbreak of Parkinson's. Guess what? It's likely none of the above. It's an inflammatory response syndrome that was initiated by being exposed to buildings wet for more than two days, and not dried out properly. There was no energy and no electricity to do the drying out. So these people are getting sick and staying sick.

SS: Are people sick in New Orleans as a result of Katrina and water-damaged buildings?

RS: Absolutely. There's no difference. And yet these people are being looked at for allergy. Well, the problem never was allergy; it's from the mold exposure.

SS: Feels like there needs to be a medical school specializing in the new environment diseases. Today's doctors are stymied, and antibiotics and antifungals are about all they have to treat this with; it seems to me you have a much more sophisticated protocol. Do you have a clinic, or do you have a consult business? Do you educate other doctors?

RS: A little bit of each. I retired from patient care back in January of 2013, but I do phone consults and connect these patients with the right treatments.

SS: If I hadn't watched this cognitive issue firsthand, I would never have truly understood it; my brilliant granddaughter, a straight-A student, temporarily lost her ability to think because of mold and Lyme.

RS: The problems I see with Lyme are underdiagnosis and overdiagnosis. I have published the symptoms of Lyme, mold, and *Pfiesteria,* and frankly they all present about the same. You can't sort out Lyme by symptoms. Until we were able to find results with lab findings, C3A, and NeuroQuant, we couldn't sort out Lyme from mold just by lab abnormalities. There is no question Lyme creates an inflammatory response syndrome. About 23 percent of the HLA haplotypes we see in Lyme syndrome (which are not the same as that in mold) are real.

SS: Are antibiotics ever the answer with Lyme?

RS: When I look at those who get an acute episode of Lyme and don't have the HLA gene, they are able to clear up very nicely with antibiotics.

With infectious disease 80 percent of the people get better, but the 20 percent that don't get better have an HLA problem and they have the inflammatory issues running parallel with it.

SS: That explains why the treatments vary. What works for some doesn't seem to kill it with others. No changing genetics. And it seems all those who carry the HLA gene are not created equal. So that's the puzzle . . . the detective work. There's no set treatment; it's individualized. Replacing hormones is a similar "art." Each person is different and has different requirements.

RS: There are a few people I've seen in my practice who have benefited from intravenous antibiotics. But having seen nearly two thousand Lyme patients, those on IV antibiotics who get well are in the distinct minority, because for the others, the Lyme has not really been eradicated. What is not factored in are the priming events for those who carry HLA. Is Lyme disease one of those? Yes, it is.

SS: Is die-off of internal toxins by a variety of means a positive indicator that you're making progress?

RS: No, it means you're killing one population without creating the nets that will let some other run of related organisms into the body. When we look at people with Lyme who've been treated with antibiotics for a long time, the antibiotic resistance patterns are the most complicated ones I've ever seen.

SS: Where I live in Malibu, the hills are alive; deer are on the lawn at Pepperdine University and people sit on the lawn and those deer have Lyme ticks. We have a lot of people in this coastal area who've got Lyme; the rich ones have concierge doctors with nurses coming to their homes to administer IV antibiotics a couple times a day and they all have the same reaction. A little better at first, then massive gut problems, gut pain, gut disturbances, overgrowth of bacteria, then candida, yeast, leaky gut. Now autoimmune issues are activated, then the feet start turning up mimicking MS; then inability to sleep, leg and foot pain accompanied by depression, sadness, and hopelessness. No one seems to know what to do.

For starters my thinking is, why aren't these doctors at least giving commensurate amounts of probiotics to rebalance the GI ecosystem?

RS: Yes, of course probiotics. But what you're describing is a common occurrence in people being treated for Lyme with one symptom, but with other symptoms developing inflammatory pathways. When we look at peripheral neuropathy and chronic pain syndromes, it could be MSH deficiency, or if they start having tremors, it could be they need to look at TGF beta-1. When cognitive issues progress, the answer could be in the information provided by NeuroQuant. In areas like Malibu, you have ocean mold to deal with. In the desert, it's also possible because you have indoor plumbing. Or is your air conditioner running all the time? So no area is exempt and what is often diagnosed as Lyme could be mold.

SS: So before people get mold and/or Lyme, they should be really cognizant of their air-conditioning ducts and units, keeping them clean and changing filters, right?

RS: Yes, those are all important if you don't have excessive humidity. If you have humidity over 50 percent, we see growth of organisms like *Wallemia*, which loves 60 to 80 percent water saturation; it is the most common problem you find in HVAC systems. The problem with *Wallemia*, especially if you've got fiberglass-based ductwork, is that it is able to grow into the middle of the ductwork.

Wallemia sebi is a brown mold commonly found in indoor air dust, soil, and dried and salty foods (bread, cakes, sugar, dried fish, dates, bacon, and jams).

SS: Is there a way to build a mold-free home?

RS: No. There is no such thing as a mold-free home. But what you can do is to build a home that does not let moisture and toxigenic fungi and bacteria get a foothold.

SS: So what do you do, go outside and wash? Get an outhouse? Just have no indoor plumbing at all?

RS: Look at it another way; what's going to be easier for water to get into, a ceiling that has six or seven gables and three or four openings and a nice big elaborate doorway, or a simple 12-pitch roof with shingles on it? So the roof should be simple and easy. How about the cladding of the house itself? Would you rather have wood siding or would you rather have this fake stucco? I mean you can make pretty homes with stucco, but it's the most difficult substance to get proper seals around windows and doors.

SS: Mold, awful as it is, is a fascinating subject. And I do think when you said 50 percent of people are experiencing mold symptoms and have no idea this could be their problem, that's more than an epidemic. That's bigger than cancer.

RS: And this is the can of worms no one wants to open up. If people knew what I know about homes and their right to a safe home or a safe rental or a safe school, or a safe college for God's sake, the amount of money that would be spent either closing those facilities down, or fixing them up, is beyond the world's gross national product. But there is a responsibility to health issues that are not being addressed, and medical schools are not addressing these new issues.

SS: Sounds like the FDA! Ha ha.

Thanks for all this valuable information. It's a huge ocean liner to turn around, but you have much to teach with your tremendous insight developed from being on the front line. Your knowledge allows people to be able to piece together the puzzle of their own lives. Keep on with your great work.

RS: Thanks. On the tough days when bad things are happening, your words will bring welcome solace. All I can tell you is that it's people like you who will carry the message to the masses.

GO FROM *TOX*-SICK TO NOT SICK

1. A NeuroQuant is an MRI software program for the brain. The company is located in San Diego.

REMEDY PRICE: Approximately $89 for the test and results.

2. Suspect mold's an issue for you?

REMEDY: To look up symptoms of mold toxicity, go to SurvivingMold.com, Dr. Shoemaker's website.

3. If you've a problem with high cholesterol, particularly LDL, try an inflammagen binder:

REMEDY: Cholestyramine and Welchol are used by Dr. Shoemaker for this issue.

4. To fight mold, the remedy is to do the following:
   • Eliminate anything that could be harboring mold spores.
   • Stop all water intrusion so the building envelopes are cleared and watertight.
   • Get rid of porous materials.
   • Clean nonporous materials, and, usually, get rid of your carpets.
   • Install a HEPA filter and then and only then you can start using particular fogging solutions. The good ones that work have Borax in them.

5. If you're worried about a genetic sensitivity to mold, there are tests you can take.

REMEDY: Determine HLA-DR based on work from these labs: Labcore, ARUP, and Quest.

6. Toxins are affecting our brains.

REMEDY: Magnetic resonance spectroscopy (MRS) provides the ability to look at the chemical makeup of people's brains. To fight the toxins, you need to know what is in there!

CHAPTER 8

PROTECTING YOUR HOME, FAMILY, AND WORKPLACE

WE'VE TALKED ABOUT WHAT WE NEED TO DO TO PROTECT EVERY organ system in the body, as well as general steps to protect yourself, including, in our last chapter, what to do to protect you and your loved ones from the newest toxic threat, mold.

But what do you do about the rest of your environment? If you need convincing that it's worth doing (I can't imagine you're not already convinced), keep reading. The stats that follow are pretty shocking:

- The U.S. Environmental Protection Agency (EPA) ranks poor indoor air quality among the top five environmental risks to public health. Interestingly, five out of ten Americans are not aware of this fact.
- The EPA found the levels of air pollution inside the home can be two to five times higher (and sometimes even 100 times higher) than outdoor levels.
- An EPA study concluded that the toxic chemicals in household cleaners are three times more likely to cause cancer than outdoor air.
- A study comparing women who work outside the home with women who work at home found a 54 percent higher risk of developing cancer in women who work at home. The study concluded that this is a direct result of the chemicals in household products.
- Cleaning substances are the third-most-common reason for exposure to poison in adults.

- Fifty-one percent of the human exposures to poison in 2006 involved children under six years old.
- Unintentional ingestion of toxic household chemicals is associated with an annual average of 39 deaths to children under age five, and an estimated 87,700 children treated in hospital emergency rooms. These poisoning incidents resulted in an estimated societal cost of almost $2.3 billion.

When a product becomes trendy or appealing to consumers, manufacturers respond. It's why over the last few years, you've probably noticed a proliferation of "all-natural" this, "organic" that, and "green" as far as the eye can see, whether on food packaging, cleaning product labels, clothing, or furniture.

It can be difficult—almost impossible—for the average person to make sense of it all, and to distinguish between the good, the bad, and the truly awful. After all, the terms "all-natural" and "organic" can easily refer to substances that are indeed both natural and organic— and also bad for your health.

The interview that follows will give you a decoder ring to protect yourself, your home, and your family.

BOXING 'EM OUT:
AN INTERVIEW WITH WALTER CRINNION, N.D.

Dr. Walter Crinnion is one of America's foremost authorities on environmental medicine. A naturopathic physician, he is the director of the Environmental Medicine Center of Excellence at the Southwest College of Naturopathic Medicine in Arizona and chair of the Environmental Medicine Department. Naturopathic doctors, N.D.s, have the freedom to treat with natural remedies and protocols, which gives him more opportunity to explore the full scope of natural cures and protocols. He is passionate and encouraged by the success he has had with his patients. He feels that in spite of the massive toxic assault, people who make the changes as outlined in this interview can get well. Dr. Crinnion's book, Clean, Green & Lean, *is an education, an eye-opener, and a mind-opener.*

SS: Thank you for your time, Dr. Crinnion. You are an environmental N.D. How did you choose this specialty?

WC: Thank you, Suzanne. Actually, I would say the specialty chose me instead. I was attracted to naturopathic medicine because it's focused on natural remedies and is based on a number of principles, including *Tolle causum*, or treat the cause, and *Vis medicatrix naturae*, or the healing power of nature. For instance, in naturopathic medicine we don't believe that people get a headache because their blood is deficient in aspirin; instead, we look for the cause of the headache and treat that. When I started my practice, I was plagued with migraines that began when I was a medical student. I came to find out they were an adverse food reaction to the little bit of milk on my cereal every morning. I was getting migraines twice a week from dairy five days a week; I wasn't deficient in acetaminophen. Eliminating the dairy eliminated the migraines (and some other health issues as well).

This experience helped to frame my approach to my patients. I was able to help many of my patients be free of chronic health problems by identifying and having them remove the foods they were reacting to from their diets. I saw fatigue, brain fog, arthritis, hay fever, asthma, weight problems, ADHD, intestinal problems, and chronic skin problems all go away with this approach. It was magic, but it was also hard for them to do.

SS: But no one wants to stay off their favorite foods forever. How do you deal with that?

WC: Right. Who wants to go without their latte and their doughnut? As a naturopathic doc I continued to work on treating the cause. I had found that patients' health problems were caused by an adverse reaction to certain foods (usually their favorite foods that they ate at least three times weekly). But then I had to look for the causes of why they were reactive. Poor digestion and an imbalance of the flora in the intestines, as well as a compromised intestinal lining, were all underlying causes of reacting to foods. But an overload of toxicants is another and can also lead to all of those other intestinal "causes." So I decided to address the old naturopathic idea of "liver toxicity" and worked to reduce my patients' toxicant loads to hopefully get them over their adverse food reactions. As I started cleansing regimens with my patients, I saw them starting to get better in more ways than I imagined. As a result of my developing a major focus on cleansing, a whole new group of patients started coming to me who were chemically reactive and had tremendous problems with chronic illnesses, immune problems, and neurological problems. Soon I saw that these individuals who had "flunked out" of clinic after clinic and treatment after treatment began to get better. They had reversals of major illnesses (called "spontaneous remissions") and had returns to health that were amazing to watch. I got used to hearing "Doc, I feel twenty years younger." After cleansing, many of my patients would lose weight with no dietary change. Their abnormal blood values would normalize, and other health problems that we did not address would also evaporate. I began to see that the health problems associated with aging, which we typically think of as inevitable, really were not (associated with aging or inevitable). I started to realize that these health problems were more associated with the addition of more environmental toxicants to the body than to adding birthdays to the résumé.

SS: That must have been very rewarding for you.

WC: It was, but now the playing field has changed. When I started my practice, I could get people over a strep throat in a weekend with a homeopathic dilution of echinacea and a homeopathic combination tablet #255 from Boericke and Tafel (homeopathic suppliers), which they don't make anymore.

But now patients are coming in with colds and flus that are lasting for three to five months no matter how many immune supportive treatments one does. It's not that the virus or bacteria are getting more virulent, it's that our immune systems are more suppressed. And it is not just me who has been noticing this. In the last decade or so I have had docs flocking to my six-month environmental training program because they are finding it basically impossible to practice alternative medicine without addressing their patients' toxicant burdens. Our load of common environmental toxicants has become a major cause of illness as well as an obstacle to cure.

In my years as a physician there have been numerous fungal-, viral-, or bacterial-associated chronic infections (candida, chronic Epstein-Barr, etc.). These chronic infections were thought to be the main cause of a host of chronic health problems (Lyme disease is the big one now). But what's the real cause? The cause is that we have suppressed immune systems that are unable to fight these organisms off when they first show up. I have seen this play out for years, but there is now enough published research on this phenomenon of "immunotoxicity" that I can show you step-by-step how it happens.

SS: Is that how you got into environmental medicine?

WC: Yes, environmental medicine is about trying to find the *cause* of chronic ill health in patients and recognizing that the answers lie in a whole different paradigm than standard alternative medicine.

The pioneers of alternative medicine include Drs. Jonathan Wright, Alan Gaby, and Joe Pizzorno. They taught a generation of docs the methods of finding what nutrient the body needed to regain its ability to heal itself. The basic principle was to find the substance or substances that the body needed to right itself. Alternative medicine is still focused on what natural compound can be added to your body to help you regain your health. But environmental medicine asks a different question; what needs to be removed from the body so that the natural self-healing ability of the body can do its job?

SS: That's an interesting question.

WC: Yes, it's a totally different question. I used to call my practice the caboose on the train of health because people came to me who had been to many different standard allopathic and alternative practitioners but hadn't been helped because everybody was trying to *add* something to them. When I get patients with boxes of supplements and meds that they tried unsuccessfully, I know that the most likely cause of their chronic problems lies in the environmental medical field. Why? Because no one looks there. If the cause was a deficiency of a nutrient or supplement, they would have been better long ago. M.D.s hand out pharmaceuticals and alternative docs give a supplement, but none of them was looking for what was poisoning the system.

SS: In general, what was the main poison?

WC: The majority of them are toxicants, which are things that are man-made: DDTs, solvents, plasticizers, et cetera. Toxins are compounds produced by living things like rattlesnakes, black widows, and molds (mycotoxins that are the new bad boy on the street). According to the Centers for Disease Control reports, 104 common environmental toxicants are found in pretty much everyone in this country. The CDC's researchers have not yet started measuring mycotoxins. Keep in mind that the 104 compounds they have found in all of us are out of only 212 they have measured so far! That is close to 50 percent. With over 3,500 chemical toxicants being in "high use" in this country, if 50 percent of all those chemicals will be found in us, well, that is terrifying.

SS: Are they both (toxins and mycotoxins) prevalent?

WC: Yes, the biggest problem inside people's homes making them sick is the mold toxins. If someone moves into a certain house and slowly everybody in the house is getting sick, it's usually mold; in fact, ninety-eight times out of a hundred it's mold, and these mycotoxins affect a number of systems in the body. Mold damages the part of each cell that makes energy; it's called the mitochondria. And, in addition to these toxins, a huge number of chemical and heavy metal toxicants are present in our home air, our personal care products, our food, and our water.

SS: Are you talking about the toxins in the body or in the home itself or the toxins people are breathing and putting on their bodies?

WC: I'm talking about what is in their blood or urine. Using the CDC information I put the name of those 104 chemical toxicants into the PubMed database and found that all those chemicals found ubiquitously in U.S. residents all damage mitochondrial function.

SS: Is that why there is an epidemic of chronically fatigued people and those who simply lack energy?

WC: Yes, when the mitochondria are under this tremendous burden of toxicant (and mycotoxin) attack, they cannot produce enough ATP for proper function of the body. It affects proper cellular function as well as overall energy; do you know of anyone these days who doesn't complain of being fatigued?

When you don't make enough ATP, you're going to have trouble with all parts of your body, and certainly your digestive ability. The lining of the intestine is particularly vulnerable because those cells turn over rapidly and they require energy to make new cells. Mitochondrial suppression is also key to most of the other big systemic problems like immunotoxicity, neurologic toxicity, and endocrine toxicity.

ATP is adenosine triphosphate. It's the way the molecule is structured, which makes for easy energy storage and transportation, hence its significant role in metabolism.

SS: Immuno being the immune system, endocrine being your hormone system?

WC: Correct, and mitochondrial suppression causes multiple problems in the endocrine system, from infertility to diabetes. When I was starting my practice in the early '80s, I had a lot of young women in their midtwenties who were married and couldn't conceive. Basically I cleaned up their diet, started them on multiple vitamins, and six months later they were pregnant. That approach hasn't worked in the last twenty years because of our increasing toxicant burden. You just can't conceive if you have a toxic load. One of the major ways toxicity shows up is in infertility; and, sadly, with each generation our newborns start off with a greater load of toxicants than their mothers because the mom passes a portion of her toxic load to her children.

SS: I think this point is greatly misunderstood, that the toxic burden of the mother, including the state of her GI ecosystem, gets passed on to the child.

WC: Yes, there are numerous studies looking at that, the amount of toxicants that our children are exposed to in utero. Each generation starts with a greater load. My mother was born in 1918, but DDT was not introduced until 1945, so she did not receive a load of toxicants from her mother and only had a few decades of exposure before my sister and I were born. Our generation inherited a portion of that small toxic load from our mothers, and then we added to it every day with additional exposures. If I were a woman, then I would have passed a portion of that toxic load to my daughters, so they would start with a higher load than I would have had and so on. The load of toxicants to today's fetuses is huge; a recent study showed over a hundred chemical toxicants present in their cord blood. That's why today the rates of childhood brain tumors, autism, and ADHD have all skyrocketed. When I started my practice, the patients who came to see me would be thirty- to fifty-year-olds who had just developed chemical sensitivities. Now I get three-year-olds with chemical sensitivity because they have that big of a burden in their body already.

SS: It's shocking and overwhelming for young mothers today; my own grandchildren are suffering with ADHD, OCD, asthma, and more and they grew up on organic foods. So is it exposure from the environment?

WC: Yes, and also from their mothers' toxic load. Scientists just did six studies in the Los Angeles area that found that the closer a mom lived to a busy roadway, the higher her children's rates of autism. Just by proximity to a roadway, and ADHD's pretty much the same. Kids get the majority of their toxicant load from their mothers and we build on that from the air they breathe, which is primarily indoor air, but all indoor air starts from the outside pollution. Add to it furnishings, toxic household cleaners, plasticizers, et cetera, and if there's mold, you can easily see how it adds up.

SS: A lot of people complain of feeling allergic in their cars; is that just more toxic exposure?

WC: Yes, you get exposed to a combination of all the outdoor air plus the solvents offgassing from the car itself.

Asthma is clearly an environmental toxic burden issue, which explains why the rates of asthma and allergy have been skyrocketing for the last thirty years worldwide. These conditions are strongly associated with environmental toxicants, and the biggest association with asthma are exhaust particles filling urban areas such as the Phoenix Valley, Los Angeles, actually pretty much everywhere. Diesel exhaust particles are the absolute worst ones when it comes to causing illness, and biodiesel produces even more of the nastiest particles. When people live close to busy roadways, they get that much more of that exposure and then they get overloaded very rapidly. Outdoor air pollution from vehicular exhaust dramatically increases rates of autism. But were you to purchase a thousand-dollar air filter and put it in a couple's bedroom, it would not only improve their chances to conceive a child, but dramatically drop their chances of having a child who's autistic.

SS: You mean asthma?

WC: Sadly, I mean autism (exhaust particles also cause allergies), but recently there have been a handful of studies that have clearly shown that the greater the exposure levels of vehicular exhaust to expectant mothers, the greater the risk of having an autistic child. Further, as vehicular exhaust exposures continue after delivery, the autism can get more severe.

SS: That is very dramatic information. The fetus is so vulnerable to the toxic assault. On the upside, you are saying that for a mere thousand dollars for an air purifier you could dramatically improve health and conception? Are you talking about the HEPA filter?

WC: Yes, there are the HEPA filters; but you have to get a good-quality one. That's why I like the IQ Air, Austin Air, or Blue Air; these are the top three.

SS: Is this something that can be installed in a car also?

WC: The only company I know that has a car air purifier is E.L. Foust in Illinois. Some of my patients, the really highly chemically reactive ones, have used it, and they found that they needed to go out and get the car started and leave it running for fifteen minutes before getting in the car. If they don't get it started on cleaning the air inside the car before they start driving, it just isn't able to keep up.

SS: Are the materials used in cars outgassing?

WC: Absolutely. There was an interesting study done in Australia looking at new-car smell that found it was full of solvents that are neurotoxic. These are brain toxins, including the exhaust coming out of the tailpipe. Solvents, neurotoxins, are all scary because about half of the population is deficient in a phase two enzyme in their liver— glutathione S-transferase (GST)—which is responsible for clearing toxins inside of the bloodstream. People who have that genetic difference, called a "null genotype," do not clear solvents out very well. These are the people who get very brain foggy when they're around solvents. If you figure half the population on the L.A. freeways around you are of the null genotype, it means they're not clearing out solvents, which means they are full of neurotoxins. It's just like being drunk, and so (a word of caution) don't expect other people on the roadway to drive correctly.

SS: It's funny, but it's tragic simultaneously, isn't it?

WC: And could be fatally tragic. I've had patients come to my office where I've run a blood test for solvents and they come back with five or six solvents and fairly high levels in their blood. I tell them, you've got to take extra care when driving because you are literally impaired.

SS: How about wall-to-wall carpeting, what's in that?

WC: Have you ever pulled carpeting out of a house? If so, you will know how dirty and nasty it was; not only dirty but so much dirt under the carpet, and under the carpet pad. That dirt wasn't there when workers installed the carpet and pad; carpeting is the dirtiest thing to do to a house because it holds dirt and toxicants in the fiber. Ninety-eight percent of the toxicants in your home are bound to dust and then fabric fibers, carpeting, upholstery, and drapery. In the '80s, the TEAM (Total Environmental Assessment Methodology) studies found that high levels of household toxicants were in dust, and often the carpet was the absolute worst offender. We are not even including all the chemicals inherent in carpeting to make it stain resistant and wrinkle resistant. Most of the toxins in the carpet are chemicals that are neurotoxins.

SS: Does this affect the brain?

WC: Yes, of course, it affects the brain.

SS: Are toxins making people . . . crazy?

WC: Yes, but no one wants to recognize it. Recently there was a study looking at the rate of violent crime; researchers found when they took out the lead in paint and gasoline, the crime rate dropped. Studies show that elevated lead levels alter behaviors. This is published and well documented, called the adverse effect of lead on the crime rate.

SS: Is it only lead or is it also what people are eating and what they are using to clean their houses?

WC: Pollution and toxins are responsible for so many of our health and emotional problems such as heart disease. We find that whenever the outdoor air pollution levels go up, more people show up at emergency rooms with heart attacks. It's documented all over the world.

SS: What's that pathway?

WC: Primarily the inflammatory pathway; toxins are pro-inflammatory agents, but they also alter the ability of the cells that line the blood vessels (endothelial cells) to adapt, so people develop health issues.

SS: What a dilemma. The lining of our blood vessels are under attack. We know the lining of our GI tracts are under attack, and leaky gut is leading to the toxic attack on our brains; once these toxins get into the brain, what does that do to the HPA (the hypothalamus/pituitary/adrenal axis)?

WC: Yes, that's the endocrine effect on the adrenal glands primarily, but many toxicants also affect the thyroid. And a great number of the toxicants are clearly associated with obesity and type 2 diabetes.

SS: It's not that individuals are overeating, it's what they're eating?

WC: Correct. Polychlorinated biphenyls (PCBs), chlorinated pesticides, and many other common toxicants, which all damage mitochondrial function, have been shown to greatly increase one's risk of developing type 2 diabetes. I have an appendix in the back of my book *Clean, Green & Lean* where I discuss and show (among many other things) that the rates of diabetes in the last twenty years in the U.S. parallel the increase in the consumption of farmed salmon, which is horribly high in PCBs—and our current main source of exposure to these nasty compounds.

SS: Yet salmon is hailed as healthy with high rates of essential fatty acids. People need to understand that wild-caught salmon is clean, and farm-raised salmon is toxic. I find when I go to a restaurant these days, it's like working my way through a minefield, just trying to find something to eat. I don't want to eat beef that's not grass fed, nor do I want to eat farm-raised fish, or GMO food; it's rare to find a restaurant that has any organic offerings, why is that?

WC: I hope that changes, because it should be easier for us to go to a grocery store or a restaurant and buy healthy.

SS: Do you think people have to demand, as in supply and demand?

Most people are eating many of their weekly meals in restaurants. Why are we seeing young girls with bloated stomachs? I call them chemical bellies. Friends of mine who are entertainers live on the road, eat on the road, eat fast food, and so many of them complain to me about their bloated stomachs and stomach discomfort. These symptoms are a language, aren't they?

WC: That's a lot of questions in one. [Laughs]

SS: Sorry! [Laughs]

WC: With immunotoxicity, your immune system gets imbalanced and you start developing allergies and autoimmunity and lose the ability to fight off viruses and bacteria, so the body develops conditions and diseases. You might get chronic infections, your GI tract may become compromised, and you may experience bloating. In addition, as I said, we are all loaded with at least a hundred environmental chemicals that reduce our energy productive ability. The production of digestive enzymes and stomach hydrochloric acid requires a huge amount of energy. If you were to make a pie chart of where the energy expenditures of your body went, the biggest piece would be digestive ability. So, with our burden of mitochondrial toxins, we just are not able to digest things right. And, as it turns out, the common use of acid blockers for heartburn increases the likelihood of having "small intestinal bacterial overgrowth," which results in bloating from eating any carbohydrates.

SS: Do toxicants make infections difficult to control because of our body's inability to detox?

WC: Of course; infections are more difficult to control: Lyme disease, herpes, Epstein-Barr virus, yeast, so many others. Asthma shows up first in many people, but it can also be allergies as well, and one of the big food reactions now is gluten. So the question gets asked: Are these conditions and allergies really more common now than they were back in the '50s? Or is it just that we're more aware of it and we are looking for these conditions everywhere, as in, is it a witch hunt?

If you go back, there is a study where scientists froze the blood from people in the '50s and got permission to test for a gluten antibody. They also used blood from a similar group of persons in a current study. They found gluten intolerance, gluten allergy, or antibodies against gluten are twice as common now as in the 1950s. Just as allergies are going up, so is gluten intolerance, because we are all toxically burdened.

SS: And you believe that allergies and gluten intolerances are the accumulation of many different toxins and intoxicants?

WC: Correct. In fact, at CDC.gov they have an environmental health page called the *Fourth National Report on Human Exposure to Environmental Chemicals* (which I was referring to earlier), and its Excel spreadsheet lists all the toxicants that the CDC has listed as present in everyone's body, meaning they are ubiquitous throughout the population. I had been focusing on things like PCBs and DDT and persistent organic pollutants, but I hadn't paid attention to many of the other ones. Turns out that over 80 percent of the toxicants rolling around in our bloodstream are not the persistent DDT or PCBs, but the nonpersistent compounds, compounds that if we stopped exposing ourselves, our blood and urine would be clear of them in two weeks. As I write in my book, "If people learn to have a clean home and watch their diets, they could drop the circulating level of toxicants in their bodies by close to eighty percent within two to three weeks."

SS: I would think this will be very encouraging to my readers. Two to three weeks is not overwhelming. So many feel so out of control and helpless, but does this mean you've got to get rid of all fabric, all carpet, all drapes? For the average person that's very daunting. Is it necessary to go to that extent?

WC: Carpet, yes. Get all the carpets out of your house.

SS: I saw in your book the list of chemical agents that are in carpets; it's long!

A partial list of chemicals in carpets, from Dr. Crinnion's book *Clean, Green & Lean*:

Acetonitrile	Octadecenyl amine
Azulene	1-chloronaphthalene
Benzene	1-ethyl-3-propylbenzene
Biphenyl	1-methyl-4-tridecene
Butadiene	1,2,4-trimethylbenzene
Cyclopentadiene-ethenyl-3-ethelene	1,3,5-cycloheptatriene
	1,2,3-trimethylbenzene
Diphenyl ether	Oxarium
Dodecane	Phthalic acid esters
Ethylzylene	Polyacrylates
5-methyltridecane	Styrene
Formaldehyde	Tetradecene
4-phenylcyclohexane	Trichloroethylene (TCE)
Hexadecanol	Toluene
Hexamethylene triamine	2-butyloctanol-1
Isocyanates	2-methylnaphthalene
Methacrylic acid	2,3,7-trimethyldecane
Methyl methacrylate	Undecane,2,6,dimethyl

WC: And that is just a partial list.

SS: I'm aware when my husband walks into any room with carpeting, his eyes get red and watery, his sinuses bother him, his tongue swells, and he generally starts not feeling well. Is that an allergic attack?

WC: It is either allergy or a chemical overload reaction. As far as draperies and fabric, I feel it's most important to go for the big guns. Carpeting is a big gun. But if you bring in a service to vacuum out your ductwork, and put in high-quality pleated air filters so that it grabs the dust before it gets into those pipes, that usually eliminates the worst contaminants.

SS: What are high-quality air filters?

WC: They are pleated paper filters, the kind that look like an accordion, inside of a cardboard holder, often with a metal support mesh. They cost more than the cheap ones that look like spun fiberglass, but those are basically worthless.

SS: So the dust would stick to that?

WC: Yes, the high-quality pleated ones are like HEPA filters in and of themselves; they grab more dust, and the key to reducing the toxic load that you're breathing in is going to be in controlling what is in your home. You can't control the outside air, but you can control your inside air. These filters cost about ten dollars and they work. But home air systems are not designed to clear the smallest particles out of the air. If you put a truly high efficiency filter in your furnace, it will burn out the motor, repeatedly! So, in addition to the pleated filters, you will need a good air purifier in the home. If you take those two steps, you will be miles ahead of the game. Just by living in a cleaner home, as the months pass, you are going to be much healthier. Just by making these simple changes.

SS: But of course now you still have to deal with what's in the body itself, the liver, the tissue?

WC: Yes, of course. Cleaning the air in your home is one step, but you also have to include personal care products because of the enormous amounts of phthalates or plasticizers. For food: You avoid the dirty dozen, the twelve most toxic fruits and vegetables, because those have the organophosphate pesticides in them, which are neurotoxicants.

Go to the EWG's website for the full list at ewg.org.

SS: You can't just wash them off?

WC: You can if you use either an acid or alkaline wash to remove over 95 percent of most pesticides. Many people have water alkalinizers that make drinking water alkaline. If you soak your vegetables and fruits (even the organic ones) in alkaline water, you'll be amazed at what gets removed. Then avoid farm-raised salmon, canned sardines (the next highest in PCBs after salmon), and high-mercury fish.

If you have already taken care of your home air, avoid toxicant-laden personal care products. With these dietary and product changes, your levels of toxicants are going to be 80 percent lower within three weeks.

SS: I've heard from other environmental docs that by the time patients come to your office, they've been to twenty different doctors; what is the overriding main complaint of people who show up at your front door?

WC: I see a lot of autoimmunity, chemical sensitivity, fibromyalgia, chronic fatigue, and some cancers. But the main complaint is often neurologic; their brains aren't working anymore. Not only do they have cognition, memory, and reasoning issues, but also chronic neurologic problems as well. I am finding a lot of Parkinson-like problems showing up.

SS: What is that, tremors, tics, spasms?

WC: Yes, an alarming amount of tremors, especially in postmenopausal women. I'm finding about ten years or so after they've hit menopause, their increased bone turnover releases a lot of lead from their bones. And now that lead gets dumped into their tissues and results in Parkinson-like problems and other issues.

SS: Is that why you see older people who have the "shakes"?

WC: It is quite likely, yes.

SS: Is that reversible?

WC: It can be. I have seen it reversed more than once.

SS: How would you do that?

WC: Two ways: First we chelate to pull the lead from their tissues, and then we do IVs or IV therapy with a compound called glutathione.

SS: Glutathione is the body's master antioxidant?

WC: Yes, and the toxicants rob glutathione from the body. That is why both the immune system and your mitochondria get imbalanced. Parkinson's is one of those things recognized as a dysfunction of the mitochondria in your body, and glutathione is one of the main nutrient compounds inside the mitochondria.

SS: Where does CoQ10 play into that?

WC: CoQ10 is the other nutrient that is actually found inside the mitochondria.

SS: So CoQ10 can be replaced by supplementation?

WC: Yes, as well as a host of other antioxidants. Once CoQ10 and glutathione are begun, and the level of lead in the soft tissue begins to drop, my patients start doing much better.

SS: You think the Parkinson's-like symptoms have lead as their main culprit?

WC: I'm finding in my practice that it's lead more than other things, although I have also found solvents are part of the problem. Dr. How-ard Hu published in a standard medical journal that the greater the lifetime exposure to lead, the greater the risk of Parkinsonism.

SS: That's profound. People hear about lead and lead pipes, but women get constant exposure to lead from their lipstick. Everything I've read about lead says its effects are devastating.

WC: There are many effects; lead is one of the other main causes of high blood pressure.

SS: So if your doctor says you have high blood pressure, you should ask to be checked for lead levels in your body?

WC: Yes. It's generally a blood test. Standard lab values for lead are for acute lead poisoning in an industrial setting, but you can get high blood pressure at levels far lower than that. So I recommend a urine test for heavy metals from two samples of urine: the first morning urine, and then take a mobilizing agent for heavy metals, and then check it again. The baseline level will reveal your current exposure and then after a chelation, you get a better idea of what the body bur-den of lead is.

SS: Can people get well?

WC: Oh yes.

SS: Are you well?

WC: Oh yes. I'm one of the rare environmental doctors who did not get into this field because my own health was devastated by chem-icals. I got into it wanting to help patients, and this is the path I was led toward. Through cleansings I've seen ALS get better, Parkinson's get better. But the best outcomes I've seen with cleansing is for auto-immunity.

SS: You're talking about MS, fibromyalgia, lupus?

WC: Yes, lupus, Hashimoto's thyroiditis, rheumatoid arthritis, all these crippling, chronic illnesses. Suzanne, for years, I was deal-ing with these conditions daily and wondering why I wasn't reading about their association with environmental toxicants in the medical literature. I kept wondering . . . am I in my own version of the *Emperor's New Clothes*? In the last five years, articles linking toxicants with autoimmune conditions are finally starting to be published in the environmental medicine journals.

SS: What is the protocol to treat someone with Hashimoto's thyroiditis, lupus, or any of these autoimmune diseases?

WC: You treat the burden on the immune system.

SS: Do you treat each person the same or is each person different because the toxic cocktail has different effects with each person?

WC: Genetics play into it somewhat, but mainly we see the same toxic load in people. It varies in that one person will have a clear immunotoxicity history with asthma and allergies for decades and then autoimmunity shows up. The next person with the same load might have brain fog and neurologic problems, or the next one might have primarily endocrine/hormonal-related disorders. The catchphrase for the last twenty years has been, "Genetics points the gun, but the environment pulls the trigger." Just having the genetic predisposition to ANY disease is not enough by itself to bring the disease on. One also needs the right environment, which our current toxic lifestyle obviously provides in spades.

SS: If you carry the HLA gene, making you more susceptible to toxins and chemicals than the next person, are you the first to go down?

WC: Not everybody with the HLA marker has autoimmunity. It comes down to the amount of each person's toxic burden. Genetics points the gun, but you have to have something else that helps it pull the trigger.

SS: How are you pulling these toxicants out of bodies?

WC: The first step is don't put any more in!

SS: As in toxins and toxicants?

WC: Yes; find the greatest exposure sources and stop it. Plug the hole in the side of the boat before you start bailing. If you do that, then within a few weeks you can cut your level of circulating toxicants in your body by close to 80 percent. That's pretty doggone good.

The formula for reducing a person's toxicant load is basic cleaning of the air in the home and cleaning up one's food. After you reduce the amount coming in, then increase the amount going out. The most efficient means I have found to dramatically drop one's burden in a very short period of time is to use colonic irrigations.

Colonics have been around forever and they are literally the butt of the joke. The Rodney Dangerfield of medical treatments, they get absolutely no respect, but, oh my God, do they work. It's important with colonic irrigations to use filtered water. For autoimmunity, or anyone with lupus, colonics will eventually wash the lupus away.

SS: Initially, would they have to do them every day, once a week, twice a week?

WC: I like to have my toxic patients do five colonics in the first two weeks. My preference is three the first week and two the second. If they did one a week for five weeks, they would see nothing, nothing; but if they do five in two weeks, they will usually say by the end of the first week, wow, I'm better.

SS: The orthodox answer to these mystery illnesses is antibiotics, antifungals, amphetamines, steroids, antidepressants. What's that doing to people?

WC: In Seattle, they have a public health hospital called Harbor View. A number of years ago Harbor View put in a clinic for chemically sensitive people, and I met with the two doctors who were running it. I explained my whole program to them and they were quite amazed. I said, what's your treatment? I was expecting some type of comprehensive protocol, but they only gave antidepressants.

Unfortunately, antidepressants actually make chemical sensitivity worse, because they slow down the ability of the liver to clear environmental chemicals out of the blood. If someone is chemically sensitive, they are compromised already. So anything that suppresses that function even more is going to make them worse. This is why most chemically reactive people don't do well on antidepressants or antibiotics.

SS: In orthodox medicine, antibiotics are rarely (if ever) prescribed along with probiotics; what's your thought on that?

WC: Antibiotics that are broad spectrum knock out a whole host of other intestinal bacteria and most of them healthy, *Lactobacillus* and *Bifidobacterium*. If you're not replenishing these bacteria, it alters the balance of the ecosystem. Your intestinal flora are supposed to live in synergy, but if some of them are knocked out, then the balance becomes disordered and you will start having chronic problems. Hospitalized patients on antibiotics often end up with horrible clostridia overgrowth and severe diarrhea. That's real bad news.

SS: What do you mean?

WC: Several things are going on at once. The flora in your intestine is a huge determining factor in whether you're going to be sick. Autism is now associated with a gut flora imbalance (insufficient levels of *Bacillus fragilis*). In animal models of autism, when *Bacillus fragilis* is provided supplementally, the animals show improvement in their GI function as well as in some of the mental aspects.

SS: Don't you think that it's the same for not only autism, but also ADD, ADHD, OCD, bipolar, even schizophrenia? Doesn't it *all* start in the GI tract?

WC: The woman who influenced me to go into natural medicine, Grace Bliss, used to say all the time, "All disease starts in the colon." Now all the research into the microbiome is proving her true. Neurologically, there is a clear gut/brain interaction going on. We know that in human models the right kind of probiotic helps improve mood, anxiety, and depression. It all improves with the right kind of probiotic.

SS: How important in today's world is it for everyone to take a probiotic?

WC: Correcting bacterial imbalance in your GI system with probiotics can reverse the immune imbalance. That will take care of allergies, autoimmunity, and an inability to fight off infections.

SS: Can you overtake probiotics?

WC: Not if you're taking the right ones.

SS: Can you explain the difference between prebiotics and probiotics?

WC: Prebiotics are nondigestible plant fibers. If you're eating a plant-based diet—vegetables, grains, beans—you have the fuel for probiotics to live and grow and thrive. But if you are eating the standard American low-fiber diet and you are taking probiotics, it's a waste. I think you've heard the phrase "pissing in the wind." You can put them there, but they don't grow because they have to have something to eat.

One particular study put animals on the basic Western diet and watched their microbiome. Then they changed to a high-plant-fiber diet, and within one day their microbiome began to change. One day.

A microbiome is "the ecological community of commen-
sal, symbiotic, and pathogenic microorganisms that literally
share our body space."

Pamela Reed Gibson, in charge of the national support group for
chemically sensitive people in the United States, sent out to all her
members a communication that asked them to list every supplement
and medication they'd taken to try to help with their chemical sensitivities and answer if it made things worse, better, or no change. It
was published in *Environmental Health Perspectives*, which I think is the
finest environmental medical journal on the planet, and it's published
by the U.S. government, available online, totally free at ehponline
.org. She found that antidepressants make people worse, but the one
supplement that helped more than anything was acidophilus. That
tells me that probiotics are much more powerful than we know.

No, the biggest deal in helping chemically sensitive persons is to
find the exposure source, stop it, and then begin increasing their ability to clear toxicants out (with colonics). But if they can drink alkaline
water to clear their urine, it will help dramatically as well.

SS: Who should be drinking alkaline water?

WC: Installing an alkalinizer on your faucet is a worthwhile investment. Chronic disease and environmental toxic burden are both associated with acidic urine. When your urine is acidic, you urinate out
all your magnesium and you recycle (suck back into the bloodstream)
a huge number of toxicants that are trying to leave. Alkalinizing your
urine reverses both of those issues.

Everything you can do to clear the toxins in your body is going
to help. People can also use a little baking soda in water (1 teaspoon)
every day to alkalinize, and if you are eating more plant-based than
meat foods, your urine will be more alkaline.

SS: I'm a proponent of healthy dietary fats, are you?

WC: Yes, they're called essential fatty acids because they're essential to life.

SS: Most people are terrified of the word *butter* and terrified of red
meat; can you make any argument for them? You tend more toward a
plant-based diet?

WC: I eat wild Alaskan red salmon, some chicken, and occasionally a little red meat. It's the oils that are significant. Anti-inflammatory oils are good: olive, flax, and others. Bad oils are pro-inflammatory.

SS: Inflammation is crucial to understand as the cause of heart disease and so many other conditions and diseases.

WC: People just have to be smart and conscious about what they eat and how it makes them feel. If they start paying attention to that, plus what they drink, what they breathe, and—no small thing—what they read, watch, and listen to, it allows them to feel better and become more centered and present.

SS: Antibiotics, antidepressants, the prevalence of amphetamines— what is this overuse of drugs doing to people, considering that everyone carries within them some amount of toxic load, from mild to severe?

WC: Well, as I said at the beginning, I'm a naturopathic physician, so the first thing I think about is what's the cause? The cause isn't a deficiency of a neuroactive pharmaceutical.

Instead you have to ask why all these conditions are happening. Research points to environmental toxicants for many chronic problems. Air pollution and organophosphates are a big deal in terms of ADHD, autism, asthma, hypertension, and other problems. The sources for most organophosphate pesticides are the dirty dozen fruits and vegetables. These pesticides kill the bugs by knocking out the nervous system. Organophosphates do it by neutralizing an enzyme in the nerves that clears neurotransmitter chemicals out of the junctions between the nerve cells. When the neurotransmitters do not get cleared, the cell just keeps firing and firing and firing and firing. Sound like ADD to you? Now kids with high levels of these organophosphates have greater problems with ADHD, which is no surprise. But most kids get exposed from the dirty dozen fruits and vegetables, and if you look at those, the dirty dozen fruits and vegetables are what we eat most of the time: apples, peaches, Chilean grapes, celery, cherries. The more they consume, the higher their urine level of organophosphate pesticides.

SS: So what's good for us actually becomes bad because of man's contamination?

WC: Soaking your fresh food, all of it, in alkaline water will help greatly and is very important. By reducing your intake of toxicants, you keep from adding to the daily load on each cell in your body.

SS: Why do you think so many people are serotonin deficient?

WC: In my practice, I find that when I ask the parents of those with ADD and ADHD if there are any blood relatives who had a problem with alcohol, they all say yes. So far 100 percent of all my serotonin-deficient patients have a bloodline connection to alcoholism or brain disorders such as ADD, ADHD, because it's all part of the same issue. Low serotonin is very, very common in alcoholics and alcoholic bloodlines. Then of course add in our chronically stressed lifestyles, which also lowers serotonin levels, and you see where the problem begins. Mercury burden, which we all have to some extent, also lowers serotonin levels and is associated with a variety of neurologic symptoms like depression and anxiety. With all these factors you can see that serotonin is under attack from many directions.

SS: And serotonin deficiency causes addictive cravings. So is that why everyone is resorting to something, be it drugs, alcohol, sugar, prescription drugs, to give them the hit?

WC: Yes, exactly.

SS: What I'm hearing you say is we can get well if we change our environment, soak our food in alkaline water to remove contaminants, pay attention to the dust in our environment, clean out our ventilation ducts, air conditioners, et cetera, change our skin care and makeup products, and change out our household cleaners.

WC: Yes, all of that would be ideal. But if I was going to choose a single method of cleansing after avoidance of the toxins, it would be colonics. They will reduce the level of circulating toxicants.

SS: Colonic irrigation, because it goes up farther than a regular enema?

WC: I believe that is right. I can't document that it lowers the circulating level from measurements, but I can tell you from watching hundreds and hundreds of patients who have done colonics, it clearly lowers their circulating level of toxins. Saunas are good also—they clear some toxicants from the skin—but all the fat pads that are inside the body, rather than right under the skin, dump their toxicants into the bloodstream. This results in increased circulating levels of persistent pollutants, which is why many of those with severe chemical sensitivity will have an increase in symptoms with saunas. I tell the chemically sensitive patients we want to open the fire doors before the crowd starts running for the exits, meaning start on colonic irrigation as the first step to get the circulating level of toxicants lower.

SS: Colonic first and then when your toxic load seems to have diminished, then you can do infrared sauna?

WC: Yes, regular sauna or infrared. With regular saunas you can sweat out heavy metals, but also exercising until you sweat helps move heavy metals. It doesn't matter, really, the heat source. Dr. Stephen Genuis in Edmonton, Canada, has done a series of studies called the BUS studies for blood, urine, and sweat. His conclusions are that it doesn't matter what method you use to sweat, it's just important that it happens.

SS: I imagine nature had a pretty good plan. Do you agree with grounding?

WC: A lot of people with chemical sensitivities can end up getting electrical sensitivity as well, where they react to EMF (electromagnetic field) levels. I have found grounding to be very beneficial for individuals with this issue.

SS: What about EMFs? In California, the EMF grid is complete. What happens when we live in a world of electromagnetic frequencies along with the radiation from cell phones and Wi-Fi?

WC: This is not a good experiment we are doing with our population.

SS: Creating more brain issues?

WC: Yes, definitely.

SS: Do you ever get overwhelmed in your practice?

WC: No, I'm very hopeful. When people do the simple steps of avoidance and cleansing their bodies, they are able to heal themselves and then they get better. I've seen it hundreds of times. The one area that I'm getting concerned about is the generational effect.

SS: Meaning this generation begets the next and it gets worse?

WC: Yes, this is starting to concern me because research has been clearly showing that when kids are exposed in utero to certain toxicants, they have lifelong effects, and I am not sure that cleansing would give them the same health benefits that I can easily achieve with their parents.

SS: I guess also gynecologists could help with this so that when a woman becomes pregnant or wants to become pregnant, she'd learn that cleaning up her body and getting her ecosystem in balance is absolutely crucial.

WC: Yes. Every year I do a conference called Annual Updates in Environmental Medicine. Two years ago the conference focused on the effect of toxicants on pregnancy and childhood health outcomes. We ended up producing a consensus statement that *preconception* care should be a matter of course for all women who are wanting to conceive. Every fertility and gyn doc should be providing it, although I would bet that 99 percent would not know what advice to give or what testing to do.

SS: Seems to me that it would give the baby a real fighting chance as it enters this toxic world.

WC: It would make a huge difference for millions of children, and probably change the financial burden on schools and families as well. While preconception care is not common I have found that many young moms are quite focused on organic foods and cleaner home air when they bring their babies home. Another simple action that I recommend is that the new mothers take powdered bifidobacteria and put it on their breasts right around the nipple. Babies are always sucking on your fingers, so a little powder bifidobacteria on the finger is another way, and they like it, because of the milky flavor. Bifidobacteria has a wonderful health-promoting effect on all humans, children especially.

SS: I'm glad to hear that you feel hopeful about the future.

WC: Yes, absolutely. When I teach other teachers and students about combating the environment with this new approach to medicine, I tell them that clean living can reverse all these issues. Again, genetics point the gun, but the environment pulls the trigger. If you deal with your toxic burden and take the steps to cleanse, the problems go away.

These are new illnesses—chemical sensitivities, fibromyalgia, chronic fatigue—all of which are associated with one's chemical burden. Suzanne, I am beyond thrilled that you are taking up this banner. I've dedicated my life to trying to get this information out to people.

It will be so inspiring to people reading this to know that they're not crazy, it's not all in their heads, they're not hypochondriacs, and that, in fact, they are ill and it's not an illness that can be fixed with the usual doctor's arsenal.

When patients come to my office, as they sit in the chair and tell me everything going on with them, often I finish their sentences. When I explain the biochemical reason for all their chronic health problems, they go through a half a box of Kleenex, because they've been told by other docs that it was all in their heads and they have begun to think they might be crazy. I'm able to say, "No, you're not crazy. I can explain exactly why you're experiencing what you're experiencing and I can tell you what to do to get out of it."

SS: Imagine what that means to someone who has gone from doctor to doctor. Where do patients find you?

WC: I left practice to teach other docs how to do this medicine. I have a list of docs who have trained with me on my website (drcrinnion.com). However, I do have a very limited phone consult practice through Naturopathic Specialists LLC in Scottsdale, Arizona, at (480) 990-1111. I am also the chief science officer for Enzymedica, a company that makes digestive enzymes and GI supplements.

SS: Thank you, Dr. Crinnion. It's been my pleasure.

GO FROM *TOX*-SICK TO NOT SICK

1. Asthma is strongly associated with environmental toxicants.

   REMEDY: Purchase a HEPA filter, or IQ Air, Austin Air, or Blue Air air filter (price approx. $1,000). Try E.L. Foust, a company in Illinois, for a car air purifier if particularly sensitive.

2. Ninety-eight percent of home toxicants are bound to dust, fabric fibers, carpeting, upholstery, and drapery.

   REMEDY: Get the carpet out of your house and have a service in to clean out your air ducts.

3. Personal and home-care products are replete with enormous amounts of phthalates and plasticizers.

   REMEDY: Use only organic personal and home-care products.

4. Avoid the "dirty dozen," the twelve most toxic fruits and vegetables, because they have organophosphate pesticides in them, which are neurotoxicants.

   REMEDY: Use either an acid or alkaline wash to remove over 95 percent of most pesticides on your food. Soak vegetables and fruits (even organic ones) in alkaline water. Avoid farm-raised salmon, canned sardines (the next highest in PCBs after salmon), and high-mercury fish.

5. Tremors can develop in postmenopausal women, because of a release of lead from their bones that gets dumped into their tissues and results in Parkinson-like problems and other issues.

   REMEDY: Use chelation to pull the lead from their tissues, and then IV therapy with glutathione, plus CoQ10 supplementation.

6. The most efficient means to dramatically drop one's toxic burden in a very short period of time are colonic irrigations.

REMEDY: Dr. Crinnion's top pick for a single method of cleansing after avoidance of toxins is colonics because they reduce the levels of circulating toxicants.

7. Chronic disease and the environmental toxic burden are both associated with an acidic urine.

REMEDY: Install an alkalinizer on your faucet; it is a worthwhile investment. Drinking alkalinized water will alkalinize your urine and reverse both of these issues.

PART III

COMING CLEAN

PROTOCOLS FOR OPTIMAL HEALTH

CHAPTER 9

THE DETOX BASICS

THE SECRET TO SURVIVAL IN TODAY'S WORLD IS TO GET YOUR BODY so chemically cleaned out and primed with nutrients that it heals itself. This is the how-to part of your crash course in curing whatever ails you, as you heal your insides by ridding your body of the toxins.

YOUR 9-POINT DETOX CHECKLIST

Here are some first steps in minimizing this toxic soup from damaging our bodies. None are hard, all are important.

- Reduce your consumption of processed foods.
- Never microwave in plastic bottles, Tupperware, or any plastic containers.
- Keep leftovers in glass containers in refrigerators. Plastic bags leach toxins.
- Buy juice, milk, and so on in glass bottles.
- Put reverse osmosis filters on your water faucets and change filters every three months.
- Consume sufficient vegetables daily.
- Take supplements daily (see "The Protocol," next).
- Use high-quality oil: olive oil, coconut oil, flaxseed oil.
- Use toxin-free organic household cleaners.

THE PROTOCOL: SUPPLEMENTS FOR SURVIVAL

This next section is the protocol, a miniature handbook in itself of the supplements identified to target your particular areas of health concern. Are you mainly concerned about toxicity in your body? Or do you have a family history of heart disease? Read on to see what supplements you feel would best support your health and wellness issues. Not many of us like to "down" handfuls of supplements on a daily basis. In a perfect world there would be no necessity; even using the argument "my grandparents never took supplements" no longer holds water. When I installed our cherished organic garden on the property, I realized finding uncontaminated soil was like finding diamonds. Even those who sold organic soil had caveats. I installed the best-quality organic soil I could source, set up a purified water system, use only organic plants and organic seeds, and hope the acid rain and nearby GMO intoxication downwind in the Coachella Valley will not contaminate my food. These things are airborne, no matter how hard I try to keep my garden clean.

Even with this, I know that the nutrition I go out of my way to obtain for myself and my family may not provide everything my body needs in today's world. So what to do? Enter supplements. Oprah asked me to lay out the supplements I take on a daily basis on my kitchen table. Yes, it looked daunting, and, yes, I take a lot, but I am a health writer and I've had cancer, so I take my body "fuel" very seriously. The result for me is robust health and a body that works perfectly. Do I enjoy downing all these supplements daily? Of course not, but I try to think of what each one does as I take it and imagine it going to work.

It's overwhelming to walk into a store and look at a shelf of products trying to decide what supplements to take. To give you some guidance, I've asked my friends at Forever Health (ForeverHealth .com) and Life Extension (LifeExtension.com/tox-sick) to lay out a comprehensive explanation of the supplements that are most important for surviving and thriving in today's toxic, polluted world. With their expertise they will highlight the essential supplements for health and navigating the toxic world we inhabit.

GET 'EM OUT!

You've read a lot so far about keeping environmental toxins out of your body. But it is of critical importance to understand the role supplementation plays in protecting you against toxins you cannot avoid. I always feel privileged that Life Extension's team of doctors and scientists provides you, my readers, with the most cutting-edge information on the value of supplementation.

No matter how hard we try to stay away from environmental contaminants, our bodies will endure some adverse chemical exposure capable of damaging our cellular DNA, what are known as mutagens. The good news is that there are proven measures to protect your DNA from the toxins we are inevitably exposed to. After the discussion of gene mutation that follows, we'll look at what top scientists reveal as simple ways you can avoid becoming a victim of the toxic world we must now survive in . . . but that we also want to thrive in!

WHAT CAUSES GENES TO MUTATE?

Before I reveal how easy it is to defend your DNA against mutagens (those agents or chemicals that change our genetics), and get them out of your body, I want to explain the importance of what you're really guarding. Our cells thrive and stay cancer-free because of the *genes* located in our DNA. Our very existence is dependent on these genes properly regulating every cellular event.

Healthy young cells have relatively perfect genes. Aging and environmental factors cause genes to mutate, resulting in cellular disorder. Genetic mutations create a host of diseases ranging from cancer to neurological impairment. As gene mutations accumulate, our body loses its ability to sustain life.

Human studies show that about 70 percent of gene mutation is environmentally driven and thus relatively controllable based on what we eat, whether we smoke, exposure to environmental toxins, radiation, and so on.

The most prevalent cause of environmental gene mutation is the food we eat every day. While certain foods are particularly toxic, even foods regarded as safe can result in the body being exposed to small amounts of carcinogens. A consistent scientific finding is that **people who consume the most calories have significantly higher incidences of cancer**. There are several mechanisms that explain why overeating causes cancer, but one reason is that more gene mutations occur in response to higher food intake.

Overcooked foods also inflict massive damage to our genes. A group at the University of Minnesota reported that women who eat very well-done hamburgers have a 50 percent greater risk of breast cancer than women who eat them rare or medium. The famous Iowa Women's Health Study found that women who consistently eat well-done steak, hamburgers, and bacon have a 4.62-fold increased risk of breast cancer. Cooking foods at high temperatures causes the formation of gene-mutating heterocyclic amines. That's one reason why deep-fried foods are so dangerous to eat. Heterocyclic amines have been linked to prostate, breast, colorectal, esophageal, lung, liver, and other cancers. While health-conscious people try to avoid foods that are known carcinogens, even grilled salmon contains a potent dose of gene-mutating heterocyclic amines.

Although one can reduce exposure to them, it may be impossible to keep them from forming in your body. That's because enzymatic activities that naturally occur in the liver can inadvertently manufacture these amines from otherwise harmless organic compounds.

Heterocyclic amines are a major cause of disease, yet they are not the only dietary culprit involved in gene mutation. Other mutagenic agents found in food are nitrosamine preservatives, aflatoxin molds, and pesticide-herbicide residues.

Since avoiding all dietary carcinogens is impossible, identifying methods to protect genes against mutation is critical. And that's what this chapter will do for you.

PREVENTING GENE MUTATION

The first lines of defense then are antimutagenic agents that have been identified in fruits and vegetables; the most potent are the indole-3-carbinols, the chlorophylls, and chlorophyllin.

Chlorophyllin

Chlorophyllin is the water-soluble form of chlorophyll that has been tested as an antimutagenic agent for decades.

Chlorophyllin can cross cell membranes and blood-brain barriers while chlorophyll itself cannot. Chlorophyllin even enters into the mitochondria, the energy-producing organelles of the cell where the majority of free radicals are produced. Chlorophyllin quenches all the major free radicals, and protects mitochondria from a variety of external chemical, biological, and radiation threats.

Curcumin

Another very effective antimutagen is curcumin, a phytonutrient derived from the Indian spice turmeric, a primary ingredient in curry.

Turmeric has played an important role in the traditional Indian Ayurvedic system of holistic medicine for centuries. A member of the ginger family, turmeric has a reputation for lowering inflammation and healing various conditions ranging from ulcers to arthritis.

In the last decade, scientists have discovered that curcumin can also help protect against the multitude of mutagens in our environment. A study at India's Panjab University explored the benefits of curcumin and two of its analogs in counteracting the effects of seven of these heterocyclic amines. The researchers found that curcumin inhibited mutations by as much as 80 percent against all the tested mutagens in cooked food. Several studies have found that curcumin supplementation can reduce the likelihood of colon cancer. In a year-long study of rats at the American Health Foundation, the results indicated that dietary administration of curcumin significantly inhibited the incidence of all colon cancer tumors (both invasive and noninvasive). The curcumin regimen also suppressed the size of the average colon tumor by 57 percent compared to the control diet.

Curcumin has proven its effectiveness against other types of cancer as well. Two studies at Thailand's Chiang Mai University found that dietary curcumin reduced skin tumor formation in mice. More of the mice ingesting curcumin remained free of tumors than mice in the control group, and those that did develop tumors had fewer and smaller ones than the controls. Curcumin intake also significantly decreased the expression of cancer-causing genes. Laboratory experiments demonstrate that the herb boosts the effectiveness of the anticancer drug vinblastine against drug-resistant human cervical cancer cells and inhibits the growth of breast cancer cells. With positive results such as these, more long-term human studies are clearly warranted to confirm curcumin's benefits in cancer treatment.

Wasabi

Wasabi japonica is a member of the cruciferous family of vegetables, which includes cabbage, broccoli, cauliflower, bok choy, horseradish, and several other plants. These vegetables add crunch and flavor to meals and have long been recognized as important parts of a healthy diet because of their fiber content. Recent research has revealed, however, that there is much more to them than mere fiber. They contain high levels of potent cancer-protecting compounds called glucosinolates, a group of compounds that are converted to isothiocyanates. It is the isothiocyanates that give these vegetables their sharp flavors. Wasabi, the green, pungent horseradish typically served with sushi, is one of the most potent sources of isothiocyanates among all plant species.

The isothiocyanates do more than add flavor to a meal. A Japanese study found that a wasabi isothiocyanate has significant antioxidant actions. According to the authors, this phytochemical also has an inhibitory effect on the growth of food-poisoning bacteria and fungi, and showed anti-mutagenic activity against a common carcinogen found in broiled fish and meat.

Broccoli and Its Extract

Broccoli is a plentiful source of glucosinolates, which are also converted enzymatically into isothiocyanates. In the body, the isothiocyanates in broccoli boost production of several detoxification enzymes, enhance antioxidant status, and protect animals against chemically induced cancer. As a result, nutritionists often recommend consuming broccoli and similar vegetables at least three times a week. Concentrated extracts of broccoli enable you to boost your intake of these beneficial compounds even more.

One of the primary isothiocyanates in broccoli is sulforaphane. In numerous studies, this plant chemical has demonstrated powerful anticarcinogenic actions. In a laboratory experiment with mouse liver cancer cells, sulforaphane increased two detoxification enzymes, glutathione S-transferase and quinine reductase. The authors concluded that sulforaphane's ability to elevate these enzymes may be a significant component of broccoli's anticancer action.

Broccoli's benefits do not end there. A study of vegetables found that broccoli produced the greatest protective effect against several mutagenic chemicals, and it also stimulated the proliferation of noncancerous cells. Another experiment at Johns Hopkins found that the sulforaphane in broccoli is a potent agent against the *H. pylori* bacterium, which causes ulcers and increases the risk of stomach cancer. A study performed at the same time showed that sulforaphane also blocked stomach tumors in mice exposed to mutagenic chemicals. According to the researchers, these multiple benefits resulted from increased production of Phase II detoxification and antioxidant enzymes.

MAXIMIZING PROTECTION AGAINST MUTAGENS

It has become increasingly difficult to protect our health from toxic chemicals, including pesticides, that are part of the air we breathe, the water we drink, and the food we eat. Providing the body with defensive agents such as curcumin, chlorophyllin, wasabi, and broccoli extract can maximize protection against DNA damage, thus making an important contribution to optimal health and longevity.

I am pleased to announce that you can now easily obtain this scientifically validated protection against environmental toxins. My friends at Forever Health have combined them all into a low-cost formula appropriately called Healthy Genes Formula. The recommended dose is one capsule of the Healthy Genes Formula before at least two meals of the day.

CELLULAR HEALTH SUPPORT

When you're sick, your cells are too. The toxins we are regularly exposed to infiltrate our bodies and cause damage on the cellular level. When enough cellular damage takes place, your body stops working efficiently and you might get sick, experience a lack of energy, have trouble digesting your food, or, worst of all, experience cellular mutations potentially leading to cancer.

Although we don't often consider our individual cells when we're not feeling well, it's those cells that are taking the brunt of the toxic assault. We have to do everything we can to protect them from the ravages of our modern, toxic world.

One of the most important ways that toxins harm us is by damaging the powerhouses of cells—the mitochondria. Mitochondria convert sugars into ATP (adenosine triphosphate) that cells use for energy. Mitochondria are exquisitely sensitive to environmental toxins, and when mitochondrial dysfunction occurs, cells are less capable of producing the energy they need to carry out their normal activities.

In fact, environmental toxins and medications impair mitochondrial function through several mechanisms of action that vary with individual agents. Mechanisms include inhibition of the electron transport chain, impaired mitochondrial protein transport, increased development of free radicals, inhibition of mitochondrial DNA replication, or a combination of these.

Scientists are now linking environmental interactions with the mitochondria to an array of metabolic and age-related conditions, including cancer, autism, type 2 diabetes, Alzheimer's disease, Parkinson's disease, and cardiovascular illness.

Studies show that mitochondria are vulnerable to a number of environmental toxins, such as polycyclic aromatic hydrocarbons and heavy metals. Moreover, mitochondria contain enzymes that can turn otherwise nontoxic compounds into toxic ones; this is the case with certain mycotoxins. To make matters worse, the specialized DNA in mitochondria is more vulnerable than standard cellular DNA to damage by some toxins. Thus, it's critical that we supplement with agents that help support mitochondrial function, like coenzyme Q10 and lipoic acid.

There are several supplements that can help your cells stand up to the stress of constant toxic exposure and continue functioning at peak performance. We're going to outline a few of the most important supplements for cellular health in this section. These include resveratrol, quercetin, pterostilbene, and EGCG (from green tea); coenzyme Q10 (CoQ10); R-lipoic acid; vitamins C and E; and beneficial berries like blueberry and açaí.

Resveratrol

We've all heard about the health benefits of red wine. The good health of the people of the Mediterranean region has been partially attributed to their regular consumption of moderate amounts of red wine. Folks who eat a Mediterranean-style diet have lower rates of heart disease and cancer, and even appear to live longer than the rest of us. Of course, the wine isn't the only reason these people are so healthy (they also eat a lot of omega-3 fatty acids and healthy plant foods), but studies have shown that some components in wine do indeed exert plenty of health benefits.

Enter resveratrol. This hard-to-pronounce plant chemical is found in red wine and has been shown to combat a number of health problems that catch up with us as we age—cancer, heart disease, osteoporosis, and memory loss to name a few. Resveratrol supports cellular health in many ways, including antimutagenic activity, reduction of oxidative stress, suppression of inflammation, mitochondrial protection, and modulation of toxin metabolism.

Right, so I need resveratrol; I'll just drink more wine. Not so fast. There actually isn't that much resveratrol in a normal serving of wine, so you'd have to drink a whole lot of wine to get much of it, which isn't going to help you stay healthy. The good news is that purified resveratrol is available as a supplement. It's best to find a resveratrol product that contains *trans*-resveratrol, as this is the form that's usually used in studies. Also, resveratrol works well when it is combined with other healthy plant chemicals such as quercetin and pterostilbene.

Green Tea

The health benefits of green tea have been extolled for years, but it's worth mentioning this power-packed plant again here.

The active constituents in green tea are powerful antioxidants called polyphenols (catechins) and flavonols. Several catechins are present in green tea and account for the bulk of favorable research reports. Epigallocatechin gallate (EGCG) is the most powerful of these catechins.

Green tea extracts prevent DNA damage through their antioxidant properties, and they also trigger innate DNA repair mechanisms to quickly patch up damage before it is transmitted to new cells. In human studies, consumption of green tea or its polyphenols rapidly reduce DNA damage throughout the body. In mice treated with chemicals that cause skin cancer, topical application or oral administration of green tea both protected against tumor formation. Another animal study showed that green tea reduced the mutagenicity of tobacco.

What makes green tea extract such an important nutrient are the large volumes of published scientific findings that validate its multiple biological benefits. Green tea compounds uniquely enhance Phase I and Phase II detoxification in the liver. Green tea extracts are also highly antimutagenic. When green tea components were combined with standard mutagens, they were found to be highly protective in validated tests, while protecting against chromosome breaks in other lab tests. Other important findings involve studies showing that green tea extract helps maintain cellular DNA and membrane structural integrity. Decades of research suggests green tea inhibits the development of cancer.

R-Lipoic Acid

Lipoic acid is one of the most potent, versatile, and longer-acting antioxidant vitamins known. Lipoic acid possesses the unique ability to work in both water-soluble and fat-soluble environments in the body. This ubiquitous property means that lipoic acid has access to all parts of our cells to neutralize damaging free radicals, which are implicated in many age-related diseases. Being able to navigate cellular membranes throughout the body also means that lipoic acid can also cross the blood-brain barrier to exert its protective effects on neurological tissue.

Lipoic acid is a vital "cofactor" for enzymatic reactions within the mitochondria, helping to optimize energy conversion. It possesses active properties that specifically slow mitochondrial aging by preventing release of mutagenic oxidants. Other research reveals lipoic acid's ability to alleviate mitochondrial dysfunction in aging cells (thus improving mitochondrial function). In addition, lipoic acid has been shown to prevent chemically induced genotoxicity in a dose dependent fashion.

Lipoic acid may also protect the body against toxic metal contaminants found in the environment and food supply. This multifunctional agent works by chelating these dangerous agents, such as arsenic, cadmium, lead, and mercury, and rendering them inactive so that they can be removed by the body. In animal studies, lipoic acid has been shown to provide protection against arsenic poisoning and to safeguard the liver against the effects of cadmium exposure. Another study also showed that lipoic acid helped protect the delicate nervous system against the harmful effects of mercury poisoning.

Lipoic acid comes in two "mirror image" forms labeled "R" and "S." Only the R form is produced and used by life processes. Newer precision techniques allow production of a pure R-lipoic acid, which has a much higher potency. A dose of pure R-lipoic acid provides twice the active ingredient as a typical R/S-alpha lipoic acid supplement, simply because the whole dose consists of the active "R" molecule. Look for the "R" label to ensure that you are getting the most potent form of this valuable nutrient.

Coenzyme Q10 (CoQ10)

CoQ10 is an essential coenzyme that, when added to the diet, acts as a fuel additive to optimize mitochondrial performance, extracting the most energy with the least damage. CoQ10's beneficial effects on the mitochondria are especially important in the context of environmental toxicity. Mitochondria are known to be exquisitely sensitive to environmental toxicants and mitochondrial dysfunction has been associated with an array of age-related conditions such as cancer, autism, type 2 diabetes, Alzheimer's disease, Parkinson's disease, and cardiovascular illness.

CoQ10 is well known for its heart and vascular health benefits. By helping the cellular powerhouses known as mitochondria burn fuel more effectively, CoQ10 is able to protect not only the heart but every cell in your body.

That's why scientists are growing increasingly fascinated with the role of CoQ10 in tissues beyond the cardiovascular system. There is evidence for CoQ10's protective effects in the nervous system, in asthma and chronic lung disease, in diabetes and the metabolic syndrome, on ocular health, and even on the aging immune system.

Most excitingly, there's early support for the idea that CoQ10 supplementation can extend the life span of both primitive animals and mammals, laying the groundwork for a similar pro-longevity effect in humans.

Be sure you are using the right form of CoQ10—ubiquinol. Scientific studies show that ubiquinol absorbs up to eight times greater than the typical ubiquinone form of CoQ10, and higher levels of ubiquinol remain in the blood far longer than ubiquinone. In studies measuring exercise-induced fatigue, ubiquinol was 90 percent more effective than ubiquinone. In middle-aged mice, ubiquinol was shown to be 40 percent more effective in slowing measurements of aging compared to ubiquinone.

Vitamin C

Even though humans cannot synthesize vitamin C, every tissue and cell in our body needs this nutrient for healthy growth and repair. Vitamin C is essential for eight major enzyme systems on which life depends. Vitamin C is also antimutagenic and has been shown to be especially protective against the genotoxic effects of ionizing radiation. Another important way vitamin C is protective is through inhibiting the formation of N-nitroso compounds. Increased levels of N-nitroso compounds are formed with the consumption of red meat and are associated with higher gastrointestinal cancer incidence.

Nitrosamines can be formed within the body following ingestion of nitrates/nitrites via reactions within the oral cavity and gastrointestinal tract. This is a concern in the context of nitrate-preserved meats. Fortunately, vitamin C strongly inhibits the formation of nitrosamines. In fact, the U.S. Department of Agriculture mandates that meat manufacturers incorporate vitamin C into certain processed meat products to combat the formation of nitrosamines during the cooking process.

Maintaining optimal levels of vitamin C is difficult because it is water soluble and cannot be stored in the body. This inability to maintain high vitamin C levels is recognized by researchers as limiting its potential benefit, especially with regard to chronic illness.

Fortunately, a method has been discovered to increase the speed at which vitamin C is absorbed. Two botanical compounds, piperine and dihydroquercetin, can improve your body's utilization of vitamin C.

When choosing a vitamin C product, aim for one that contains piperine and dihydroquercetin so that you get the most from your supplement.

Berry Extracts and Anthocyanins

One of the best ways to support cellular health is to eat plenty of antioxidant-rich berries each day. In general, the more deeply pigmented a fruit or vegetable is, the more nutritional value it has. In particular, deep purple, red, and blue pigments are a sign of the presence of powerful antioxidants known as anthocyanins. Anthocyanin-rich berries and fruits have been shown to be active against some of today's most common diseases, including cancer, cardiovascular disease, Alzheimer's disease, and diabetes. Anthocyanins help regulate detoxification of environmental toxins and carcinogens and can protect the DNA in your cells from free-radical damage. Bioactive extracts of berries also appear to inhibit cancer-promoting pathways within cells.

Pomegranate is a powerful superfruit with antimutagenic properties. Research has found strong antimutagenic activity at various concentrations. Pomegranate has been shown in preclinical research to prevent brain damage by reducing aluminum accumulation. The superfruit also prevented chemically induced gene toxicity.

Açaí is rich in anthocyanins and has been shown to inhibit the growth of chemically induced tumors in preclinical research. Raspberries also contain beneficial phytochemicals. In one study, raspberry extract reduced the incidence of liver nodules that formed in rats exposed to a liver-damaging toxin.

Anthocyanins and other exceptionally active phytonutrients are not limited to berries.

Blue corn, also known as purple corn, is botanically identical to yellow corn but with one important difference. Its deep blue-purple color is the result of its rich anthocyanin content—with a concentration equal to, or greater than, the anthocyanin concentration of blueberries. Blue corn possesses antimutagenic effects, reducing expression of genes involved in the proliferation of tumor cells.

DOSAGE SUGGESTIONS FOR DNA PROTECTION AND OVERALL CELLULAR SUPPORT		
Nutrient or Intervention	Typical Daily Dose	Suggested Products
Chlorophyllin	20 mg once or twice daily with meals	Forever Health Healthy Genes Formula
Turmeric extract (providing curcumin)	240 mg up to three times daily with meals	
Wasabi	50 mg once or twice daily with meals	
Broccoli extract	225 mg once or twice daily with meals	
Resveratrol	250 mg	Forever Health Resveratrol
Quercetin	60 mg	
Pterostilbene	0.5 mg	
Green tea	725 mg daily without food	Forever Health Green Tea
R-lipoic acid	240 mg once or twice daily	Life Extension Super R-Lipoic Acid
CoQ10 as ubiquinol	50–200 mg (Also, consider CoQ10 blood testing to optimize dose.)	Forever Health CoQ10 Mitochondrial Support Complex
Vitamin C	500 mg once or twice daily	Life Extension Fast-C® with Dihydroquercetin
Berry, açaí, pomegranate extract blend	Once or twice daily take 500 mg açaí and 200 mg antioxidant fruit blend	Life Extension Enhanced Berry Complete with Açaí

To support healthy cells and genes, Forever Health has created a convenient Cellular Support Kit for my readers with many of the recommended ingredients listed in the previous table: chlorophyllin, turmeric extract, wasabi, broccoli extract, resveratrol, quercetin, and pterostilbene.

LIVER SUPPORT

The human body is truly a miraculous thing. It never ceases to amaze me with its complexity and elegance. Take the liver, for example. It is the largest organ inside your body and has at least five hundred life-sustaining functions. Intricate systems of enzymes are constantly working overtime in the liver to remove toxins. Optimal liver function is critical to all aspects of health. Maintaining robust liver capacity ensures our body will effectively rid itself of heavy metals, pollutants, and other toxins.

Unfortunately, liver function declines with aging. Left unchecked, toxic overload can lead to conditions ranging from cirrhosis and hepatitis to nonalcoholic fatty liver disease and even cancer. If all of the liver's detoxification systems aren't operating at peak performance, toxic chemicals can slip through our defenses and permeate our bodies. That's why it's so important to take supplements that keep your liver up to snuff.

In this section, we'll mention some key liver support ingredients that are practically essential in our toxic world. These include milk thistle, selenium, N-acetyl cysteine (NAC), schisandra fruit extract, melon pulp concentrate, cruciferous vegetable extracts, and vitamin C.

Cruciferous Vegetable Extracts

Extracts from cruciferous vegetables—such as broccoli, cauliflower, cabbage, and Brussels sprouts—can help promote liver detoxification and maintain healthy hormone levels.

Extracts of broccoli, watercress, and rosemary provide isothiocyanates, carnosic acid, and carnosol—bioactive compounds that have a multitude of favorable effects on estrogen metabolism and cell division. Glucosinolates from cruciferous vegetables protect against the carcinogenic compounds created by cooking meat at high temperature. Apigenin, a powerful plant flavonoid, boosts cell protection, while cabbage extract, a natural source of benzyl isothiocyanate (BITC), maintains cell health. BITC has been shown in several studies to exert anticancer activity.

Milk Thistle

Milk thistle has been used for over two thousand years. It supports liver detoxification and even helps liver cells regenerate. Studies confirm that milk thistle can protect liver function and prevent liver damage.

Extracts from milk thistle (*Silybum marianum*) have been used for centuries for their preventive and therapeutic properties in liver diseases. Modern science has identified the specific components in milk thistle extracts responsible for these protective effects, one being *silymarin*.

Silymarin is a potent antioxidant and anti-inflammatory, which helps it fight the root causes of liver disease. Further research has identified a specific molecule, *silybin*, as the most active component in silymarin. Another compound in milk thistle, *isosilybin*, also keeps cells healthy. Milk thistle has been shown to fight several types of cancer including liver, colon, skin, and prostate and activate a cell-signaling pathway that helps regulate lipid and glucose metabolism. Isosilybin actually consists of two chemical cousins, called "isomers." These are isosilybin A and isosilybin B, and both are beneficial.

These milk thistle components are very protective against the chemical insults we face on a daily basis. They have been shown to counteract toxicity from a wide variety of toxic substances, including ethanol, organic solvents, pharmaceuticals, and mushroom-based poisons or mycotoxins. Milk thistle, for instance, produces superior survival rates from *Amanita phalloides* mushroom poisoning, compared with standard treatment.

Look for a milk thistle product standardized to silymarin and silybin along with isosilybin A and B.

Glutathione

Glutathione is the most abundant antioxidant molecule naturally produced in the body. It is a powerful regulator of oxidative stress and immune system function. Glutathione is especially important in the liver, where it helps detoxify free radicals generated by toxin exposure and is active in Phase I and Phase II detoxification processes. It also has been shown to prevent toxin-induced liver damage through a mechanism involving changing the liver cell's response to injury. Moreover, glutathione is critical for the detoxification of several carcinogens.

Experts recommend taking a glutathione supplement each day. Life Extension makes one that combines glutathione with vitamin C and the amino acid cysteine. I like this formula because vitamin C and cysteine help promote glutathione synthesis.

Selenium

The mineral selenium is essential for health. It is involved in the recycling of glutathione and is an important cofactor in several free-radical detoxification pathways. Selenium is especially important for liver health. And one study showed that taking a selenium supplement every day reduced the risk of liver cancer. Likewise, animal studies have shown that selenium depletion can lead to liver damage caused by toxins and that selenium supplementation can counter these effects.

There are several forms of selenium available as supplements. I suggest a product that combines multiple forms, including Se-methyl-L-selenocysteine, L-selenomethionine, and sodium selenite.

N-acetyl Cysteine

Another molecule that replenishes the natural antioxidant glutathione is N-acetyl cysteine (NAC), a versatile sulfur-rich compound that was first used to prevent liver damage following acetaminophen poisoning. It rapidly restores depleted glutathione to normal levels, sparing liver cells from the effects of oxidant damage.

In humans, the combination of NAC (1,200 mg/day) with the

antidiabetic drug metformin (850–1,000 mg/day) improved liver appearance and reduced fibrosis in patients with nonalcoholic fatty liver disease. And stunning findings in a 2009 preclinical study revealed that NAC could stimulate regeneration of healthy liver cells in animals that had part of their livers removed! The researchers in that study observed that NAC supported glutathione levels, and they postulated that the resulting reduction in oxidative stress accounted for the good outcome. In addition, NAC has been shown to combat the detrimental effects of toxic notrosative compounds formed during radiation therapy in an animal model.

Schisandra Fruit Extract and Melon Concentrate

One of the biggest threats to liver health is lipid peroxidation. This is a process where fat in the liver (and elsewhere) turns rancid due to the continuous assault from free radicals. Over time, this process can make us more vulnerable to liver injury.

A purified concentrate from the *Cucumis melo* melon has been found to be rich in superoxide dismutase (SOD), a key enzyme in your body's mitochondrial oxidant protection system. Melon-derived SOD quickly converts primary free oxygen radicals into hydrogen peroxide.

That hydrogen peroxide must be rapidly converted into water to complete the mitochondrial oxidant detoxification process. Schisandra fruit extract complements melon pulp concentrate by stimulating a liver mitochondrial antioxidant enzyme, glutathione peroxidase, which converts hydrogen peroxide to water.

DOSAGE SUGGESTIONS FOR LIVER SUPPORT			
Nutrient or Intervention		Typical Daily Dose	Suggested Products
Cruciferous vegetable ingredients	Indole-3-carbinol (I3C)	80 mg once or twice daily	Forever Health Cruciferous Detox Formula
	Di-indolyl-methane (DIM)	14 mg once or twice daily	
	Broccoli concentrate (standardized to glucosinolates)	400 mg once or twice daily	
	Watercress	50 mg once or twice daily	
	Cabbage extract	25 mg once or twice daily	
Milk thistle (phosopholipid blend)		380 mg twice daily	Forever Health Milk Thistle
Glutathione, L-cysteine, and vitamin C		One to three times daily take 50 mg L-glutathione, 200 mg L-cysteine, and 500 mg vitamin C	Forever Health Amino-Antioxidant Support
Selenium (as Se-Methyl-L-selenocysteine, SelenoPure™, L-selenomethionine, sodium selenite)		200 mcg daily with food	Life Extension Super Selenium Complex
N-acetyl-cysteine		600 mg one to three times daily	Life Extension N-Acetyle-L-Cysteine
Schisandra extract		250 mg	Life Extension Liver Efficiency Formula
Melon pulp concentrate (providing superoxide dismutase) (SOD)		10 mg (providing 140 IU of SOD)	

To aid in detox and support a healthy liver system, Forever Health has created a Healthy Liver Kit for my readers with many of the recommended ingredients listed in the previous table: cruciferous vegetable extracts, milk thistle, and glutathione, L-cysteine, and vitamin C.

BRAIN AND NEUROLOGICAL SUPPORT

It's easy to dismiss periodic brain fog as a consequence of getting older. But research suggests that environmental toxins could be a major cause of problems with memory, learning, and cognition.

We've already discussed several supplements to help protect our cells and our livers from the toxins that abound in our environment. In this section, we'll outline some supplements that can help support your brain and neurological system; these sites are often a target for the damaging effects of environmental toxins. Important nutrients to consider include omega-3 fatty acids, magnesium-L-threonate, the hormone pregnenolone, alpha-glycerylphosphorylcholine (A-GPC), and phosphatidylserine (PS).

Omega-3 Fatty Acids

Today's diet contains far greater amounts of omega-6 fatty acids and less of omega-3 fatty acids than before large-scale, industrialized food production was the norm. Omega-3 fatty acids help combat inflammation, and they're good for cardiovascular health too. In contrast, omega-6 fatty acids are pro-inflammatory. Studies have shown that a high ratio of omega-6 to omega-3 fatty acids promotes the development of many killer diseases, including cancer and cardiovascular disease.

In contrast, appropriate levels of omega-3, relative to omega-6, may help reduce the toxicity of some medications. By their potent beneficial effects on chronic inflammation and autoimmunity, adequate fish-derived omega-3 levels may allow patients to reduce their reliance on medications that can tax the body's detoxification pathways. A high omega-3 fish oil has been compared to a high omega-6 corn oil and shown an ability to protect against the cancer-inducing effects of a carcinogenic chemical used extensively in colon cancer research.

Brain health and cognitive function can also suffer as a result of low omega-3 intake. In one study, researchers assessed serum phospholipid levels in 280 middle-aged, healthy volunteers, which were then correlated to cognitive function. It was found that people with the highest serum levels of DHA performed significantly better in multiple areas of cognition than people with lower DHA levels.

It's hard to avoid excess omega-6 fats and get enough omega-3s through diet alone given the state of our current food supply. That's why supplementing with high-quality omega-3 fatty acids is especially important. Fish oil supplements are one of the best ways to get plenty of omega-3 fatty acids, but not just any product will do. Look for a fish oil product that contains eicosapentaenoic acid (EPA) and docosahexaenoic acid (DHA) along with olive extract and sesame lignans. The sesame lignans are important because they help keep the fish oil stable, and the olive oil complements the cardiovascular benefits of fish oil. To make sure your fish oil product doesn't contain high levels of toxins, look for a five-star International Fish Oil Standards (IFOS) rating on the label. The five-star IFOS rating means that the product has passed thorough testing for dangerous toxins.

Pregnenolone

As a result of normal aging, key hormone levels decline. One result of this is a detrimental impact on memory and cognitive function. Scientists believe that the hormone pregnenolone has vast potential for maintaining healthy cognitive function and may be "the most potent memory enhancer yet reported."

Pregnenolone is the first hormone in the pathway that generates a host of key neurohormones in the brain that are known to affect nerve cell growth and to modulate various moods. Pregnenolone affects a wide range of nervous system functions and has been shown to reduce the risk of dementia and improve memory, as well as alleviate anxiety and fight depression.

The formation of memory is still one of the most fascinating functions of the brain. Scientists are learning more each day about how molecules and memories interact. There is strong evidence that pregnenolone levels diminish with advancing age and that restoring these levels may help alleviate deteriorating brain function.

What is more, pregnenolone is able to activate memory-formation pathways independently of the chemical glutamate. While glutamate in the right amount is essential for normal brain function, it can contribute to overexcitation and overstimulation of neurons, and this may contribute to degenerative diseases like Alzheimer's. Thus pregnenolone may be exerting its positive effects on brain function and memory as a result of its ability to protect from the excitotoxic effect of glutamate.

Work with your physician to determine whether this is something that might be useful to your unique hormonal needs. You can test your levels of pregnenolone and other hormones by ordering a blood test from Life Extension. They offer comprehensive hormone blood testing for both men and women.

Vinpocetine

A compound called vinpocetine, derived from the common periwinkle plant, has shown great promise in improving blood flow in the brain and restoring lost cognitive abilities. Vinpocetine appears to work by inhibiting the action of an enzyme called phosphodiesterase 1 (PDE1), resulting in relaxation of cerebral blood vessel walls and increased cerebral blood flow. Additionally, vinpocetine helps support cerebral glucose metabolism by enhancing glucose supply to brain tissue.

Gastrodin

For thousands of years, Chinese doctors have used gastrodin, extracted from the root of the exotic orchid *Gastrodia elata*, for a range of cognitive problems from vertigo and headaches to paralysis and seizures.

Scientists today are discovering that gastrodin acts as a broad-spectrum "brain shield" that protects against various factors that cause age-related degradation of our mental processes. Gastrodia extract appears to protect the brain partly by protecting it from toxins, free radicals, and inflammation, all of which may play a role in neurodegenerative conditions such as Parkinson's disease.

What has researchers excited are new findings showing that gastrodin has *regenerative properties* that include rebalancing neurotransmitters, improving blood flow, decreasing memory loss, protecting brain functions during a stroke, and potentially reducing the risk of Alzheimer's and Parkinson's. In short, gastrodin provides unparalleled, multifactorial brain protection in both extreme and everyday conditions.

DOSAGE SUGGESTIONS FOR BRAIN AND NEUROLOGICAL SUPPORT		
Nutrient or Intervention	Typical Daily Dose	Suggested Products
Gastrodin	300 mg	Life Extension Brain Shield® Gastrodin®
Vinpocetine	10 mg one to three times daily with meals	Life Extension Vinpocetine
Phosphatidylserine (PS)	100 mg	Life Extension Cognitex® Basics
Alpha-glycerylphosphorylcholine (GPC)	600 mg	
Omega-3 fatty acids	700 mg EPA twice daily with food 500 mg DHA twice daily with food	Forever Health Omega-3 Fish Oil Complex
Pregnenolone	Best determined by blood testing; 50 mg one to four times daily	Forever Health Pregnenolone

DIGESTIVE AND GASTROINTESTINAL SUPPORT

In this section we're going to cover some of the most important supplements you can take to help keep your gut in great shape. We'll talk about probiotics, digestive enzymes, fiber, and L-glutamine.

Probiotics

The digestive tract begins with the mouth, runs through the stomach and intestines, and ends at the anus. And it is actually separated from the inside of your body by powerful defense systems that help keep toxins and other harmful substances from entering systemic circulation. One of the most important gut-body barriers is the one formed by the good bacteria in your intestines. These beneficial bacteria help break down toxins so they can be excreted instead of being absorbed and causing problems.

It's easy to take the good bacteria in your gut for granted while you're healthy. But in today's toxic environment, we ought to be thinking more about these beneficial bugs. Poor diet, lifestyle choices, and environmental factors can cause the balance of good and bad bacteria in the gut to shift toward an unhealthy state. This opens up the door to toxins in the food we eat. This is why I take a high-quality probiotic every day. Supplementation with probiotics can help restore the healthy balance of good and bad bacteria in your gut and help keep the toxins we encounter in our food from being taken up by our bodies. (And I show you how to make your own, too; see page 287 for more.)

Digestive Enzymes

In youth, digestive enzymes break down ingested food into vital proteins, fats, and carbohydrates to provide optimal nutrition for the body. But with aging and illness, the body's digestive functions deteriorate, leading to gas, bloating, partially digested food, nutritional deficiencies, and even inflammatory conditions.

Age-related digestive problems needn't become significant health issues, given that supplemental digestive enzymes—many derived from plants—can help replace the enzymes produced in youth. These modern digestion-assistance preparations offer natural enzymes that, when taken with meals, can enhance the digestive process.

Fiber

Dietary fiber has myriad health benefits, but most Americans' diet is markedly deficient in fiber. This is unfortunate, because fiber is a highly effective toxin absorber within the digestive tract. Fiber can bind or dilute cancer-causing compounds in the digestive tract; prevent the formation of cancer-causing toxins from bile; promote the formation of anticancer short-chain fatty acids; and decrease the amount of time toxins from food spend in contact with the gut lining. Some compounds in fiber may have additional anticancer effects. Adequate dietary fiber has anti-inflammatory and immunity-improving characteristics and is essential for the proper health of the microbial residents of the digestive tract, known as the gut microbiome.

L-Glutamine

Glutamine, an amino acid, is the preferred fuel of enterocytes, the cells that form the delicate and metabolically active lining of the digestive tract. During stressful episodes, the body's need for glutamine increases, and this is especially true for the digestive tract. It is a highly versatile amino acid that also plays a role in detoxification and immunity. In fact, L-glutamine supplementation can help preserve the lining of the digestive tract. By maintaining normal gastrointestinal permeability, it can prevent or help reverse leaky gut syndrome. Because food-borne toxins are more easily able to enter the bloodstream through a more permeable gastrointestinal tract lining, L-glutamine supplementation may help protect the body from the negative consequences of allergens, microbes, and toxins in food.

DOSAGE SUGGESTIONS FOR DIGESTIVE AND GASTROINTESTINAL SUPPORT		
Nutrient or Intervention	Typical Daily Dose	Suggested Products
Probiotics including *L. acidophilus, B. lactis, L. paracasei, L. rhamnosus, B. bifidum/lacis, B. longum*	15 billion CFU	Forever Health Probiotic
Digestive enzyme blend	With each meal take 290 mg vegetarian digestive enzyme blend and 400 mg pancreatin alternative 8x blend	Forever Health Digestive Enzymes
Fiber	With 8 to 16 oz of water take 3,000 mg psyllium, 875 mg guar gum, and 875 mg apple pectin twice daily with meals	Life Extension Fiber Food Caps
L-glutamine	2000 mg	Life Extension L-Glutamine Powder

For your convenience, Forever Health has created a Healthy Digestion Kit for my readers.

CARDIOVASCULAR SUPPORT

Constant exposure to toxins creates ideal conditions for damaging inflammatory and oxidative reactions inside our bodies. This can cause particles of our LDL cholesterol to become oxidized. One dangerous consequence of this is the buildup of plaque in our arteries, which can rupture and cause a heart attack or stroke. Dr. Sinatra's interview explains why our Lp(a) number is so crucial (see page 159).

We can combat some of the vascular repercussions of pro-inflammatory toxins by taking supplements that help keep the walls of our blood vessels in good shape. In this section I'm going to outline some of the most important supplements to take for cardiovascular health, including B vitamins, pomegranate, magnesium, and potassium.

B Vitamins

B vitamins are essential for cardiovascular health because they help rid the body of a toxic metabolic by-product called homocysteine. Homocysteine is an amino acid that inflicts damage to the inner arterial lining (endothelium) and other cells of the body. Studies have shown that high homocysteine levels can increase the risk of stroke and heart attack.

To safely lower homocysteine, use vitamins B_{12} and B_6 and the active form of folate (5-methyltetrahyrofolate).

Magnesium and Potassium

The minerals magnesium and potassium are extremely important for heart health. They both help keep the heart beating in a normal rhythm. But many of us don't get enough magnesium and potassium from diet alone. I recommend taking magnesium and potassium each day.

Pomegranate

Pomegranate is rich in powerful antioxidant molecules that can help offset the oxidative stress induced by toxins. Research shows that pomegranate confers unprecedented cardiovascular protection by restoring the health of the cells that line the insides of our blood vessels, lowering blood pressure, and protecting low-density lipoprotein (LDL) from damaging oxidation. Pomegranate extract has proven its ability to protect the heart from a damaging cardiotoxin that is used in cancer treatment, doxorubicin. Doxorubicin damages the heart at least in part through its generation of free radicals. Pomegranate extract has the unique ability to boost one of the body's essential internal detoxification and antioxidant enzymes, superoxide dismutase. Super-oxide dismutase plays an important role in protecting the body from environmental toxins.

In addition, scientific evidence indicates pomegranate flower extract and seed oil uniquely complement conventional pomegranate fruit extract's capacity to combat multiple diseases of aging.

Look for a pomegranate supplement that is standardized to punicalagins and contains extracts of pomegranate flower and seed, as well as the fruit.

Probiotics—for Your Heart

Intriguing evidence shows that a certain probiotic organism can boost heart health. One strain of probiotic in particular—*Lactobacillus reuteri* 30242—favorably modulates several cardiovascular risk factors, including cholesterol, CRP, fibrinogen, apoB-100, and vitamin D.

Don't Forget CoQ10 and Fish Oil!

There are a few nutrients that deserve a double mention in this chapter. I've already talked about CoQ10 (in the form of ubiquinol) and omega-3 fatty acids elsewhere, but these two are also of the utmost importance for cardiovascular health.

DOSAGE SUGGESTIONS FOR CARDIOVASCULAR SUPPORT		
Nutrient or Intervention	Typical Daily Dose	Suggested Products
Omega-3 fatty acids	700 mg EPA and 500 mg DHA twice daily with food	Forever Health Omega-3 Fish Oil Complex
Vitamin B$_6$	250 mg with food	Life Extension Homocysteine Resist
Vitamin B$_{12}$	500 mcg with food	
Active form of folic acid 5-methyltetrahydrofolate (5-MTHF)	400 mcg	
Magnesium (as magnesium oxide, citrate, succinate, TRAACS® magnesium lysyl glycinate chelate)	500 mg one to three times daily	Life Extension Magnesium Caps
Pomegranate extract	537 mg	Life Extension Full-Spectrum Pomegranate™
L. reuteri NCIMB 30242	2.5 billion CFU twice daily	Life Extension FlorAssist® Heart Health
CoQ10 as ubiquinol	100 mg or more depending on blood test results	Forever Health CoQ10 Mitochondrial Support Complex

HORMONAL SUPPORT

Hormonal support is crucial. Lab testing for hormonal deficiencies is essential and can be done either through ForeverHealth.com or Life Extension, www.lef.org/tox-sick. Testing will determine your hormonal deficiencies (for women and men) and will indicate to your qualified doctor (again, find one at ForeverHealth.com) the amount determined just for you with your individualized complement of hormones. As I've said many times, my previous books on hormones are comprehensive and will explain hormones extensively, if you have any questions. To see the full array of my many books on hormones and replacement, go to SuzanneSomers.com.

But there now are other factors that could impact your replacement and the following supplements can be used in conjunction with BHRT. Environmental toxins can impact our bodies in sly, subtle ways. For example, several common toxins, like bisphenol A and phthalates, may disrupt hormone signaling. Some environmental endocrine disruptors can interact directly with the estrogen receptors in our bodies or interfere with natural estrogen production and metabolism. So those hot flashes and menopausal symptoms may be related to environmental toxins!

To support your hormones in a toxic environment, you can take natural products that help support healthy function, including DHEA, Norway spruce lignan extract, vitex, and hops extract.

DHEA

DHEA is produced by the adrenal glands. It serves as a precursor to the hormones testosterone and estrogen. In the past several years alone, significant scientific substantiation of DHEA's antiaging effects has emerged. Its neuroprotective effects are now recognized as being vital in protecting memory and reducing depressive symptoms as we age. DHEA modulates immunity in a coordinated fashion, boosting resistance to infection while quelling dangerous inflammation. DHEA supports cardiovascular health and activates genes that prevent cardiovascular risk factors, including diabetes and obesity. DHEA also enhances bone health by improving mineralization to reduce fracture risk. The hormone is intimately involved in improving quality of life and bolstering sexual arousal, while dramatically improving the appearance of healthy, youthful skin. Supplementing with DHEA may favorably alter gene expression to inhibit multiple factors implicated in metabolic syndrome; boost bone strength; enhance cognitive function and memory; and ward off osteoarthritis.

You can test your levels of DHEA and other hormones by ordering a blood test from Life Extension. They offer comprehensive hormone blood testing for both men and women.

Norway Spruce Lignan Extract

The Norway spruce (*Picea abies*) produces abundant quantities of the plant lignan *7-hydroxymatairesinol*, or HMR. In the digestive tract, HMR is converted to an active compound called enterolactone. Both HMR and enterolactone are mild phytoestrogens, and as such, offer additional support for women undergoing menopausal transition.

In one important study, menopausal women supplemented with HMR lignan for eight weeks. The supplement was readily absorbed and distributed in the women's bodies, raising 7-HMR levels in the blood. The study found HMR lignan was able to produce about a 50 percent reduction in the mean number of weekly hot flashes, from 28 to 14.3.

Vitex

Vitex agnus-castus (chasteberry) contains compounds in both the berry and the leaf that have been shown to induce relief of common menopausal symptoms. Studies attribute these effects to activation of estrogen receptors, indicating that the plant has beneficial phytoestrogen properties.

Hops Extract

Hops are the female flowers of the hop plant (*Humulus lupulus*). Their bitter, floral taste has been used for centuries as a flavoring and natural preservative in beer. But they also contain specialized glands that secrete natural bioactive molecules that offer benefits for human health.

Among these compounds is the molecule 8-prenylnaringenin (8-PN), which research suggests is a very effective *phytoestrogen* (plant-derived estrogen-like molecule). These estrogenic properties make hops and 8-PN extremely attractive for use during menopause, when estrogen levels drop and produce an array of unpleasant symptoms.

The estrogenic properties of hops extracts, and particularly of 8-PN, are known to alleviate menopausal symptoms and disorders, including osteoporosis, hot flashes, and low sex drive. 8-PN also has the benefit of being rapidly and almost completely absorbed after being orally consumed.

DOSAGE SUGGESTIONS FOR HORMONAL SUPPORT		
Nutrient or Intervention	Typical Daily Dose	Suggested Products
DHEA	Best determined by blood testing. Generally, 25–75 mg in the morning.	Forever Health DHEA
Norway spruce lignan extract	56 mg	Life Extension Natural Estrogen
Vitex	20 mg	
Hops extract	120 mg	

ROUNDING IT ALL OUT—MULTIVITAMINS AND VITAMIN D

Throughout this chapter we've reviewed several supplemental nutrients that are important for specific purposes. But there are two others that are all-important for your overall health and can't be easily categorized: a comprehensive multivitamin and vitamin D.

Vitamin D

Just a few years ago, vitamin D was simply known as the "bone vitamin." But data now show that nearly every tissue and cell type in the body has receptors for vitamin D. As a result of this discovery, we now know that much higher doses are required for optimal functioning. This discovery has radically changed how we understand the role of vitamin D in the body.

Unless your vitamin D levels are optimal, you are opening the door to a host of disorders, ranging from heart disease and Alzheimer's to weak bones and diabetes.

In fact, even if you have normal blood sugar today, a vitamin D deficiency makes you 91 percent more likely to progress to insulin resistance, or "prediabetes," and it more than doubles your risk for progressing to active, type 2 diabetes.

Vitamin D and its receptors play a surprisingly important role in the body's detoxification systems for both internally created and environmental toxins. An example of this role as it relates to internal toxins is that the vitamin D receptor is also a receptor for a type of bile that is a liver toxin, which can promote colon cancer. When activated by vitamin D, the receptor activates an enzyme that detoxifies this bile compound in the liver and intestines, which may explain why vitamin D appears protective against colon cancer.

Unfortunately, vitamin D deficiency is a global epidemic. An estimated 1 billion people do not have adequate vitamin D levels. And 64 percent of Americans don't have enough vitamin D to keep all their tissues operating at peak capacity.

The results of this deficiency are catastrophic. Studies have now shown that vitamin D deficiency is associated with increased risk of a long list of diseases that span all systems in the body. In fact, low levels of vitamin D are associated with an almost twentyfold increased risk of non-Alzheimer's dementia!

Vitamin D testing is very important: without testing your levels of vitamin D, you won't be able to optimize your supplement dosage. You can order a vitamin D blood test from Life Extension.

Multivitamins

Evidence shows that the nutritional content of fruits and vegetables has declined significantly since the 1950s. So even if we're eating all the right foods, we might still not be getting all the right nutrients. That's why it's so important to round out any supplement plan with a comprehensive multivitamin that contains not only vitamins and minerals but also other natural compounds like plant extracts rich in phytochemicals that help protect our cells from free-radical damage and inflammation.

Studies have shown that multivitamin supplementation confers meaningful benefits. In one comprehensive review, there was a trend for reduced risk of death from any cause among multivitamin users compared with control subjects. Other evidence suggests multivitamin use might even improve some aspects of memory and prevent cancer in some individuals.

MULTIVITAMINS AND VITAMIN D		
Nutrient or Intervention	Typical Daily Dose	Suggested Products
High-potency, comprehensive multivitamin	Per label instructions	Forever Health Complete Multivitamin with Minerals
Vitamin D$_3$	Typically 5,000–8,000 IU depending on blood test results	Life Extension Vitamin D$_3$

WHERE TO FIND RECOMMENDED SUPPLEMENTS AND REMEDIES

At SuzanneSomers.com, you will find many options for supplements, as well as links to ForeverHealth.com and Life Extension.com/tox-sick. Forever Health offers many of the recommended ingredients in this section. Their high-quality products are selected for purity and potency. If you are overwhelmed by the numerous suggestions, start with the kits they have put together for my readers.

Another trusted source for vitamins, supplements, and testing needs is Life Extension, an organization dedicated to rigorous medical science. You can reach them by calling toll-free at 1-866-585-1398 or logging on to www.lef.org/tox-sick. Readers of my book will receive special discounted pricing on all the supplements mentioned in this chapter. Call or visit now and also receive a free issue of *Life Extension*® magazine and a catalog of their latest products.

FOOD, GLORIOUS FOOD

Taking an assortment of powerful antioxidants can prevent free-radical damage. But don't forget the food! Eat a diet that includes nutrient-dense vegetables and a few fruits (mainly berries) . . . and of course healthy fats.

A good diet should include broccoli, Brussels sprouts, cabbage, greens, onions, garlic, ginger, celery, shallots, and kale. Blending them together is the best way to get the full benefit of nutrients (throw in an apple or a banana to make it taste better). Also drink at least six to eight 12-ounce glasses of pure water each day. Avoid fluoridated water like *the plague.*

Many of the things and appliances that were designed to make our lives easier and better have worked against us. Giving up favorite foods is always hard at first. I love sugar. That was very difficult for me. I had such cravings, but today I don't think about it at all. Instead, every time I put on a dress from yesterday that fits perfectly today and is not tight at the waist or tight through the abdomen, or that I don't have to be afraid to sit down in because my stomach will bulge over, I become thankful. Sugar was a "happy meal" for the mold, yeast, and bacterial overgrowth in my intestines. I had to give it up to get well. Sugar and carbs were my obstacles to good health. I thought I was doing everything right, but it wasn't until I decided to go cold turkey and give them up that I started seeing and feeling results. I feel lucky because eventually sugar would have had a negative effect on my health, maybe even causing a return of cancer, so I forced myself to give it up, and the result is that I feel better all the time. My stomach is flat again and I like the way my body looks at age sixty-eight.

When you factor into the equation that healthy fats are good for you and incorporate them into your diet regularly, you will find, like me, that you're always satiated. If I am craving something (anything), where I once would have gone for sugar or carbs, I now get myself a piece of cheese, or I have a slice of my fabulous toasted seed bread slathered with organic sweet butter.

Enjoy, but Remember: There Is No Free Lunch

Eating fats is not a free-for-all! It's important to understand *how* to eat fats and *what* kinds of fats are healthy and what you can eat them with. If you are thinking about hot toast with melted butter dripping down the sides, I have to put an end to that fantasy right now. Eating butter *with* carbs is a problem. These two together will be accepted by the body as sugar. This combination will work against you (and make you fat). To heal your abdominal pain and bloating, healthy fats need to be added to your diet, but you cannot have carbs with them for now . . . or at all depending on your health.

Carbs are sugar. Remember the little bad guys in your gut? They are begging for sugar and in order to heal, you have to starve the little bad guys (bacteria) to death. Consider this a war that you are going to win!

So, no to toast with butter, but, yes, toss your steamed vegetables in as much butter and sea salt or olive oil as you desire. Put a pat of butter on that seared, grass-fed steak at the end to melt into the juices. This is the way to eat your fats, making the good food that your body needs delicious as well as satiating.

Soon you will find you can easily walk away from the dinner table without even thinking about sugary foods. The object is to heal, and to do that, you must consume healthy fats and eliminate carbs and sugar until the problem goes away. Plus eating fats without carbs allows you to eat until you are full or satiated. For those of you who have followed my Somersizing programs over the years, you already know the joys of a nice wedge of cheddar in the afternoon, when you normally might have gone to the vending machine to get some sugary, chemical-laden foods loaded with dangerous trans fats. And I promise, eating this way, you will never have to feel hungry.

When I say healthy fats, I am talking about *organic* animal fats: grass-fed meats, organic cheeses, butter, dairy (if you are not allergic).

What I am *not* talking about are the standard American dietary fats, including hydrogenated fats, margarine, trans fats, unhealthy vegetable oils that are processed with chemicals for shelf life and color stabilization. I am not talking about nasty fast-food fats; those are harmful, even deadly.

Not All Sat Fats Are Equal

It's important to note that all saturated fats are not created equal. The operative word here is *created*. Because some saturated fats occur naturally, while other fats are artificially manipulated into a saturated state through the man-made process called hydrogenation.

Hydrogenation manipulates vegetable and seed oils by adding hydrogen atoms while heating the oil, producing a rancid, thickened substance that really only benefits processed food shelf life and big business profits. It is generally agreed upon that hydrogenation does *nothing* good for your health.

These manipulated saturated fats are also called trans fats, and you should avoid them like the plague. Extra-virgin olive oil is the best monounsaturated fat and works great as a salad dressing. However, as Dr. Sinatra told me, olive oil should not be used for cooking. Due to its chemical structure, heat makes olive oil susceptible to oxidative damage. So for cooking, I use coconut oil most of the time. Omega-6 vegetable oils such as soy, corn, and safflower oils produce a variety of very toxic chemicals, as well as form trans fats. Frying destroys the antioxidants in oil, actually oxidizing the oil, which causes even worse problems for your body than trans fats. The only oil that is stable enough to withstand the heat of cooking is coconut oil.

LET'S REVIEW

To achieve peak health you should

    • Change your diet so that it includes organic healthy fats: grass-fed animal protein, wild-caught salmon, organic butter, cream, and dairy products.
    • Eat healthy oils containing essential fatty acids, such as olive oil, flaxseed oil, coconut oil.
    • Eliminate all processed foods.
    • Eliminate all sugar until you are healed.
    • Eliminate all carbs until you are healed.
    • Supplement for survival with what it is you require from The Protocol.

Make these changes along with the supplementation we discussed and your gut will begin to work correctly, your brain will become sharp again, and you'll get skinnier, healthier, and happier.

Keeping a Healthy Heart

Remember, cholesterol is not the problem; inflammation is the problem, and inflammation is part of the aging process. So as we get older we have to work harder.

To check for your inflammation levels ask your doctor to order the highly sensitive CRP (C-reactive protein) blood test to determine your inflammation levels.

And above all avoid the major source of oxidized oil, which is what most fast-food restaurants use: omega-6 oils. Another source of oxidized (used and damaged) oils (the list continues) is foods that are processed with polyunsaturated vegetable oils, which are a major ingredient in most fast foods and are highly regarded as foods that lead to high levels of *inflammation*: a minute on your lips is a fast track to your heart attack. It goes on: most bottled salad dressings also contain oxidized oils, even if the label says extra-virgin olive oil.

Again, it comes back to the FOOD. The food you choose determines your health and outcome. Choosing healthy fats and healthy oils—virgin organic coconut oil, extra-virgin organic olive oil, flaxseed oil, organic butter—is "heart protective" and *inflammation* lowering. Processed fats and trans fats are dangerous to your health and heart.

MAKING YOUR OWN PROBIOTICS

Remember, you cannot heal your body without probiotic supplementation because probiotics are ESSENTIAL for health!

They are your army; without them your effort to heal is not going to work. I'll say it again: Commit to taking daily probiotics for the rest of your life. The environment is working against all of us, toxins are everywhere, chemicals are in all the food except organic. So be smart. You have the power to heal yourself.

Fermented foods go way back in history, when people "fermented" their foods most likely because refrigeration was nonexistent. For thousands of years people fermented milk, producing the first yogurts and kefir; they also fermented some fruits, vegetables, beans, fish, meats, and even cereals. Fermenting food improves its taste, makes food more digestible, and preserves it. Many cultures around the world routinely consume beneficial bacteria in fermented foods like sauerkraut, fermented fish, grains, and fermented soy beans.

I regularly make my own yogurt and homemade sauerkraut from homegrown cabbages. Both of these foods are easy to prepare and are an easy and delectable way to prepare your stomach for digestion. What follows are my personal recipes for each. Store-bought yogurt is questionable due to transport problems and time spent without refrigeration. As in, for instance, how long did the cases of packaged yogurt sit in the store parking lot?

Fermented foods aside, the easiest way to replace missing gut flora is supplementation.

Sauerkraut—Better Than the Dog It Comes With

In America, sauerkraut is something we sometimes eat with our chemical-laden hot dog piled on a white nutrition-less Wonder bun made from grains most likely genetically modified and bleached with other chemicals to make that flour "whiter than white."

It originated, though, with German immigrants who came to America and brought their old-world recipes, serving German sausage with homemade sauerkraut. Over the years that lovely first introduction degenerated into those dangerous hot dogs filled with nitrates and God knows whatever other chemicals that we chow down. And whereas sauerkraut was once given as an option with your hot dog, now it is rarely offered, probably for economics. We are happy with the white bun, the chemical dog, and mustard.

Sauerkraut is regularly eaten today in Germany, Russia, Poland, Eastern Europe, and many other countries. There is a reason these cultures have had fermented foods, in particular sauerkraut, in their diets, going back hundreds of years. Nature did not know that in modern times we would have refrigeration. To survive, these cultures needed to be able to preserve certain foods to have nutrition available in the harsh winter months when growing was impossible. That and the fact that cabbages grow abundantly in this part of the world made for the perfect match.

It was a natural course of life to find a way to save these foods for winter survival. But nature also had a plan, and that was to keep the GI tract healthy and balanced by constantly replacing probiotics with foods like sauerkraut. It is unlikely that restoring the GI tract to a perfect balance of microflora was ever given a thought; instead this was simply a smart staple for meals served along with preserved meats and fish.

Sauerkraut is a wonderful healing remedy for the digestive tract, full of digestive enzymes, probiotic bacteria, vitamins, and minerals. Eating it with meats will improve digestion, as it has a strong ability to stimulate stomach acid production. This helps people like me with low stomach acid. (Anyone who has had radiation for breast cancer was probably not told that radiation inhibits your body's ability to manufacture stomach acid [hydrochloric acid] for LIFE! And hydrochloric acid [HCL] is crucial to digest your food.)

A few tablespoons of sauerkraut ten to fifteen minutes before meals will seriously aid digestion. Regular intake of sauerkraut will assist greatly in relieving gas, bloating, constipation, and general stomach discomfort; and it is the best way to restore microflora balance in the GI tract and heal a distressed or damaged GI tract.

Dr. Natasha Campbell-McBride says, "For children, adding 1 to 3 tablespoons of the sauerkraut juice into their meals will greatly help to offset the damage already done to their fragile GI tracts from the chemicals and processed foods that are so available and damaging in today's world."

My recipes for sauerkraut and yogurt follow. Need I recommend that the ingredients you use be organic? No sense making something so healthy and then contaminating it with pesticides, chemicals, and GMOs. FYI: There is a difference between fermented foods and pickled foods. Pickled foods are made with vinegar. Fermented foods are pickled by the creation of lactic acid by the fermentation process: pickled foods have vinegar (acetic acid) added to create an acid environment for food preservation. So all fermented foods are pickled, but not all pickled foods are fermented. Your body can metabolize the lactic acid of fermented foods well but will not do well with vinegar-containing pickles.

SUZANNE'S SAUERKRAUT
  1 medium white or red cabbage, thinly sliced (or a mix of red and
    white)
  2 tablespoons good-quality sea salt*
  1 tablespoon caraway seeds
  Whole bulb of garlic, peeled and smashed
  ¼ teaspoon fresh or dried rosemary (fresh is best)
  ¼ teaspoon red pepper flakes

*Salt is essential as it will draw the juice from the cabbage during the kneading. In addition, salt will stifle the putrefactive microbes in the initial stages of fermentation until the fermenting bacteria produce enough lactic acid to kill the pathogens.

Combine all the ingredients in a large bowl. Knead the mixture well with clean hands until a lot of the juice comes out. If the cabbage is not juicy enough, add a little water. Pack this mixture into a suitable glass or enamel bowl, pressing it firmly so there is no air trapped and the cabbage is drowned in its own juice.

Fermentation is an anaerobic process; if the cabbage is exposed to air, or your container is not clean, it will rot instead of ferment. Place a plate on top of the cabbage (the plate should be slightly smaller than the opening of the bowl; this gap will allow the fermentation gases to escape). On top of the plate place something heavy enough to keep the cabbage constantly submerged in its juice. Cover the whole thing with a kitchen towel and keep it in the dark.

Let sit about 2 to 3 weeks. Then enjoy. It will keep in an airtight container in the fridge for 3 months.

Williams-Sonoma sells a jar that is perfect for making excellent sauerkraut. I found with mine that, after putting the cabbage mixture in the dark glass container, if I put a heavy, clean weight, such as a clean brick, on it, it will hold down the cabbage so it is airtight. You can also use a bag of water, triple bagged in Ziplocs, on top to hold down the cabbage so it is airtight. Be careful that you use more than one Ziploc bag; otherwise the salt and fermentation can "eat" through it. Triple bagging will fix the problem. Don't forget to leave about two inches of space in the jar at the top, as the cabbage will expand during fermentation.

If you are able to find an organic Ziploc bag—does that exist?—let me know.

That's it. Easy, old-world simplicity! I'm sure in cabbage season in Eastern Europe during our parents' generation, kitchens were filled with women making their own tasty sauerkraut. As with all old-world recipes, each woman most likely had her own version. Experiment; it's fun. You can season yours any way you desire. I found the flavors I added above to make a delicious tasty treat, and I now crave this sauerkraut every day. (The body knows what it needs.) As soon as I started incorporating homemade sauerkraut into my daily diet, I felt better and my bloating and discomfort became less and less by the day.

Yummy Yogurt

Another ages-old phenomenon was finding a way to preserve milk when refrigeration was not available in the home. As with so many old-world recipes, they usually came from a sense of practicality. Milk was prized and it makes sense that people needed to find a way to "keep it" when they didn't have modern-day conveniences.

If you have never made your own yogurt, you are in for a special treat. When you learn how to make natural probiotic yogurt at home, you'll never want store-bought! Making yogurt is very easy and the flavor is delicious. Natural homemade yogurt is rich in good probiotic bacteria and can help improve the immune system as well as aid digestion. Also probiotic foods and probiotic supplements have been shown to be effective in helping people to lose belly fat.

You can purchase a yogurt maker (I bought mine from Williams-Sonoma, but any gourmet kitchen supply store will have one). If you don't have a yogurt maker, then use the method below to keep the milk mixture warm. Yogurt makers are handy because they provide a convenient way to maintain the right temperature for the yogurt to develop; however, yogurt can easily be made without the use of a special yogurt maker.

NATURAL PROBIOTIC YOGURT

2 tablespoons freeze-dried bacteria culture or plain (unflavored) yogurt with active-live cultures (this is your starter)
1 quart organic milk (either goat or cow)*
⅓ cup nonfat dry milk

You can use any kind of milk you like: whole milk, soy milk (but only if it is organic), raw milk, powdered dry milk (organic only), goat's milk. The only kind of milk that doesn't work is ultra-high pasteurized because it is processed at such high temperatures that the proteins and bacteria necessary to turn the milk into yogurt are broken down. Experiment with different types of milk for different flavors and texture.

Remove the starter from the refrigerator and allow it to come to room temperature while you prepare the milk; this will ensure that it is not too cold when you add it to the warm milk mixture. (Your first batch of homemade yogurt will require either a freeze-dried bacteria culture or a purchased yogurt "starter," such as a plain [unflavored] yogurt with live-active bacteria. Once you have made your own yogurt, you will be able to use a little of your previous batch to inoculate the next batch.)

Heat the milk to 185°F, either very carefully on the burner or by using a double boiler. If you do not have a double boiler, you can create one by placing a bowl or small pan on top of another pan that will hold the water. Be sure to watch the milk carefully so that it does not scorch. Stir occasionally. If you place the pan directly on a burner, you will want to slowly and continuously stir.

Note: If you are using raw milk that has not been pasteurized or processed in any other way, you don't need to heat it. You can just skip this step. Raw milk has its own bacterial population, so the fermentation is not going to be as controlled as with using heated milk. That means your yogurt may turn out to be more liquid or lumpy or sour than you expect.

Remove the milk from the heat and cool to 110°F. You can lower the temperature quickly and evenly by placing the pan in a cool water bath and stirring occasionally. Do not allow the milk to cool too much; watch carefully and proceed with the next step when the temperature reaches 110°F.

Stir in the nonfat dry milk. This will not only enhance the nutritional quality of the yogurt but it will also help it to thicken. Stir in the yogurt culture or freeze-dried bacteria culture starter. Ferment the yogurt for at least 24 hours or as long as 2 days. After fermentation is complete, move your yogurt to a clean glass jar, cover, and refrigerate.

By using cream instead of milk you can make crème fraîche or sour cream. (For 1 cup of cream use one packet of commercial starter, or ½ cup of live yogurt from your original batch.)

Homemade yogurt tends to be thinner than the commercially prepared yogurts. This is because most commercial brands include thickening agents such as starch, gum, pectin, or gelatin. Without these additional thickeners, your yogurt will naturally be somewhat thinner in consistency. For a thicker consistency, after combining ingredients, place cheesecloth in a colander and place the colander in a large bowl; pour the yogurt into the colander and put a plate on top of it.

Set in the refrigerator and let the whey drain out of the yogurt. If you let the yogurt drain for a couple of hours, you will end up with Greek yogurt; if you leave it overnight, the yogurt will be very thick, almost like cream cheese. Adjust the thickness by how long you leave the yogurt to drain. If it becomes too thick, you can also stir some whey back in to lighten it up some.

HOW TOXIC ARE YOU? GET TESTED

If you are concerned about your "toxic burden," ask your doctor to prescribe the Estronex Urine Test. This will show levels of tricothecenes (chemical levels) such as pesticides, cadmium, mercury, heavy metals, diesel fumes, and many more. For genetic testing, go to ForeverHealth.com.

CLEANING HOUSE—SAFE PRODUCTS AND PROTECTORS

Skin Care

The skin is the largest organ in the body. If you were to look at your skin under a microscope, you would see what look like big holes, which are what we know as pores. Think of that visual every time you rub a lotion or potion on your skin that is chemically based.

I became cognizant of this problem in trying to lower my own personal toxic burden. I no longer wanted to actively add to my toxicity through chemical-based body and skin care products regardless of how expensive or how magical the claims they make.

I tried organic product after product. I liked the idea, but none of them were doing the job as I would have liked. That's when I decided to develop my own line. I work with a formulator who is as passionate as I am, and together we have created an organic, certified toxic-free line that surpasses anything I have ever used from any high-end department store.

Did you know that almost all the makeup you've been using all these years has plastic as a main ingredient? With this book, you can begin to see the devastation chemicals are causing to the human body. And did you also know most lipsticks have lead in them? Lead is extremely toxic to the brain and bones; and the list goes on.

My makeup is filled with "good for you" ingredients, with lipsticks that are creamy and gorgeous, with no lead and no chemicals, mascara with no chemicals, and no GLUE! Yes, the mascara that is so hard to take off after a long night has GLUE in it. Imagine.

All my makeup is from nature. It's a feel-good feeling to wear it, and best of all, it beats all the chemical products makeup artists have been using on my face all these years.

Hair Care

One day I was in my shower and looked at the dozens of hair care products I had lined up on the bench: shampoos, extrarich shampoos, conditioners, extrarich conditioners, then hair masks, and extra-, extrarich conditioners. I had spent thousands on hair care products throughout the years, all of which eventually dried out my hair because of their toxic chemicals.

So once again, I went back to my formulator, and through trial and error we came up with the greatest shampoo and conditioner I've ever used. Now in my shower I have two bottles: shampoo and conditioner, both by Suzanne Organics.

When you put it all together, you will see how using toxic-free products for skin, body, hair, and face eliminates a huge portion of the toxins from your everyday life. If the solution to environmental illness and stress on the body is detoxification, then this is a huge way to start diminishing your toxic burden, all the while getting healthier and more beautiful. I now have people ordering my products from all over the world.

Your Nontoxic Household

What is the point of eating clean, consuming grass-fed or wild-caught protein, avoiding GMOs and pesticides, putting reverse osmosis filters on your faucets and showers, eliminating chlorine from your swimming pools and instead using saline or ozone as purifiers, if you are going to clean your house with dangerous toxins?

What is the point of switching from skin care with chemicals and dangerous parabens to organic, nontoxic formulations, if your home is going to be a haven for chemicals coming from your household cleaners?

The solution is to go organic in every aspect of your life. This is how you will survive and get well. I hear over and over, "But it doesn't get things white enough." Or "It's not strong enough." Well, there are now such products that are safe and do the job perfectly.

Cleaning House

If you haven't cared about this aspect until now, here is why it's a good idea to switch over to nontoxic cleaning agents:

- One out of every three chemical cleaning products contains ingredients known to cause human health or environmental problems.
- Commercial cleaning companies are under no legal obligation to research how their products might harm human health.

Which leads me to this: How can *you* find the best, healthiest, and safest cleaning products to use in your home? Here are some helpful hints for what to look for, regardless of a product's name, labeling, or database rating:

- Packaging should have full disclosure of *all* ingredients.
- Ingredients should be derived from plants and minerals.
- Products must not contain petroleum-derived or petro-chemical ingredients.
- Labels should stipulate the origin of fragrance and whether it is naturally derived or not.
- All ingredients should be biodegradable.
- Products must have no animal testing or animal-derived ingredients.
- Finished products must be safe for septic tanks and gray water.
- Products must not be corrosive.
- Products must not contain compounds that cause or contribute to the creation of greenhouse gases or ozone depletion.

- Products must be free of any known human carcinogens, mutagens, teratogens, and endocrine disruptors.

At SuzanneSomers.com you can purchase toxic-free skin care, makeup, and household cleaners. Because of the importance of making this critical change in my personal sphere to protect myself and my family from the environmental toxic assault, my company has devoted years to devising a line of quality products.

Baby Care

When a mother takes her newborn from the hospital, she is usually given a parting gift of well-known baby products: lotions and powders and ointments. Most hospitals are given these "gifts" from well-known traditional baby product companies, and all of these products are laden with chemicals. For many, the first ingredient is sodium laureth sulphate. Any time you see the letters -eth inserted into a word, it is a code for chemicals. Stay away from it. Imagine, taking a little baby, already toxic from the inherited toxins through the mother's exposure to the environment, and then further contaminating the baby with more chemicals, all in the name of trying to do something good for him or her.

Take a few minutes to look up these chemicals so you understand the dangers and what to avoid:

- Sodium hydroxymethylglycinate: Current research indicates this ingredient may turn into formaldehyde in the body. If true, this would be a particular concern if found in a moisturizer, which is designed to permeate the skin.
- Bis-PEG/PPG-16/16 dimethicone: Restricted in the use and manufacturing of cosmetics. Not safe for use on injured or damaged skin.
- Disodium EDTA (different from chelating EDTA as referenced in Dr. Gordon's interview): EDTA is used in calcium and sodium compounds to preserve food; and to promote the color, texture, and flavor of food.
- Benzyl alcohol: This compound is used as a preservative. The

problem with it is that young children cannot metabolize benzyl alcohol into hippuric acid using benzoic acid, which can result in an accumulation of chiefly benzoic acid. The side effects that have been described as a result of this substance accumulating in the central nervous system include metabolic acidosis, vasodilation, paralysis, epileptic seizures, respiratory depression, and death.

Rx for EMFs

The goal is to eliminate or reduce the exposure to everything electrical in the areas where you spend the most time. The less radiation in your environment, the more your body will have an opportunity to recover from the assault that it has to endure while being in today's public areas with Wi-Fi and other EMF exposures. The more you can eliminate these contaminants from your life, the better off you and your family will be.

- The first thing you can do is refuse to have the utility company install the new smart meter in your home. Unfortunately, there will be a small monthly fine (which annoys me), but it's worth it to eliminate an electromagnetic grid covering your whole house.
- Do not sleep with your laptop, cell phone, or computer. Most people recharge their phones and laptops next to the bed. You can be sure you are getting EMFs and rads all during your sleep. Imagine what it is doing to your brain and the brains of your children.
- At work, ask not to have your seat or desk near walls that have PBX phone systems, banks of computer servers, or high-voltage electrical services. You can be "hit" through windows. If there is a choice, choose to sit next to a wall to reduce the exposure from outside sources.
- Grounding provides the body the return of the normal electrical charge on the blood cells, which allows them to separate and go back to their normal disklike shape. This can occur within a half hour of grounding. I use a grounding sheet on my bed

nightly. For more information you can go to grounded.com and click through to the shop cart for earthing. Obtain a grounding mat to place under your feet while working on your computer at home and work.

- Daily walking provides grounding for EMF release and corrections in your body. Walking either on fresh-cut (unsprayed) lawn, dirt, ground, or sand daily will provide tremendous health benefits in addition to exercise.
- In your kitchen: do not use microwave ovens. Radiation can leak through the door. The FDA advises not to stand against or directly in front of the oven while it is operating; that should tell you something!
- Home environments can be investigated if you hire a biological environmental building inspector. Costs vary but suffice it to say it is not inexpensive. It depends on your exposure and the information you need to know to be able to determine how much a part EMFs are playing in your downgraded health.
- Order a sterling silver, EMF-protective pendant to wear daily.

Cell Phones: Turning the Dangers Off

- If your cell phone has a speaker or a hands-free speaker, use it rather than holding it next to your head. There are air tube headsets that can also increase the distance from the phone. Wireless earpieces like Bluetooth put out less radiation, but people are wearing the devices for hours each day and creating an antenna on the side of their heads. Your brain tissue is still being exposed, which disrupts cell activity and glucose metabolism, increasing the risk of cancer to those areas.
- When your distance from a cell tower is farther away, you have to use more power to make the connection. In this case you take the full "hit." Try to only use your cell phone if four bars of reception are indicated.
- Don't carry your cell phone in your pants or breast pocket. Anywhere you carry this device becomes an antenna, bringing up its signal to the body parts in that area. Young boys who are placing cell phones in their pockets are risking becoming infertile.

- Pregnant women should keep their cell phones or wireless devices away from their bodies, especially around the stomach area.

Cell phones are something we seemingly can't live without. But they are also potentially dangerous. They now have GPS (global positioning systems) designed to transmit periodically to update their location, even when turned off. Amazingly, the only way to stop this pulsing is to take the battery out, which is a nuisance. The greatest protection is an inexpensive chip made by LifeWave. I highly recommend the Matrix 2 chip for your iPhone to protect you from electromagnetic radiation by 98 percent (go to SuzanneSomers.com, and click on LifeWave). Unfortunately, at present there is no chip for your laptop, computer, or iPad. The LifeWave Company is working on it, though, so the future holds promise.

- Don't use your cell phone as your alarm clock unless it has the Matrix 2 chip.
- Children's brains are more susceptible to radiation, so kids should not be given cell phones and tablets unless their phones have a Matrix 2 chip. Without it, cell phones are hazardous for them, and confirmed EMF exposure (such as that experienced with smart meters) will have an impact on their future health.

CHAPTER 10

ADVANCED TECHNIQUES

FOR SO LONG MANY OF US HAVE CARRIED OUR INDIVIDUAL TOXIC burdens and the conditions that come with them. They are now just part of how we always feel: fatigued, sluggish, uncomfortable, bloated, depressed, with headaches, rashes, acne, brain fog, and so much more. Once you clear the toxins out of the body, everything will start working better: the brain will start functioning at optimum again and hormones can become balanced. Once cleared of this TOX-sickness, you will realize how much toxicity has dragged down your quality of life. It's as though you get a brand-new shot at life.

Here are some advanced techniques and strategies to explore with your physician that will help get you to full healing.

COCONUT OIL DETOX

The coconut can be viewed as nature's medicine chest. The products derived from it—meat, oil, milk, and water—can be used to nourish the body, prevent disease, heal injuries, and overcome sickness.

Coconut oil is unique. Unlike most other dietary oils, it gives multiple nutritional and medicinal properties. Coconut oil is a healthy oil because it is composed of medium-chain fatty acids (MCFAs or MCTs), and they are what give it its remarkable nutritional and medicinal properties. There has been a prejudice about coconut oil until recently. It got a bad rap its first time out due to a general misunderstanding of saturated fats. Coconut oil has been proven to digest more easily and can provide a quick and easy source of nutrition without taxing the enzyme systems of the body.

When coconut oil is added into the diet, it enhances the absorption of minerals such as magnesium and calcium, some of the B vitamins, the fat-soluble vitamins (A, D, E, K, and beta-carotene), and some amino acids. Coconut oil in your diet can help keep you alert and gives a quick energy boost, and unlike caffeine, the effects of coconut oil can last many hours, yet you don't develop a dependence on it.

With raw, virgin, organic coconut oil there is no cooking, pasteurization, fumigation, hydrogenation, or other artificial process involved. This is all about harvesting the coconut meat, drying it, and then pressing out the oils to be captured, filtered, and packaged. It is probably the most natural process you can find for consuming coconut oil other than picking and eating the coconut yourself. It's important to note *hydrogenated* coconut oil is harmful; use only virgin, organic coconut oil.

In addition, coconut oil has a surprisingly long shelf life—up to several years on the shelf due to its ability to naturally resist oxidation. When stored in the refrigerator, it is naturally a solid. When warmed in ambient room temperature, it becomes a liquid.

I take four teaspoons of virgin, organic coconut oil daily for four reasons: first and foremost it is a great daily detox; second, it is a great source of omega-3 essential fatty acids; third, it provides great benefit to healing the intestinal tract and building up the barrier wall; and, fourth, it's a great source of energy.

My housekeeper of many years is from Sri Lanka. She was the first person to introduce me to coconut oil. I too had been misinformed and thought it was a heart clogger. But she started cooking vegetables with it and they tasted better; then occasionally she would treat me with her fabulous chicken curry using coconut oil. I started reading up on the benefits and was impressed. She would tell me how her culture used coconut oil for just about everything: burns, cuts, snakebites, hair oil, and skin oil; in fact, learning of its many benefits for skin is in large part why my Suzanne Organics skin care has coconut oil as a main ingredient in many of the lotions and hair care products. It makes everything shiny and soft. When applied topically, it has been found to have antiaging, regenerative effects.

Coconut oil has actually been shown to help optimize body weight, which can dramatically reduce your risk of developing type 2 diabetes. But besides weight loss, boosting your metabolic rate will improve your energy, accelerate healing, and improve your overall immune function. And several studies have now shown that MCTs can enhance physical or athletic performance. And finally, as we have already discussed, coconut oil is incredibly good for your heart.

As you know by now, detoxification is essential in today's world. And guess what else coconut is good for? Coconut oil is a great (and simple) way to detox. But because it requires not eating anything for three days, please check with your qualified doctor to see if your body can tolerate this protocol.

To Do the Detox

A coconut oil cleanse is a very simple detoxification method that replaces regular food with coconut oil, usually for about three days or less, whatever you can handle. Talk to your physician and begin there. Start your day with two tablespoons of coconut oil and take one to two tablespoons throughout the day as necessary, up to twelve tablespoons total each day.

Take the coconut oil plain if you enjoy it that way, but if you can't tolerate swallowing the oil straight, you can mix it with warm lemon water or plain organic yogurt if necessary. You can use Somersweet all-natural sweetener or stevia if you'd like to sweeten the lemon water or yogurt, but no sugar should be consumed during the cleanse.

The best kind of coconut oil to use to detoxify is organic, raw, extra-virgin coconut oil (check my website for an upcoming line of Suzanne Organics coconut products that use organic raw coconut oil). Do not use anything but virgin organic coconut oil, which is completely unrefined, cold-pressed, unbleached, and not deodorized. This ensures you are getting the maximum natural benefits from your coconut oil.

I happen to love the taste of coconut oil, but some people can't handle it at first (it's an acquired taste). I visualize all the goodness it is doing for me and I actually look forward to my four teaspoons a day. If you have never taken coconut oil before, then you'll want to let your body adjust by slowly incorporating it into your diet before trying a coconut oil detox.

Start with one-half to one teaspoon, three times per day. Gradually work your way up to one to three tablespoons four times daily before you start your detox. It may take two weeks to work up to the full amount. When you feel comfortable eating this much coconut oil, then you should be ready to start a coconut oil detox.

Some people will experience "die-off" symptoms when they begin a coconut oil detox. These symptoms are often flulike, including headaches, joint stiffness, dizziness, and foggy thinking. This is good. It means it is working. Depending on your individual toxic burden, your die-off will be commensurate with your discomfort or lack thereof. Die-off may not feel so good, but it's a sign that your body is ridding itself of harmful toxins like fungal organisms. Die-off symptoms usually only last for three to five days, but you can ease them by gradually introducing coconut oil to your diet before doing a detox.

During a coconut oil detox, it's important to drink plenty (at least eight glasses daily) of filtered water to nourish the body and facilitate cleansing benefits.

Here is a recipe for a delicious drink that can replenish you during a cleanse:

1 cup pure lemon juice
6 cups filtered water
1 teaspoon sea salt

The lemon juice has cleansing properties, and the sea salt replaces minerals that may be lost during a cleanse. Add Somersweet or stevia for a sweeter taste, but do not sweeten with any kind of sugar.

Remember, if you have medical conditions or if you are on prescription medications, it's important to talk with your physician before trying a coconut oil cleanse.

> If you fail to plan, you are planning to fail!

COFFEE AND BENTONITE ENEMAS

Enemas have been around as a means of detoxification for almost four thousand years. One of the earliest medical textbooks ever discovered, the Ebers Papyrus, found in the sands of Egypt, shows that physicians of long ago were already using enemas to help the body cleanse itself and fight off disease. In India, Ayurvedic medicine also utilizes detoxification methods, including colon cleansing, to treat many chronic conditions and to prevent illness. Enemas are such a powerful healing tool, they are the main weapon in Dr. Gonzalez's arsenal for his very sick cancer patients. Depending upon the severity and stage of his patients' illnesses, anywhere from two to ten enemas a day may be prescribed.

I personally met with many of his patients, all of whom had stage IV cancers who have now been alive anywhere from ten to twenty-two years after their diagnosis, because they constantly detox the junk out of their livers, daily. Coffee enemas, in the simplest explanation, stimulate the liver (as though it was being tickled and squeezed), thereby forcing out the chemicals.

People are very uncomfortable with the idea of inserting coffee and/or bentonite into their rectums. It's an uncomfortable area of the body to discuss. But enemas have been a medicinal, natural remedy for health since the time of Cleopatra. In this era of toxicity, cleansing the liver is of the utmost importance. I urge you to get over the awkwardness of this protocol and consider giving them a try. I have to say the feeling after a detox of this sort is to feel "light as air." There are remarkable beauty benefits as well: shiny hair, clear skin, clear eyes, less wrinkling, weight loss.

To Do the Coffee Enema

- Use organic coffee only (doesn't make sense to detox with toxins).
- Make sure the coffee is sufficiently cooled off. Hot coffee could be pretty uncomfortable, so you have to factor this into your daily schedule. Making your coffee the night before is a good idea.
- Fill an enema bag with a pint (or more) depending on what you can hold with cool coffee.
- Lie on the floor on your left side and hold the coffee in your rectum for ten minutes.
- Repeat the process for enema #2 immediately after enema #1 and hold for another ten minutes.

You will get a better detox doing two enemas back-to-back. Check with your physician as to what's best for you.

It's twenty minutes out of your day; you will feel fantastic and soon you will crave doing them every day. Your skin will be clearer, your energy will be better, you will be thinner, and there will be an overall feeling of well-being.

There are some theories on the dangers of electrolyte imbalance from coffee enemas that I wanted to clear up. I asked Dr. Gonzalez his thoughts, which I share below:

Over the past thirty-four years I have investigated every published report alleging so-called dangers of coffee enemas, including electrolyte imbalance. The classic article was in *JAMA* in 1980 that reported "two deaths" from coffee enemas due to electrolyte imbalance.

The first case was an elderly woman who developed severe gastroenteritis with frequent vomiting and diarrhea. On her own with no supervision she started doing coffee enemas at the rate of four an hour. After eight hours, thirty-two coffee enemas, frequent vomiting, and diarrhea, she had a seizure and died from electrolyte imbalance that the authors, pathologists at the coroner's office in Seattle, blamed on the coffee enemas. They deliberately ignored the copious vomiting and diarrhea as contributory to make enemas the culprit. And of course no one should do thirty-two enemas in eight hours—especially true when one is vomiting and has diarrhea, which both cause electrolyte disturbance!

The second case was a tragic young woman with stage IV breast cancer into the liver, brain, and bone, who had failed chemotherapy, more chemo, etc. She ended up in Mexico at an alternative medical clinic, not identified, that recommended coffee enemas. She returned home, did her coffee enemas, juicing, and dies. The Seattle coroner tries to blame the coffee enemas, even though it turns out there was absolutely no evidence of electrolyte imbalance in this case.

The coroner's office held a press conference announcing proof coffee enemas are dangerous. I investigated both cases and wrote to the Seattle coroner disputing their claims of danger. They didn't answer, despite repeated registered-mail attempts. I called repeatedly, but they wouldn't take my calls.

I have reviewed several other cases that are equally questionable. In my thirty-three years of study, I have found three cases of death bizarrely and inappropriately attributed to the use of coffee enemas in the medical literature, three in thirty-four years. Remember, aspirin kills 600 to 1,000 people a year, and everyone is okay with that.

During my Kelley investigation I interviewed over a thousand of Dr. Kelley's patients, some of whom at the time of my study had been doing coffee enemas daily for ten or more years, and never found a case of electrolyte imbalance. I have been doing them for thirty-three years myself, have hundreds of patients on the enemas for periods of up to twenty-seven years, and have not once seen a case of electrolyte imbalance related to coffee enemas.

To Do the Bentonite Enema

Bentonite very effectively draws out toxins from the intestinal tract. (Here's how to get rid of that poofy stomach.)

A single-quart bentonite (mixed with water) enema should be done regularly. Depending on your toxic burden (how sick you are feeling), you would do it every week or once a month. These are not in place of coffee enemas, but in addition to coffee enemas. You can do a bentonite after a coffee enema, but not before as the coffee would wash out the bentonite.

Bentonite is so effective at knocking out toxins that Dr. Gonzalez recommends taking a spoonful orally every day. Bentonite taken orally detoxes your intestines, whereas enemas detox the liver and the colon. At first you might experience increased bloating, but this is because the bentonite is "stirring" up the toxins and getting them ready to exit. After a while you will not experience the bloating anymore. That will be a sign you are getting well.

You can buy bentonite at Sonne's organic foods, sonnes.com.

To do the enema you add a half cup of bentonite liquid to 28 ounces of warm purified water. This should make a quart of liquid.

You insert liquid in your rectum and then lie on your left side to hold it in (same as with coffee enemas) for ten minutes and then expel by sitting on the toilet.

NANOTECHNOLOGY PATCHES

Without over-the-counter or prescribed pills for pain, sleep, and energy, what are we to do to relieve these uncomfortable conditions? In walks nanotechnology . . . nondrug remedies available right now.

The other night I had two tequilas on a night on the town. When I came home, I thought, *I hope those two drinks don't give me a headache.* In my youth I would have taken an aspirin or worse, Aleve or Advil. That's long before I understood the harmful effects of every single chemical in the body and the cumulative effect of ultimately causing a tipping point.

I have interviewed David Schmidt in many of my books. He is a genius scientist and creator of LifeWave nanotechnology pain patches, called IceWave. In the case of headache pain, you would apply one on each side of the head to alleviate pain (or possible expected pain). What I like about them is that they are nondrug patches. Result of my two tequilas? No headache. I use them for all my aches and pains. If I overdo yoga and my shoulder gives me trouble, I apply patches and, bingo, pain is nonexistent.

The miracle of these patches is complicated yet simple. In layperson's terms, the nanotechnology patches activate the infrared light in your body much like sunlight does to produce vitamin D_3. It then moves the energy (chi) around to remove the blockage, eliminates pain, and repairs in the process.

LifeWave also makes sleep patches (Silent Night), detox patches (glutathione), and repair patches (carnosine). These are excellent to wear to bed so the body can heal and repair itself from free-radical damage taken in during the day. We stop making glutathione around age forty, which is why our bodies become less resistant to disease and less able to fight off the toxins we all encounter in our everyday lives. By wearing one of these patches daily, you clean out toxins from your cells. At night I wear a patch to help my body produce carnosine, an antioxidant that repairs cell damage from free radicals. These patches are a simple way to fight the chemical onslaught. Wearing the glutathione patch can help greatly in detoxing your body. It's very simple; you wear the patch three fingers below your navel and change it every day. Along with good nutrition and eliminating outside chemicals as best you can, you will be well on your way to good health and a thin body.

LifeWave also makes energy patches that make your workout easier, as well as the Aeon patches that I wear daily to prevent disease. If I am sick, I put the Aeon patch over the area of most inflammation. All these patches have a myriad of usages, and best of all, not a single drug enters your body. To me it just makes sense.

This is another *new way* to health and has to be made public. To order, go to SuzanneSomers.com and click on LifeWave.

PEMF THERAPY

PEMF stands for pulsed electromagnetic field. In recent years, a number of scientists and inventors recognized the importance of the earth's natural pulsating magnetic field, as well as the frequencies of what is known as the Schumann resonances of the earth's ionosphere, to human health. Since the early twentieth century the earth's magnetic field has started weakening, so scientists developed a number of PEMF devices to introduce these frequencies to the body. As the frequencies are introduced, the body's flow of energy is stimulated and balanced, bringing the body into a more harmonious, energized state.

There are a variety of PEMF devices today. The Ondamed is used in my anti-aging doctor, Dr. Michael Galitzer's office regularly for every sort of energy healing: body imbalances, fungus, pain, mold, and autoimmune issues. It is such an efficient healing tool, I encourage you to ask your doctor to invest in one for his or her office.

PEMF devices utilize the principles of energy medicine. PEMF therapy is approved by the FDA for certain applications, including for stimulating bone growth, healing bone fractures, and as a complementary therapy to cervical fusion therapy.

Other health benefits of PEMF therapy include increased circulation, improved immune function, enhanced energy levels, enhanced muscle function and relief of muscle tension, enhanced oxygenation of blood and cells, reduced inflammation, improved nerve and liver function, improved detoxification, improved sleep, improved assimilation of nutrients, and overall stress relief.

Although a number of PEMF devices are designed for home use, when first exploring PEMF, I recommend you first work with a physician or other health-care expert trained in its use.

THE WRAP-UP

WELL, THAT'S IT. NOW YOU KNOW WHAT TOXINS ARE DOING TO you. Now you know why you aren't feeling well. Now you know why you are gaining weight no matter how hard you are trying to diet and exercise. Now you know the harm being done to all of us as a result of the greatest environmental assault in the history of humanity. You've read the advice of the doctors who understand this assault. And now you also know how to detox.

I hope your takeaway from this book is the realization that you can reverse the damage in your body by taking charge of your personal health and the choices you make from this moment on relative to diet and lifestyle. It all matters.

I urge you to go to ForeverHealth.com to find the doctors who are qualified to treat environmental disorders and consult on bioidentical hormone replacement. The goal of these doctors is to get you off all pharmaceutical drugs, or to at least drastically minimize your intake.

Imagine a new life of great, robust health. I have achieved this state of bliss, and I now know it can be done with perseverance. You can't "sort of" do it. You have to commit. If this information resonates, then adapt all this new knowledge into your way of life, and you will be doing yourself the ultimate favor to ensure your survival. You can achieve peak health again. You can regain your energy, your sex drive, your perfect weight, a clear brain, strong lead-free bones, a well-working GI tract. You can heal your brain through detoxification and a change of diet.

Commit to making the change to achieve peak health. Once you master your own body, you will be able to influence your family and friends. That's how grassroots change works.

Through Dr. Gonzalez, you learned where cancer comes from and how to "manage" it by detoxification of the liver and taking pancreatic enzymes to "eat the debris" whether that debris might be cancer or negative pathogens from toxicity. I have personally interviewed dozens of his patients with stage IV cancers: pancreatic, breast, ovarian, prostate, liver, lung, and others, and they are all alive and well years after diagnosis. His protocol works!

From Dr. Shoemaker, you learned that mold as a result of the toxins accumulated in water-damaged buildings does not have to reduce your life to misery. Mold is serious, and allopathic medicine has no answers. Dr. Shoemaker's protocols are magnificent in that people who commit to his program GET WELL!

With Dr. Crinnion, you learned the valuable role that naturopathic doctors play in understanding the environmental assault. He taught you to recognize what the everyday objects you live with in your home are doing to your health, including car fumes, exhaust, outgassing, formaldehyde exposure and poisoning, perfumes, and household cleaners. Each one of these toxins degrades health and can be eliminated or minimized to achieve wellness.

From Dr. Sinatra, America's leading integrative cardiologist, we learned that we have been approaching heart disease all wrong, that drugs are not the answer. The answer lies in keeping the body detoxed, along with a healthy diet heavily relying on quality organic food and healthy fats. Who knew that healthy fats were the best recipe for a healthy heart? We learned that the heart is affected by the GI tract, and whether or not your gut is healthy determines heart health. The number one killer of women is heart disease. Now we know this doesn't have to be. This is new and astounding information teaching all of us that the low-fat myth is that . . . a myth. We need healthy fats for health.

From Dr. Sherry Rogers, a doctor who has been in the trenches of environmental medicine for over forty years, we learned the truth about the effects of toxins on our health. She gave us hope that the conditions of the brain and the GI tract are indeed curable. Detoxification is so important in today's world that not taking the steps to detoxify is a sure path to death and a torturous death at that.

And finally, from Dr. Gordon you learned new protocols for removing toxic lead from the body, and we learned that lead is the most overlooked of all the toxins and is a surefire path to total body breakdown. He also taught you the ways to keep the most important gland in your body, the thyroid, clean and healthy.

We learned that the health of your mother has a lot to do with the health you inherited, but that it is not your "sentence." Understanding that the GI tract can be repaired, and that your mother's poor gut health does not have to be yours, puts you in control.

I hope that is the big takeaway from all these amazing physicians.

> YOU ARE IN CONTROL OF YOUR HEALTH BY THE CHOICES YOU MAKE REGARDING DIET AND LIFESTYLE.

Add in keeping positive with good thoughts and you can expect a long, extended life of optimal health, wisdom, and perspective. We are the next line of matriarchs and patriarchs. We have the opportunity today to change the present paradigm of health and aging. We have the opportunity to circumvent the toxic assault and learn to live in the toxic soup while remaining healthy and keeping our families healthy in the process.

You now have the opportunity to be the teacher, to change the course of health for yourself and your family.

Everyone is dreaming that true health is possible, but few believe it. Believe it!

Most people feel they are helpless and thereby hopeless. IT'S NOT TRUE!

You can do it. I did it. My husband did it, my granddaughters did it, my daughter did it, and SO CAN YOU!

Good luck, good health, long life, and much love,

SYNTHETIC CHEMICALS AND DISEASE RISK

Current evidence suggesting links between chemicals and cancer risk as well as metabolic diseases and neurodegenerative diseases is discussed below.

PROSTATE CANCER

Bisphenol A (BPA)

A 2014 observational analysis showed **higher levels of urinary BPA in prostate cancer patients than in nonprostate cancer patients, and the effect was even more profound in patients younger than age 65 years.**

> [The] study examined the association between urinary BPA levels and prostate cancer and assessed the effects of BPA on induction of centrosome abnormalities as an underlying mechanism promoting prostate carcinogenesis. The study, involving 60 urology patients, found higher levels of urinary BPA (creatinine-adjusted) in Prostate cancer patients (5.74 µg/g [95% CI; 2.63, 12.51]) than in non-Prostate cancer patients (1.43 µg/g [95% CI; 0.70, 2.88]) (p=0.012). The difference was even more significant in patients <65 years old. (Tarapore 2014, *PLoS ONE*)

Organophosphate insecticides

2013 analysis of observational data showed a significant trend for increased prostate cancer risk with increasing exposure to organophosphate insecticides. Of note, there was a **statistically significant 63% increased risk when comparing those with the highest exposure to fonofos (one of the organophosphate insecticides examined) to the nonexposed for aggressive prostate cancer.**

> Three organophosphate insecticides were significantly associated with aggressive prostate cancer: fonofos (rate ratio (RR) for the highest quartile of exposure (Q4) vs. nonexposed = 1.63, 95% confidence interval (CI): 1.22, 2.17; P(trend) < 0.001); malathion (RR for Q4 vs. nonexposed = 1.43, 95% CI: 1.08, 1.88; P(trend) = 0.04); and terbufos (RR for Q4 vs. nonexposed = 1.29, 95% CI: 1.02, 1.64; P(trend) = 0.03). (Koutros 2013, *American Journal of Epidemiology*)

Organochlorine pesticides

Data showed that **serum levels of organochloride pesticides were significantly associated with prostate cancer risk and showed as high as a fourteenfold (fourteen times) increased risk of prostate cancer associated with the highest versus the lowest levels for specific types of organochloride pesticides in serum.**

> After adjustment for other covariates, serum concentrations of beta-hexachlorocyclohexane (HCH) (p for trend = 0.02), trans-nonachlor (p for trend = 0.002), and dieldrin (p for trend = 0.04) were significantly associated with the risk of prevalent prostate cancer. Adjusted odds ratios for the second and third tertiles of detectable values were 1.46 [95% confidence interval (CI), 0.52-4.13] and 3.36 (95% CI, 1.24-9.10) for beta-HCH; 5.84 (95% CI, 1.06-32.2) and 14.1 (95% CI, 2.55-77.9) for trans-nonachlor; and 1.06 (95% CI, 0.30-3.73) and 2.74 (95% CI, 1.01-7.49) for dieldrin compared with concentrations in the lowest tertile or below the limit of detection. (Xu 2010, *Environmental Health Perspectives*)

LEUKEMIA

Polycyclic aromatic hydrocarbons (PAH)

As high as a 98% increased risk of childhood leukemia was associated with increasing concentrations of specific types of PAH in the home.

Among participants with vacuum dust, we observed positive associations between ALL risk and increasing concentrations of benzo[a] pyrene (OR perln[ng/g]=1.42, 95% CI=0.95, 2.12), dibenzo[a,h] anthracene (OR=1.98, 95% CI=1.11, 3.55), benzo[k]fluoranthene (OR=1.71, 95% CI=0.91, 3.22), indeno[1,2,3-cd]pyrene (OR=1.81, 95% CI=1.04, 3.16), and the toxic equivalence (OR=2.35, 95% CI=1.18, 4.69). The increased ALL risk among participants with vacuum dust suggests that PAH exposure may increase the risk of childhood ALL; however, reasons for the different results based on HVS3 dust samples deserve further study. (Deziel 2014, *Environmental Research*)

NON-HODGKIN'S LYMPHOMA (NHL)

Acetylcholinesterase inhibitor pesticides

There was a 216% increased risk of NHL among individuals age 40 years and younger associated with the use of two acetylcholinesterase inhibitor pesticides, and an 88% increased risk of NHL among all test subjects using five or more insecticides.

Overall, there was an increase in the risk of HL among all subjects who reported use of five or more insecticides (OR 1.88, 95% CI 0.92-3.87) and among subjects younger than 40 who reported use of two acetylcholinesterase inhibitors (OR 3.16, 95% CI 1.02-9.29). There was an elevated odds ratio associated with reported use of three or more probably carcinogenic pesticides (OR 2.47, 95% CI 1.06-5.75), but no increase in risk for use of possibly carcinogenic pesticides. The risk of HL from reported use of fungicides or any pesticides was greater for cases diagnosed before age 40 than for cases diagnosed at or after age 40. When analyses excluded proxy respondents, OR estimates strengthened in some circumstances . . . For trends by number of pesticides used, an increasing trend was of borderline significance for fungicides among those <40 years ($p = 0.06$) and significant for an inverse trend among those >40 years ($p = 0.05$). (Navaranjan 2013, *Cancer Causes Control*)

BREAST CANCER

Phthalates
Higher levels of certain types of phthalate metabolites in women were associated with as much as a 120% increased risk for breast cancer, and as much as a fourfold higher risk association with pre-menopausal women.

Phthalate metabolites were detected in at least 82% of women. The geometric mean concentrations of monoethyl phthalate (MEP) were higher in cases than in controls (169.58 vs. 106.78 microg/g creatinine). Controls showed significantly higher concentrations of mono-n-butyl phthalate, mono(2-ethyl-5-oxohexyl) phthalate, and mono(3-carboxy-propyl) phthalate (MCPP) than did the cases. After adjusting for risk factors and other phthalates, MEP urinary concentrations were positively associated with BC [odds ratio (OR), highest vs. lowest tertile = 2.20; 95% confidence interval (CI), 1.33-3.63; p for trend < 0.01]. This association became stronger when estimated for premenopausal women (OR, highest vs. lowest tertile = 4.13; 95% CI, 1.60-10.70; p for trend < 0.01). In contrast, we observed significant negative associations for monobenzyl phthalate (MBzP) and MCPP. (López-Carrillo 2010, *Environmental Health Perspectives*)

DDT, DDE, and HCB
There were significant associations between higher levels of DDT and DDE with late-onset breast cancer, and a significant association between HCB and deadly estrogen-independent breast cancer.

Significantly higher levels of DDE (1,1-bis(4-chlorophenyl)-2,2-dichloroethene) and DDT (1,1,1-trichloro-2,2-bis(4-chlorophenol)ethane) (P < 0.05) were observed in the patients with late onset of the disease which was probably due to the time of exposure. Moreover, in the patients exposed to environmental estrogens, significantly higher concentrations of DDD (1,1-bis(4-chlorophenyl)-2,2-dichloroethane) were found (P < 0.05). We also evidenced that estrogen-independent cancer was more frequent in the patients exposed to numerous risk factors in which higher levels of HCB (hexachlorobenzene), gamma-HCH (gamma-hexachlorocyclohexane), DDD and DDT in adipose tissue were detected. Breast cancer development is probably related to the accumulation of DDT and its derivatives, but the effect appears only in older patients. We postulate that environmental estrogens acting together with other risk factors might influence the progress and exacerbate the prognosis of breast cancer. (Ociepa-Zawal 2010, *Journal of Environmental Science and Health*) However, the data is conflicting with other research showing no relationship. (Raaschou-Nielsen 2005, *Cancer Epidemiology, Biomarkers & Prevention*)

RENAL (KIDNEY) CANCER

Formaldehyde, polycyclic aromatic hydrocarbons (PAH), and perchlorethylene 28%, 10%, and 9% increased association of a type of kidney cancer (Wilm's tumor) when children were prenatally exposed (during the third trimester) to formaldehyde, PAH, and perchlorethylene.

Children prenatally exposed to formaldehyde, polycyclic aromatic hydrocarbons, perchloroethylene, or acetaldehyde in the third trimester had an increased odds of Wilms' tumor per interquartile increase in concentration (odds ratio [95% confidence interval]: 1.28 [1.12 to 1.45], 1.10 [0.99 to 1.22], 1.09 [1.00 to 1.18], 1.25 [1.07 to 1.45], respectively). (Shrestha 2014, *Journal of Occupational and Environmental Medicine*)

OVARIAN CANCER

Air pollution
An increased risk of death from ovarian cancer was associated with higher levels of air pollution.

Results showed that individuals who resided in municipalities with higher levels of PM [particulate matter] 2.5, a proxy measure of PAH [polycyclic aromatic hydrocarbons], were at an increased risk of death from ovarian cancer compared to those subjects living in municipalities with the lowest PM 2.5. (Hung 2012, *Journal of Toxicology and Environmental Health*)

TESTICULAR CANCER

Polyvinyl chloride
A sevenfold increased risk of testicular cancer was associated with exposure to polyvinyl chloride.

An increased odds ratio (OR) was found for exposure to polyvinyl chloride (PVC) yielding an OR of 6.6 (95% confidence interval, 1.4-32). The risk increased further if cases with self-reported cryptorchidism or orchitis were excluded. Six of the 7 exposed cases had seminoma. Exposure to other types of plastics did not significantly increase the risk of testicular cancer.(Hardell 1997, *International Journal of Cancer*)

RESPIRATORY AND URINARY TRACT CANCERS

Polycyclic aromatic hydrocarbons (PAH)
There was a 31% increased risk of respiratory tract cancer in iron and steel foundry workers and a trend for increased risk of bladder cancer associated with aluminum production workers, industries with heavy use of PAH.

In the meta-analysis, an excess risk of respiratory tract cancers (mainly lung cancer) was found in iron and steel foundries [pooled relative risk (RR) 1.31, 95% confidence interval (CI) 1.08-1.59 from 14 studies], while a weak excess risk (pooled RR 1.08, 95% CI 0.95-1.23 from 11 studies) emerged for aluminum production. A borderline increase risk was also observed for cancer of the bladder in the aluminum production (pooled RR 1.28, 95% CI 0.98-1.68 from 10 studies) and in iron and steel foundries (pooled RR 1.38, 95% CI 1.00-1.91 from 9 studies). This updated review and meta-analysis confirm the increased risk from respiratory tract and bladder cancers in selected PAH-related occupations. It cannot be ruled out whether such excesses are due, at least in part, to possible bias or residual confounding. (Rota 2014, *Archives of Toxicology*)

ALZHEIMER'S DISEASE (AD)

DDE

There was a significant association between AD and the pesticide DDE in serum.

Elevated serum DDE levels are associated with an increased risk for AD and carriers of an APOE4 ε4 allele may be more susceptible to the effects of DDE. (Richardson 2014, *JAMA Neurology*)

DIABETES

Phthalates

There was a strong trend for development of diabetes in subjects with significantly higher levels of phthalate metabolites.

Participants with diabetes had significantly higher concentrations of di(2-ethylhexyl) pththalate (DEHP) metabolites: mono(2-ethyl-5-hydroxyhexyl) phthalate (MEHHP), mono(2-ethyl-5-oxohexyl) phthalate (MEOHP) and mono(2-ethyl-5-carboxypentyl) phthalate (MECPP) but lower levels of monobenzyl phthalate (MBzP) a metabolite of benzylbutyl phthalate, compared to participants without diabetes. Marginally significant positive associations with diabetes status were observed over tertiles with MEHHP (OR(T3 vs. T1)=2.66; 95% CI: 0.97-7.33; p for trend=0.063) and MEOHP (OR(T3 vs. T1)=2.27; 95% CI; 0.90-5.75; P for trend=0.079) even after adjusting for important confounders. (Svensson 2011, *Environmental Research*)

Arsenic

There was a significant association between increasing levels of arsenic in drinking water and diabetes development.

Over a mean follow-up of 9.7 years of 52,931 eligible subjects, there were 4,304 (8.1%) diabetes cases in total, and 3,035 (5.8%) cases of diabetes based on a stricter definition. The adjusted incidence rate ratio's per 1 μg/L increment in arsenic levels in drinking water were (IRR = 1.03; 95% CI: 1.01, 1.06) and (IRR = 1.02; 95% CI: 0.99, 1.05) for all and strict diabetes cases, respectively. . . . Long-term exposure to low-level arsenic in drinking water may contribute to development of diabetes. (Brauner 2014, *Environmental Health Perspectives*)

PARKINSON'S DISEASE

Hexachlorocyclohexane

There was **more than a fourfold association between the pesticide hexachlorocyclohexane and Parkinson's disease.**

β-Hexachlorocyclohexane (β-HCH) was more often detectable in patients with PD (76%) compared with controls (40%) and patients with Alzheimer disease (30%). The median level of β-HCH was higher in patients with PD compared with controls and patients with Alzheimer disease. There were no marked differences in detection between controls and patients with PD concerning any of the other 15 organochlorine pesticides. Finally, we observed a significant odds ratio for the presence of β-HCH in serum to predict a diagnosis of PD vs control (odds ratio, 4.39; 95% confidence interval, 1.67–11.6) and PD vs Alzheimer disease (odds ratio, 5.20), which provides further evidence for the apparent association between serum β-HCH and PD. These data suggest that β-HCH is associated with a diagnosis of PD. Further research is warranted regarding the potential role of β-HCH as a etiologic agent for some cases of PD. (Richardson 2009, *JAMA Neurology*)

ALLERGY

Air pollution and polycyclic aromatic hydrocarbons (PAH)

There showed an association of **PAH in air pollution with impaired immunity in children, including allergy.**

Collectively, these results demonstrate increased ambient PAH exposure is associated with impaired systemic immunity and epigenetic modifications in a key locus involved in atopy: FOXP3, with a higher impact on atopic children. The results suggest that increased atopic clinical symptoms in children could be linked to increased PAH exposure in air pollution. (Hew 2014, *Clinical & Experimental Allergy*)

SUPPORTIVE NUTRIENTS FOR HEPATIC (LIVER) DETOXIFICATION AND CELLULAR CHEMOPREVENTION

A multitude of studies document the beneficial effects of nutrients for chemopreventive or hepatic detoxification. A selection of studies is provided below.

Flavonoids
Flavonoids assist with hepatic detoxification, thereby providing chemopreventive effects.

> Flavones (chrysin, baicalein, and galangin), flavanones (naringenin) and isoflavones (genistein, biochanin A) inhibit the activity of aromatase (CYP19), thus decreasing estrogen biosynthesis and producing antiestrogenic effects, important in breast and prostate cancers. Activation of phase II detoxifying enzymes, such as UDP-glucuronyl transferase, glutathione S-transferase, and quinone reductase by flavonoids results in the detoxification of carcinogens and represents one mechanism of their anticarcinogenic effects. A number of flavonoids including fisetin, galangin, quercetin, kaempferol, and genistein represent potent non-competitive inhibitors of sulfotransferase 1A1 (or P-PST); this may represent an important mechanism for the chemoprevention of sulfation-induced carcinogenesis. (Moon 2006, *Toxicology in Vitro*)

Indole-3-carbinol
Indole-3-carbinol (I-3-C) has been shown to have potent anticancer as well as hepato-protective (liver-protective) effects.

> . . . the incidence and multiplicity of cancers in laboratory animal models. Based on the observation that I-3-C induced hepatocyte hypertrophy when administered orally for 13 weeks to rats, a treatment and recovery study was undertaken to test the hypothesis that the induction of hepatocyte hypertrophy and cytochrome P450 (CYP) activity by I-3-C are adaptive, reversible responses. [The researchers found increased liver weights and enhanced activity for a range of CYP enzymes.] (Crowell 2006, *Toxicology and Applied Pharmacology*)

Garlic and Tomato Extracts

Garlic and tomato constituents have been shown to reduce tumor burden and increase detoxification enzymes with known carcinogens.

From these results, we suggest that modulation of xenobiotic-metabolizing enzymes exerted by tomato and garlic combination plays a key role in mitigating the mutagenic and carcinogenic effects of DMBA. (Bhuvaneswari 2005, *Nutrition*)

Rosemary

Oral administration of *Rosmarinus officinalis L.* (Lamiaceae) prevents effects caused by chemically induced liver damage through increasing liver detoxification.

Rosmarinus officinalis increased liver cytosolic GST activity and produced an additional increment in plasma GST activity in rats treated with CCl(4). Histological evaluation showed that *Rosmarinus officinalis* partially prevented CCl(4)-induced inflammation, necrosis and vacuolation. [The authors noted that rosemary appears to improve glutathione S-transferase (GST) dependent detoxification systems.] (Sotelo-Felix 2002, *European Journal of Gastroenterology & Hepatology*)

Chlorophyllin (CHL)

CHL is known to be protective against genotoxic compounds, blocks invasion and metastasis of tumor cells, protects mitochondria, while also inducing phase II liver detoxification.

Chlorophyllin (CHL), the sodium and copper salt of chlorophyll, is capable of inhibiting the mutagenic activity of many chemical compounds. Several mechanisms have been advanced to explain the antimutagenic activity of CHL, including its antioxidant properties and its ability to form complexes with mutagens. (Ardelt 2001, *International Journal of Oncology*)

PhIP and IQ are heterocyclic amines (HCAs) that are found in cooked meat and may be risk factors for cancer. Typical chemoprevention studies have used carcinogen doses many thousand-fold higher than usual human daily intake. Therefore, we administered a low dose of [14C]PhIP and [3H]IQ and utilized accelerator mass spectrometry to quantify PhIP adducts in the liver, colon, prostate, and blood plasma and IQ adducts in the liver and blood plasma with high sensitivity. . . . CHL . . . decrease adduct formation of [14C]PhIP and [3H]IQ in rats. (Dingley 2003, *Nutrition and Cancer*)

Other studies on chlorophyllin also support these mechanisms (Thiyagarajan 2014, *Tumor Biology*; Boloor 2000, *Toxicology*; Kamat 2000, *Molecular and Cell Biology of Lipids*).

FURTHER READING

PREVENTING GENE MUTATION

Aggarwal BB, Kumar A, Bharti AC. Anticancer potential of curcumin: pre-clinical and clinical studies. *Anticancer Research* 2003; 23(1a):363–398.

Boloor KK, Kamat JP, Devasagayam TP. Chlorophyllin as a protector of mitochondrial membranes against gamma-radiation and photosensitization. *Toxicology* 2000; 155(1–3):63–71.

Brooks JD, Paton VG, Vidanes G. Potent induction of phase 2 enzymes in human prostate cells by sulforaphane. *Cancer Epidemiology, Biomarkers & Prevention: A Publication of the American Association for Cancer Research, Cosponsored by the American Society of Preventive Oncology* 2001; 10(9):949–954.

Cabrera G. Effect of five dietary antimutagens on the genotoxicity of six mutagens in the microscreen prophage-induction assay. *Environmental and Molecular Mutagenesis* 2000; 36(3):206–220.

Dashwood R, Yamane S, Larsen R. Study of the forces of stabilizing complexes between chlorophylls and heterocyclic amine mutagens. *Environmental and Molecular Mutagenesis* 1996; 27(3):211–218.

Dashwood RH. Use of transgenic and mutant animal models in the study of heterocyclic amine-induced mutagenesis and carcinogenesis. *Journal of Biochemistry and Molecular Biology* 2003; 36(1):35–42.

Doerr-O'Rourke K, Trushin N, Hecht SS, Stoner GD. Effect of phenethyl isothiocyanate on the metabolism of the tobacco-specific nitrosamine 4-(methylnitrosamino)-1-(3-pyridyl)-1-butanone by cultured rat lung tissue. *Carcinogenesis* 1991; 12(6):1029–1034.

Egner PA, Stansbury KH, Snyder EP, Rogers ME, Hintz PA, Kensler TW. Identification and characterization of chlorin e(4) ethyl ester in sera of individuals participating in the chlorophyllin chemoprevention trial. *Chemical Research in Toxicology* 2000; 13(9):900–906.

Egner PA, Wang JB, Zhu YR, et al. Chlorophyllin intervention reduces aflatoxin-DNA adducts in individuals at high risk for liver cancer. *Proceedings of the National Academy of Sciences of the United States of America* 2001; 98(25):14601–14606.

Fahey JW, Haristoy X, Dolan PM, et al. Sulforaphane inhibits extracellular, intracellular, and antibiotic-resistant strains of Helicobacter pylori and prevents benzo[a]pyrene-induced stomach tumors. *Proceedings of the National Academy of Sciences of the United States of America* 2002; 99(11): 7610–7615.

Gross GA, Gruter A. Quantitation of mutagenic/carcinogenic heterocyclic aromatic amines in food products. *Journal of Chromatography* 1992; 592(1–2):271–278.

Guengerich FP, Shimada T, Bondon A, Macdonald TL. Cytochrome P-450 oxidations and the generation of biologically reactive intermediates. *Advances in Experimental Medicine and Biology* 1991; 283:1–11.

Guo D, Schut HA, Davis CD, Snyderwine EG, Bailey GS, Dashwood RH. Protection by chlorophyllin and indole-3-carbinol against 2-amino-1-methyl-6-phenylimidazo[4,5-b]pyridine (PhIP)-induced DNA adducts and colonic aberrant crypts in the F344 rat. *Carcinogenesis* 1995; 16(12): 2931–2937.

Hecht SS. Chemoprevention by isothiocyanates. *Journal of Cellular Biochemistry* 22, Suppl. (1995):195–209.

Hernaez J, Xu M, Dashwood R. Effects of tea and chlorophyllin on the mutagenicity of N-hydroxy-IQ: studies of enzyme inhibition, molecular complex formation, and degradation/scavenging of the active metabolites. *Environmental and Molecular Mutagenesis* 1997; 30(4):468–474.

Iqbal M, Sharma SD, Okazaki Y, Fujisawa M, Okada S. Dietary supplementation of curcumin enhances antioxidant and phase II metabolizing enzymes in ddY male mice: possible role in protection against chemical carcinogenesis and toxicity. *Pharmacology & Toxicology* 2003; 92(1):33–38.

Kamat JP, Boloor KK, Devasagayam TP. Chlorophyllin as an effective antioxidant against membrane damage in vitro and ex vivo. *Biochimica et Biophysica Acta* 2000; 1487(2–3):113–127.

Kawamori T, Lubet R, Steele VE, et al. Chemopreventive effect of curcumin, a naturally occurring anti-inflammatory agent, during the promotion/progression stages of colon cancer. *Cancer Research* 1999; 59(3):597–601.

Kinae N, Masuda H, Shin IS, Furugori M, Shimoi K. Functional properties of wasabi and horseradish. *BioFactors* (Oxford, England) 2000; 13(1–4):265–269.

Limtrakul P, Anuchapreeda S, Buddhasukh D. Modulation of human multidrug-resistance MDR-1 gene by natural curcuminoids. *BMC Cancer* 2004; 4:13.

Limtrakul P, Anuchapreeda S, Lipigorngoson S, Dunn FW. Inhibition of carcinogen induced c-Ha-ras and c-fos proto-oncogenes expression by dietary curcumin. *BMC Cancer* 2001; 1:1.

Limtrakul P, Lipigorngoson S, Namwong O, Apisariyakul A, Dunn FW. Inhibitory effect of dietary curcumin on skin carcinogenesis in mice. *Cancer Letters* 1997; 116(2):197–203.

Madrigal-Bujaidar E, Velazquez-Guadarrama N, Diaz-Barriga S. Inhibitory effect of chlorophyllin on the frequency of sister chromatid exchanges produced by benzo[a]pyrene in vivo. *Mutation Research* 1997; 388(1):79–83.

Martinez A, Cambero II, Ikken Y, Marin ML, Haza AI, Morales P. Protective effect of broccoli, onion, carrot, and licorice extracts against cytotoxicity of n-nitrosamines evaluated by 3-(4,5-dimethylthiazol-2-yl)-2,5-diphenyltetrazolium bromide assay. *Journal of Agricultural and Food Chemistry* 1998; 46(2):585–589.

Mehta K, Pantazis P, McQueen T, Aggarwal BB. Antiproliferative effect of curcumin (diferuloylmethane) against human breast tumor cell lines. *Anti-cancer Drugs* 1997; 8(5):470–481.

Morimitsu Y, Hayashi K, Nakagawa Y, Horio F, Uchida K, Osawa T. Antiplatelet and anticancer isothiocyanates in Japanese domestic horseradish, wasabi. *BioFactors* (Oxford, England) 2000; 13(1–4):271–276.

Morimitsu Y, Nakagawa Y, Hayashi K, et al. A sulforaphane analogue that potently activates the Nrf2-dependent detoxification pathway. *Journal of Biological Chemistry* 2002; 277(5):3456–3463.

Morse MA, Zu H, Galati AJ, Schmidt CJ, Stoner GD. Dose-related inhibition by dietary phenethyl isothiocyanate of esophageal tumorigenesis and DNA methylation induced by N-nitrosomethylbenzylamine in rats. *Cancer Letters* 1993; 72(1–2):103–110.

Negishi T, Rai H, Hayatsu H. Antigenotoxic activity of natural chlorophylls. *Mutation Research* 1997; 376(1–2):97–100.

Nomura T, Shinoda S, Yamori T, et al. Selective sensitivity to wasabi-derived 6-(methylsulfinyl)hexyl isothiocyanate of human breast cancer and melanoma cell lines studied in vitro. *Cancer Detection and Prevention* 2005; 29(2):155–160.

Ong TM, Whong WZ, Stewart J, Brockman HE. Chlorophyllin: a potent antimutagen against environmental and dietary complex mixtures. *Mutation Research* 1986; 173(2): 111–115.

Shapiro TA, Fahey JW, Wade KL, Stephenson KK, Talalay P. Chemoprotective glucosinolates and isothiocyanates of broccoli sprouts: metabolism and excretion in humans. *Cancer Epidemiology, Biomarkers & Prevention: A Publication of the American Association for Cancer Research, Cosponsored by the American Society of Preventive Oncology* 2001; 10(5):501–508.

Sreejayan N, Rao MN. Free radical scavenging activity of curcuminoids. *Arzneimittel-Forschung* 1996; 46(2):169–171.

Sreejayan N, Rao MN. Nitric oxide scavenging by curcuminoids. *The Journal of Pharmacy and Pharmacology* 1997; 49(1):105–107.

Subramanian M, Sreejayan N, Rao MN, Devasagayam TP, Singh BB. Diminution of singlet oxygen-induced DNA damage by curcumin and related antioxidants. *Mutation Research* 1994; 311(2):249–255.

Sugie S, Okamoto K, Makita H, et al. Inhibitory effect of chlorophyllin on diethylnitrosamine and phenobarbital-induced hepatocarcinogenesis in male F344 rats. *Japanese Journal of Cancer Research: Gann* 1996; 87(10): 1045–1051.

Susan M, Rao MN. Induction of glutathione S-transferase activity by curcumin in mice. *Arzneimittel-Forschung* 1992; 42(7):962–964.

Tang X, Edenharder R. Inhibition of the mutagenicity of 2-nitrofluorene, 3-nitrofluoranthene and 1-nitropyrene by vitamins, porphyrins and related compounds, and vegetable and fruit juices and solvent extracts. *Food and Chemical Toxicology : An International Journal Published for the British Industrial Biological Research Association* 1997; 35(3–4): 373–378.

Tsunoda S, Yamamoto K, Sakamoto S, Inoue H, Nagasawa H. Effects of Sasa Health, extract of bamboo grass leaves, on spontaneous mammary tumourigenesis in SHN mice. *Anticancer Research* 1998; 18(1a):153–158.

Watanabe M, Ohata M, Hayakawa S, et al. Identification of 6-methyl-sulfinylhexyl isothiocyanate as an apoptosis-inducing component in wasabi. *Phytochemistry* 2003; 62(5):733–739.

Wei YH, Ma YS, Lee HC, Lee CF, Lu CY. Mitochondrial theory of aging matures—roles of mtDNA mutation and oxidative stress in human aging. *Zhonghua yi xue za zhi [Chinese Medical Journal, Free China ed.]* 2001; 64(5):259–270.

Xu K, Thornalley PJ. Studies on the mechanism of the inhibition of human leukaemia cell growth by dietary isothiocyanates and their cysteine adducts in vitro. *Biochemical Pharmacology* 2000; 60(2):221–231.

Zhang Y, Kensler TW, Cho CG, Posner GH, Talalay P. Anticarcinogenic activities of sulforaphane and structurally related synthetic norbornyl isothiocyanates. *Proceedings of the National Academy of Sciences of the United States of America* 1994; 91(8):3147–3150.

Zhang Y, Talalay P, Cho CG, Posner GH. A major inducer of anticarcinogenic protective enzymes from broccoli: isolation and elucidation of structure. *Proceedings of the National Academy of Sciences of the United States of America* 1992; 89(6):2399–2403.

Zheng W, Gustafson DR, Sinha R, et al. Well-done meat intake and the risk of breast cancer. *Journal of the National Cancer Institute* 1998; 90(22):1724–1729.

CELLULAR HEALTH SUPPORT

Abdel Moneim AE. Evaluating the potential role of pomegranate peel in aluminum-induced oxidative stress and histopathological alterations in brain of female rats. *Biological Trace Element Research* 2012; 150(1–3):328–336.

Alcaraz M, Armero D, Martinez-Beneyto Y, et al. Chemical genoprotection: reducing biological damage to as low as reasonably achievable levels. *Dento Maxillo Facial Radiology* 2011; 40(5):310–314.

Alexopoulos N, Vlachopoulos C, Aznaouridis K, et al. The acute effect of green tea consumption on endothelial function in healthy individuals. *European Journal of Cardiovascular Prevention and Rehabilitation: Official Journal of the European Society of Cardiology, Working Groups on Epidemiology & Prevention and Cardiac Rehabilitation and Exercise Physiology* 2008; 15(3):300–305.

Ames BN. Prevention of mutation, cancer, and other age-associated diseases by optimizing micronutrient intake. *Journal of Nucleic Acids* 2010.

Anonymous. Alpha-lipoic acid. Monograph. *Alternative Medicine Review: A Journal of Clinical Therapeutic* 2006; 11(3):232 – 237.

Anuradha B, Varalakshmi P. Protective role of DL-alpha-lipoic acid against mercury-induced neural lipid peroxidation. *Pharmacological Research: The Official Journal of the Italian Pharmacological Society* 1999; 39(1):67–80.

Aviram M, Dornfeld L. Pomegranate juice consumption inhibits serum angiotensin converting enzyme activity and reduces systolic blood pressure. *Atherosclerosis* 2001; 158(1):195–198.

Bingham SA, Pignatelli B, Pollock JR, et al. Does increased endogenous formation of N-nitroso compounds in the human colon explain the association between red meat and colon cancer? *Carcinogenesis* 1996; 17(3):515–523.

Bors W, Michel C, Schikora S. Interaction of flavonoids with ascorbate and determination of their univalent redox potentials: a pulse radiolysis study. *Free Radical Biology & Medicine* 1995; 19(1):45–52.

Boyce A, Doehmer J, Gooderham NJ. Phytoalexin resveratrol attenuates the mutagenicity of the heterocyclic amines 2-amino-1-methyl-6-phenylimidazo[4,5-b]pyridine and 2-amino-3,8-dimethylimidazo[4,5-f]quinoxaline. *Journal of Chromatography. B, Analytical Technologies in the Biomedical and Life Sciences* 2004; 802(1):217–223.

Bunkova R, Marova I, Nemec M. Antimutagenic properties of green tea. *Plant Foods for Human Nutrition* (Dordrecht, Netherlands) 2005; 60(1):25–29.

Cevallos-Casals BA, Cisneros-Zevallos L. Stoichiometric and kinetic studies of phenolic antioxidants from Andean purple corn and red-fleshed sweetpotato. *Journal of Agricultural and Food Chemistry* 2003; 51(11):3313–3319.

Chow CK. Dietary coenzyme Q10 and mitochondrial status. *Methods in Enzymology* 2004; 382:105–112.

Dellavalle CT, Xiao Q, Yang G, et al. Dietary nitrate and nitrite intake and risk of colorectal cancer in the Shanghai Women's Health Study. *International Journal of Cancer/Journal international du cancer* 2014; 134(12):2917–2926.

Dontas AS, Zerefos NS, Panagiotakos DB, Vlachou C, Valis DA.

Mediterranean diet and prevention of coronary heart disease in the elderly. *Clinical Interventions in Aging* 2007; 2(1):109–115.

Erkekoglu P, Baydar T. Evaluation of the protective effect of ascorbic acid on nitrite- and nitrosamine-induced cytotoxicity and genotoxicity in human hepatoma line. *Toxicology Mechanisms and Methods* 2010; 20(2):45–52.

Fujimoto S, Kurihara N, Hirata K, Takeda T. Effects of coenzyme Q10 administration on pulmonary function and exercise performance in patients with chronic lung diseases. *The Clinical Investigator* 1993; 71(8 Suppl):S162–166.

Fukamachi K, Imada T, Ohshima Y, Xu J, Tsuda H. Purple corn color suppresses Ras protein level and inhibits 7,12-dimethylbenz[a]anthracene-induced mammary carcinogenesis in the rat. *Cancer Science* 2008; 99(9):1841–1846.

Garrido-Maraver J, Cordero MD, Oropesa-Avila M, et al. Coenzyme q10 therapy. *Molecular Syndromology* 2014; 5(3–4):187–197.

Gazdik F, Gvozdjakova A, Nadvornikova R, et al. Decreased levels of coenzyme Q(10) in patients with bronchial asthma. *Allergy* 2002; 57(9):811–814.

Gescher A, Steward WP, Brown K. Resveratrol in the management of human cancer: how strong is the clinical evidence? *Annals of the New York Academy of Sciences* 2013; 1290:12–20.

Gvozdjakova A, Kucharska J, Gvozdjak J. [Redox therapy in mitochondrial diseases using coenzyme Q10]. *Bratislavske lekarske listy* 1994; 95(10):443–451.

Hakim IA, Harris RB, Chow HH, Dean M, Brown S, Ali IU. Effect of a 4-month tea intervention on oxidative DNA damage among heavy smokers: role of glutathione S-transferase genotypes. *Cancer Epidemiology, Biomarkers & Prevention: A Publication of the American Association for Cancer Research, Cosponsored by the American Society of Preventive Oncology* 2004; 13(2):242–249.

Henning SM, Wang P, Carpenter CL, Heber D. Epigenetic effects of green tea polyphenols in cancer. *Epigenomics* 2013; 5(6):729–741.

Jacob RA, Sotoudeh G. Vitamin C function and status in chronic disease. *Nutrition in Clinical Care: An Official Publication of Tufts University* 2002; 5(2):66–74.

Jones CM, Mes P, Myers JR. Characterization and inheritance of the Anthocyanin fruit (Aft) tomato. *The Journal of Heredity* 2003; 94(6):449–456.

Joseph JA, Denisova NA, Arendash G, et al. Blueberry supplementation enhances signaling and prevents behavioral deficits in an Alzheimer disease model. *Nutritional Neuroscience* 2003; 6(3):153–162.

Juan ME, Alfaras I, Planas JM. Colorectal cancer chemoprevention by trans-resveratrol. *Pharmacological Research: The Official Journal of the Italian Pharmacological Society* 2012; 65(6):584–591.

Karatzi K, Papamichael C, Karatzis E, et al. Postprandial improvement of endothelial function by red wine and olive oil antioxidants: a synergistic effect of components of the Mediterranean diet. *Journal of the American College of Nutrition* 2008; 27(4):448–453.

Katiyar SK. Green tea prevents non-melanoma skin cancer by enhancing DNA repair. *Archives of Biochemistry and Biophysics* 2011; 508(2):152–158.

Kim HS, Kim MH, Jeong M, et al. EGCG blocks tumor promoter-induced MMP-9 expression via suppression of MAPK and AP-1 activation in human gastric AGS cells. *Anticancer Research* 2004; 24(2b):747–753.

Krajcovicova-Kudlackova M, Dusinska M, Valachovicova M, Blazicek P, Paukova V. Products of DNA, protein and lipid oxidative damage in relation to vitamin C plasma concentration. *Physiological research/ Academia Scientiarum Bohemoslovaca* 2006; 55(2):227–231.

Kunitomo M, Yamaguchi Y, Kagota S, Otsubo K. Beneficial effect of coenzyme Q10 on increased oxidative and nitrative stress and inflammation and individual metabolic components developing in a rat model of metabolic syndrome. *Journal of Pharmacological Sciences* 2008; 107(2):128–137.

Lamuela-Raventos RM, Andres-Lacueva C. [Wine in Mediterranean Diet]. *Archivos latinoamericanos de nutricion.* 54, no. 2, Suppl. 1 (2004): 79–82.

Langova M, Pilivkova Z, Smerak P, Bartova J, Barta I. Antimutagenic effect of resveratrol. *Czech Journal of Food Sciences* 2005; 23(5): 202–208.

Littarru GP, Tiano L. Clinical aspects of coenzyme Q10: an update. *Nutrition* (Burbank, Calif.) 2010; 26(3):250–254.

Liu J. The effects and mechanisms of mitochondrial nutrient alpha-lipoic acid on improving age-associated mitochondrial and cognitive dysfunction: An overview. *Neurochemical Research* 2008; 33(1):194–203.

332 FURTHER READING

Liu J, Wang LN. Mitochondrial enhancement for neurodegenerative movement disorders: a systematic review of trials involving creatine, coenzyme Q10, idebenone and mitoquinone. *CNS Drugs* 2014; 28(1):63–68.

Liu Y, Liu M, Li B, et al. Fresh raspberry phytochemical extract inhibits hepatic lesion in a Wistar rat model. *Nutrition & Metabolism* 2010; 7:84.

Li Y, Schellhorn HE. New developments and novel therapeutic perspectives for vitamin C. *Journal of Nutrition* 2007; 137(10):2171–2184.

Loh YH, Jakszyn P, Luben RN, Mulligan AA, Mitrou PN, Khaw KT. N-Nitroso compounds and cancer incidence: the European Prospective Investigation into Cancer and Nutrition (EPIC)-Norfolk Study. *American Journal of Clinical Nutrition*. 2011; 93(5):1053–1061.

Lulli M, Witort E, Papucci L, et al. Coenzyme Q10 protects retinal cells from apoptosis induced by radiation in vitro and in vivo. *Journal of Radiation Research* 2012; 53(5):695–703.

Luo H, Tang L, Tang M, et al. Phase IIa chemoprevention trial of green tea polyphenols in high-risk individuals of liver cancer: modulation of urinary excretion of green tea polyphenols and 8-hydroxydeoxyguanosine. *Carcinogenesis* 2006; 27(2):262–268.

Maczurek A, Hager K, Kenklies M, et al. Lipoic acid as an anti-inflammatory and neuroprotective treatment for Alzheimer's disease. *Advanced Drug Delivery Reviews* 2008; 60(13–14):1463–1470.

Markley HG. CoEnzyme Q10 and riboflavin: the mitochondrial connection. *Headache 52*, Suppl. 2 (2012): 81–87.

McCarty MF, Barroso-Aranda J, Contreras F. The "rejuvenatory" impact of lipoic acid on mitochondrial function in aging rats may reflect induction and activation of PPAR-gamma coactivator-1alpha. *Medical Hypotheses* 2009; 72(1):29–33.

Meyer JN, Leung MC, Rooney JP, et al. Mitochondria as a target of environmental toxicants. *Toxicological Sciences: An Official Journal of the Society of Toxicology* 2013; 134(1): 1–17.

Mobasheri A, Shakibaei M. Osteogenic effects of resveratrol in vitro: potential for the prevention and treatment of osteoporosis. *Annals of the New York Academy of Sciences* 2013; 1290:59–66.

Morales I, Feldman S, Krieger DR, Kalman D. A Clinical evaluation comparing the bioavailability of three vitamin C supplements in healthy non-smoking males. Available at: http://www.nutraproductsinc.com/clinicals_fastC_bioavailablility_three.html. Accessed 11/11/2014. Undated.

Moyers SB, Kumar NB. Green tea polyphenols and cancer chemoprevention: multiple mechanisms and endpoints for phase II trials. *Nutrition Reviews* 2004; 62(5):204–211.

Muller L, Menzel H. Studies on the efficacy of lipoate and dihydrolipoate in the alteration of cadmium2+ toxicity in isolated hepatocytes. *Biochimica et Biophysica Acta* 1990; 1052(3):386–391.

Negi PS, Jayaprakasha BS. Antioxidant and antimutagenic activities of pomegranante peel extracts. *Food Chemistry* 2003; 80(3):393 – 397.

Orsucci D, Mancuso M, Ienco EC, LoGerfo A, Siciliano G. Targeting mitochondrial dysfunction and neurodegeneration by means of coenzyme Q10 and its analogues. *Current Medicinal Chemistry* 2011; 18(26):4053–4064.

Packer L, Cadenas E. Lipoic acid: energy metabolism and redox regulation of transcription and cell signaling. *Journal of Clinical Biochemistry and Nutrition* 2011; 48(1):26–32.

Packer L, Tritschler HJ, Wessel K. Neuroprotection by the metabolic antioxidant alpha-lipoic acid. *Free Radical Biology & Medicine* 1997; 22(1–2):359–378.

Padayatty SJ, Katz A, Wang Y, et al. Vitamin C as an antioxidant: evaluation of its role in disease prevention. *Journal of the American College of Nutrition* 2003; 22(1):18–35.

Padmalayam I. Targeting mitochondrial oxidative stress through lipoic acid synthase: a novel strategy to manage diabetic cardiovascular disease. *Cardiovascular & Hematological Agents in Medicinal Chemistry* 2012; 10(3):223–233.

Parikh S, Saneto R, Falk MJ, et al. A modern approach to the treatment of mitochondrial disease. *Current Treatment Options in Neurology* 2009; 11(6): 414–430.

Pasinetti GM, Wang J, Ho L, Zhao W, Dubner L. Roles of resveratrol and other grape-derived polyphenols in Alzheimer's disease prevention and Treatment. *Biochimica et Biophysica Acta* 2014.

Pedreschi R, Cisneros-Zevallos L. Antimutagenic and antioxidant properties of phenolic fractions from Andean purple corn (Zea mays L.). *Journal of Agricultural and Food Chemistry* 2006; 54(13):4557–4567.

Perez-Lopez FR, Chedraui P, Haya J, Cuadros JL. Effects of the Mediterranean diet on longevity and age-related morbid conditions. *Maturitas* 2009; 64(2):67–79.

Saini R. Coenzyme Q10: The essential nutrient. *Journal of Pharmacy & Bioallied Sciences* 2011; 3(3):466–467.

Salinthone S, Yadav V, Bourdette DN, Carr DW. Lipoic acid: a novel therapeutic approach for multiple sclerosis and other chronic inflammatory diseases of the CNS. *Endocrine, Metabolic & Immune Disorders Drug Targets* 2008; 8(2):132–142.

Santhosh KT, Swarnam J, Ramadasan K. Potent suppressive effect of green tea polyphenols on tobacco-induced mutagenicity. *Phytomedicine: International Journal of Phytotherapy and Phytopharmacology* 2005; 12(3):216–220.

Schmidt CW. Unraveling environmental effects on mitochondria. *Environmental Health Perspectives* 2010; 118(7): A292–A297.

Schulz C, Obermuller-Jevic UC, Hasselwander O, Bernhardt J, Biesalski HK. Comparison of the relative bioavailability of different coenzyme Q10 formulations with a novel solubilizate (Solu Q10). *International Journal of Food Sciences and Nutrition* 2006; 57(7–8):546–555.

Schwingshackl L, Hoffmann G. Adherence to Mediterranean diet and risk of cancer: a systematic review and meta-analysis of observational studies. *International Journal of Cancer/Journal international du cancer* 2014; 135(8):1884–1897.

Seeram NP. Berry fruits for cancer prevention: current status and future prospects. *Journal of Agricultural and Food Chemistry* 2008; 56(3):630–635.

Selvakumar E, Prahalathan C, Sudharsan PT, Varalakshmi P. Protective effect of lipoic acid on micronuclei induction by cyclophosphamide. *Archives of Toxicology* 2006; 80(2):115–119.

Smith JR, Thiagaraj HV, Seaver B, Parker KK. Differential activity of lipoic acid enantiomers in cell culture. *Journal of Herbal Pharmacotherapy* 2005; 5(3):43–54.

Srinivasan K. Black pepper and its pungent principle-piperine: a review of diverse physiological effects. *Critical Reviews in Food Science and Nutrition* 2007; 47(8):735–748.

Stoner GD, Wang LS, Seguin C, et al. Multiple berry types prevent N-nitrosomethylbenzylamine-induced esophageal cancer in rats. *Pharmaceutical Research* 2010; 27(6):1138–1145.

Streeper RS, Henriksen EJ, Jacob S, Hokama JY, Fogt DL, Tritschler HJ.

Differential effects of lipoic acid stereoisomers on glucose metabolism in insulin-resistant skeletal muscle. *The American Journal of Physiology* 1997; 273(1 Pt 1):E185–191.

Turkez H, Aydin E. The genoprotective activity of resveratrol on permethrin-induced genotoxic damage in cultured human lymphocytes. Available at http://www.scielo.br/scielo.php?pid=S1516 -89132013000300008&script=sci_arttext. Last updated 3/22/2012. Accessed 11/17/2014.

USDA. United States Department of Agriculture website, Topics page. Bacon and Food Safety. Available at: http://www.fsis.usda.gov/wps/ portal/fsis/topics/food-safety-education/get-answers/food-safety -fact-sheets/meat-preparation/bacon-and-food-safety/ct_index. Last updated 10/29/2013. Accessed 11/17/2014.

Valcheva-Kuzmanova S, Kuzmanov K, Mihova V, Krasnaliev I, Borisova P, Belcheva A. Antihyperlipidemic effect of Aronia melanocarpa fruit juice in rats fed a high-cholesterol diet. *Plant Foods for Human Nutrition* (Dordrecht, Netherlands) 2007; 62(1):19–24.

Valcheva-Kuzmanova S, Kuzmanov K, Tancheva S, Belcheva A. Hypoglycemic and hypolipidemic effects of Aronia melanocarpa fruit juice in streptozotocin-induced diabetic rats. *Methods and Findings in Experimental and Clinical Pharmacology* 2007; 29(2):101–105.

Villalba JM, Parrado C, Santos-Gonzalez M, Alcain FJ. Therapeutic use of coenzyme Q10 and coenzyme Q10-related compounds and formulations. *Expert Opinion on Investigational Drugs* 2010; 19(4):535–554.

Wang Y, Li X, Guo Y, Chan L, Guan X. alpha-Lipoic acid increases energy expenditure by enhancing adenosine monophosphate-activated protein kinase-peroxisome proliferator-activated receptor-gamma coactivator-1alpha signaling in the skeletal muscle of aged mice. *Metabolism: Clinical and Experimental* 2010; 59(7):967–976.

Wang ZY, Khan WA, Bickers DR, Mukhtar H. Protection against polycyclic aromatic hydrocarbon-induced skin tumor initiation in mice by green tea polyphenols. *Carcinogenesis* 1989; 10(2):411–415.

Weisel T, Baum M, Eisenbrand G, et al. An anthocyanin/polyphenolic-rich fruit juice reduces oxidative DNA damage and increases glutathione level in healthy probands. *Biotechnology Journal* 2006; 1(4):388–397.

Yan J, Fujii K, Yao J, et al. Reduced coenzyme Q10 supplementation decelerates senescence in SAMP1 mice. *Experimental Gerontology* 2006; 41(2):130–140.

Yaseen NJ, Mustafa Al-Attar MS. Assessment of mutagenic and antimutagenic effects of Punica granatum against ifosfamide induced chromosomal aberrations in male albino mice. *Iraqi Journal of Cancer and Medical Genetics* 2014; 7(1):5–10.

Yuan JH, Li YQ, Yang XY. Inhibition of epigallocatechin gallate on orthotopic colon cancer by upregulating the Nrf2-UGT1A signal pathway in nude mice. *Pharmacology* 2007; 80(4):269–278.

Zafra-Stone S, Yasmin T, Bagchi M, Chatterjee A, Vinson JA, Bagchi D. Berry anthocyanins as novel antioxidants in human health and disease prevention. *Molecular Nutrition & Food Research* 2007; 51(6):675–683.

LIVER SUPPORT

Abenavoli L, Capasso R, Milic N, Capasso F. Milk thistle in liver diseases: past, present, future. *Phytotherapy Research* 2010; 24(10):1423–1432.

A.D.A.M. *New York Times.* Alcoholic liver disease in-depth report. Available at http://www.nytimes.com/health/guides/disease/alcoholic-liver-disease/print.html. Accessed 11/11/2014.

Agrawal RC, Mehrotra N. Assessment of mutagenic potential of propoxur and its modulation by indole-3-carbinol. *Food and Chemical Toxicology: An International Journal Published for the British Industrial Biological Research Association* 1997; 35(10–11):1081–1084.

Al-Bader A, Abul H, Hussain T, Al-Moosawi M, Mathew TC, Dashti H. Selenium and liver cirrhosis. *Molecular and Cellular Biochemistry* 1998; 185(1–2):1–6.

Antony ML, Kim SH, Singh SV. Critical role of p53 upregulated modulator of apoptosis in benzyl isothiocyanate-induced apoptotic cell death. *PloS ONE* 2012; 7(2):e32267.

Aras U, Gandhi YA, Masso-Welch PA, Morris ME. Chemopreventive and anti-angiogenic effects of dietary phenethyl isothiocyanate in an N-methyl nitrosourea-induced breast cancer animal model. *Biopharmaceutics & Drug Disposition* 2013; 34(2):98–106.

Baker RD, Baker SS, LaRosa K, Whitney C, Newburger PE. Selenium regulation of glutathione peroxidase in human hepatoma cell line Hep3B. *Archives of Biochemistry and Biophysics* 1993; 304(1):53–57.

Bajt ML, Knight TR, Lemasters JJ, Jaeschke H. Acetaminophen-induced oxidant stress and cell injury in cultured mouse hepatocytes: protection by N-acetyl cysteine. *Toxicological Sciences: An Official Journal of the Society of Toxicology* 2004; 80(2):343–349.

Bosetti C, Filomeno M, Riso P, et al. Cruciferous vegetables and cancer risk in a network of case-control studies. *Annals of Oncology: Official Journal of the European Society for Medical Oncology/ESMO* 2012; 23(8):2198–2203.

Burk RF, Hill KE, Awad JA, Morrow JD, Lyons PR. Liver and kidney necrosis in selenium-deficient rats depleted of glutathione. *Laboratory Investigation: A Journal of Technical Methods and Pathology* 1995; 72(6):723–730.

Chan C, Lin HJ, Lin J. Stress-associated hormone, norepinephrine, increases proliferation and IL-6 levels of human pancreatic duct epithelial cells and can be inhibited by the dietary agent, sulforaphane. *International Journal of Oncology* 2008; 33(2):415–419.

Chang HF, Lin YH, Chu CC, Wu SJ, Tsai YH, Chao JC. Protective effects of Ginkgo biloba, Panax ginseng, and Schizandra chinensis extract on liver injury in rats. *The American Journal of Chinese Medicine* 2007; 35(6):995–1009.

Chen N, Ko M. Schisandrin B-induced glutathione antioxidant response and cardioprotection are mediated by reactive oxidant species production in rat hearts. *Biological & Pharmaceutical Bulletin* 2010; 33(5):825–829.

Chen Y, Dong H, Thompson DC, Shertzer HG, Nebert DW, Vasiliou V. Glutathione defense mechanism in liver injury: insights from animal models. *Food and Chemical Toxicology: An International Journal Published for the British Industrial Biological Research Association* 2013; 60:38–44.

Chinnakannu K, Chen D, Li Y, et al. Cell cycle–dependent effects of 3,3'-diindolylmethane on proliferation and apoptosis of prostate cancer cells. *Journal of Cellular Physiology* 2009; 219(1):94–99.

Choi EJ, Kim GH. Apigenin induces apoptosis through a mitochondria/caspase-pathway in human breast cancer MDA-MB-453 cells. *Journal of Clinical Biochemistry and Nutrition* 2009; 44(3):260–265.

Conti M, Malandrino S, Magistretti MJ. Protective activity of silipide on liver damage in rodents. *Japanese Journal of Pharmacology* 1992; 60(4):315–321.

Cornell University. What processes does the liver undergo to remove toxins? Available at http://people.cornellcollege.edu/bnowak thompson/pdfs/liverDetox.pdf. Accessed 11/17/2014.

de Oliveira CP, Simplicio FI, de Lima VM, et al. Oral administration of S-nitroso-N-acetylcysteine prevents the onset of non alcoholic fatty liver disease in rats. *World Journal of Gastroenterology* 2006; 12(12):1905–1911.

de Oliveira CP, Stefano JT, de Siqueira ER, et al. Combination of N-acetylcysteine and metformin improves histological steatosis and fibrosis in patients with non-alcoholic steatohepatitis. *Hepatology Research: The Official Journal of the Japan Society of Hepatology* 2008; 38(2):159–165.

Deep G, Gangar SC, Oberlies NH, Kroll DJ, Agarwal R. Isosilybin A induces apoptosis in human prostate cancer cells via targeting Akt, NF-kappaB, and androgen receptor signaling. *Molecular Carcinogenesis* 2010; 49(10):902–912.

Deep G, Oberlies NH, Kroll DJ, Agarwal R. Isosilybin B and isosilybin A inhibit growth, induce G1 arrest and cause apoptosis in human prostate cancer LNCaP and 22Rv1 cells. *Carcinogenesis* 2007; 28(7):1533–1542.

Deep G, Oberlies NH, Kroll DJ, Agarwal R. Isosilybin B causes androgen receptor degradation in human prostate carcinoma cells via PI3K-Akt-Mdm2-mediated pathway. *Oncogene* 2008; 27(28):3986–3998.

Eminzade S, Uraz F, Izzettin FV. Silymarin protects liver against toxic effects of anti-tuberculosis drugs in experimental animals. *Nutrition & Metabolism* 2008; 5:18.

Fan S, Yu Y, Qi M, et al. P53-mediated GSH depletion enhanced the cytotoxicity of NO in silibinin-treated human cervical carcinoma HeLa cells. *Free Radical Research* 2012; 46(9):1082–1092.

Fimognari C, Nusse M, Cesari R, Iori R, Cantelli-Forti G, Hrelia P. Growth inhibition, cell-cycle arrest and apoptosis in human T-cell leukemia by the isothiocyanate sulforaphane. *Carcinogenesis* 2002; 23(4):581–586.

Gorla N, de Ferreyra EC, Villarruel MC, de Fenos OM, Castro JA. Studies on the mechanism of glutathione prevention of carbon tetrachloride-induced liver injury. *British Journal of Experimental Pathology* 1983; 64(4):388–395.

Horn TL, Reichert MA, Bliss RL, Malejka-Giganti D. Modulations of P450 mRNA in liver and mammary gland and P450 activities and metabolism of estrogen in liver by treatment of rats with indole-3-carbinol. *Biochemical Pharmacology* 2002; 64(3):393–404.

Hwang ES, Lee HJ. Benzyl isothiocyanate inhibits metalloproteinase-2/-9 expression by suppressing the mitogen-activated protein kinase in SK-Hep1 human hepatoma cells. *Food and Chemical Toxicology: An International Journal Published for the British Industrial Biological Research Association* 2008; 46(7):2358–2364.

Ip SP, Poon MK, Che CT, Ng KH, Kong YC, Ko KM. Schisandrin B protects against carbon tetrachloride toxicity by enhancing the mitochondrial glutathione redox status in mouse liver. *Free Radical Biology & Medicine* 1996; 21(5):709–712.

Jayaraj R, Deb U, Bhaskar AS, Prasad GB, Rao PV. Hepatoprotective efficacy of certain flavonoids against microcystin induced toxicity in mice. *Environmental Toxicology* 2007; 22(5):472–479.

Jo EH, Kim SH, Ahn NS, et al. Efficacy of sulforaphane is mediated by p38 MAP kinase and caspase-7 activations in ER-positive and COX-2-expressed human breast cancer cells. *European Journal of Cancer Prevention: The Official Journal of the European Cancer Prevention Organisation (ECP)* 2007; 16(6):505–510.

Kassie F, Uhl M, Rabot S, et al. Chemoprevention of 2-amino-3-methylimidazo[4,5-f]quinoline (IQ)-induced colonic and hepatic preneoplastic lesions in the F344 rat by cruciferous vegetables administered simultaneously with the carcinogen. *Carcinogenesis* 2003; 24(2):255–261.

Kayashima T, Matsubara K. Antiangiogenic effect of carnosic acid and carnosol, neuroprotective compounds in rosemary leaves. *Bioscience, Biotechnology, and Biochemistry* 2012; 76(1):115–119.

Ketterer B, Coles B, Meyer DJ. The role of glutathione in detoxication. *Environmental Health Perspectives* 1983; 49:59–69.

Khan SI, Aumsuwan P, Khan IA, Walker LA, Dasmahapatra AK. Epigenetic events associated with breast cancer and their prevention by dietary components targeting the epigenome. *Chemical Research in Toxicology* 2012; 25(1):61–73.

Kidd P, Head K. A review of the bioavailability and clinical efficacy of milk thistle phytosome: a silybin-phosphatidylcholine complex (Siliphos). *Alternative Medicine Review: A Journal of Clinical Therapeutic* 2005; 10(3):193–203.

Kilciksiz S, Demirel C, Evirgen Ayhan S, et al. N-acetylcysteine ame-
liorates nitrosative stress on radiation-inducible damage in rat liver.
Journal of B.U.ON.: Official Journal of the Balkan Union of Oncology 2011;
16(1):154–159.

Kim SH, Sehrawat A, Singh SV. Dietary chemopreventative benzyl isothiocyanate inhibits breast cancer stem cells in vitro and in vivo. *Cancer Prevention Research* (Philadelphia, Pa.) 2013; 6(8):782–790.

Lawler JM, Demaree SR. Relationship between NADP-specific isocitrate
dehydrogenase and glutathione peroxidase in aging rat skeletal muscle. *Mechanisms of Ageing and Development* 2001; 122(3):291–304.

Lester GE, Jifon JL, Crosby KM. Superoxide dismutase activity in meso-
carp tissue from divergent Cucumis melo L. genotypes. *Plant Foods
for Human Nutrition* (Dordrecht, Netherlands) 2009; 64(3):205–211.

Li W, Zhu Y, Yan X, et al. [The prevention of primary liver cancer by selenium in high risk populations]. *Zhonghua yu fang yi xue za zhi [Chinese
journal of preventive medicine]* 2000; 34(6):336–338.

Lieber CS, Leo MA, Cao Q, Ren C, DeCarli LM. Silymarin retards the
progression of alcohol-induced hepatic fibrosis in baboons. *Journal of
Clinical Gastroenterology* 2003; 37(4):336–339.

Liu BN, Yan HQ, Wu X, et al. Apoptosis induced by benzyl isothiocyanate in gefitinib-resistant lung cancer cells is associated with Akt/
MAPK pathways and generation of reactive oxygen species. *Cell Biochemistry and Biophysics* 2013; 66(1):81–92.

Liu X, Lv K. Cruciferous vegetables intake is inversely associated with
risk of breast cancer: a meta-analysis. *Breast* (Edinburgh, Scotland)
2013; 22(3):309–313.

Loguercio C, Andreone P, Brisc C, et al. Silybin combined with phosphatidylcholine and vitamin E in patients with nonalcoholic fatty liver
disease: a randomized controlled trial. *Free Radical Biology & Medicine*
2012; 52(9):1658–1665.

Marconett CN, Singhal AK, Sundar SN, Firestone GL. Indole-3-carbinol
disrupts estrogen receptor-alpha dependent expression of insulin-like
growth factor-1 receptor and insulin receptor substrate-1 and proliferation of human breast cancer cells. *Molecular and Cellular Endocrinology* 2012; 363(1–2):74–84.

Mehta K, Van Thiel DH, Shah N, Mobarhan S. Nonalcoholic fatty liver
disease: pathogenesis and the role of antioxidants. *Nutrition Reviews*
2002; 60(9):289–293.

Millea PJ. N-acetylcysteine: multiple clinical applications. *American Family Physician* 2009; 80(3):265–269.

Moskaug JO, Carlsen H, Myhrstad MC, Blomhoff R. Polyphenols and glutathione synthesis regulation. *American Journal of Clinical Nutrition* 2005; 81(1 Suppl):277s–283s.

National Cancer Institute. Milk Thistle (PDQ®). Available at: http://www.cancer.gov/cancertopics/pdq/cam/milkthistle/Patient/page1/AllPages/Print. Updated 12/24/2013. Accessed 11/11/2014.

Nho CW, Jeffery E. The synergistic upregulation of phase II detoxification enzymes by glucosinolate breakdown products in cruciferous vegetables. *Toxicology and Applied Pharmacology* 2001; 174(2):146–152.

Ozardali I, Bitiren M, Karakilcik AZ, Zerin M, Aksoy N, Musa D. Effects of selenium on histopathological and enzymatic changes in experimental liver injury of rats. *Experimental and Toxicologic Pathology: Official Journal of the Gesellschaft fur Toxikologische Pathologie* 2004; 56(1–2):59–64.

Parkin DR, Malejka-Giganti D. Differences in the hepatic P450-dependent metabolism of estrogen and tamoxifen in response to treatment of rats with 3,3'-diindolylmethane and its parent compound indole-3-carbinol. *Cancer Detection and Prevention* 2004; 28(1):72–79.

Pferschy-Wenzig EM, Atanasov AG, Malainer C, et al. Identification of isosilybin a from milk thistle seeds as an agonist of peroxisome proliferator-activated receptor gamma. *Journal of Natural Products* 2014; 77(4):842–847.

Pradhan SC, Girish C. Hepatoprotective herbal drug, silymarin from experimental pharmacology to clinical medicine. *The Indian Journal of Medical Research* 2006; 124(5):491–504.

Prakash D, Gupta C. Glucosinolates: the phytochemicals of nutraceutical importance. *Journal of Complementary & Integrative Medicine* 2012; 9:Article 13.

Ramasamy K, Agarwal R. Multitargeted therapy of cancer by silymarin. *Cancer Letters* 2008; 269(2):352–362.

Ramirez MC, Singletary K. Regulation of estrogen receptor alpha expression in human breast cancer cells by sulforaphane. *Journal of Nutritional Biochemistry* 2009; 20(3):195–201.

Rao CV. Benzyl isothiocyanate: double trouble for breast cancer cells. *Cancer Prevention Research* (Philadelphia, Pa.) 2013; 6(8):760–763.

Ravichandran K, Velmurugan B, Gu M, Singh RP, Agarwal R. Inhibitory effect of silibinin against azoxymethane-induced colon tumorigenesis in A/J mice. *Clinical Cancer Research: An Official Journal of the American Association for Cancer Research* 2010; 16(18):4595–4606.

Richie JP, Jr., Nichenametla S, Neidig W, et al. Randomized controlled trial of oral glutathione supplementation on body stores of glutathione. *European Journal of Nutrition* 2014.

Rogan EG. The natural chemopreventive compound indole-3-carbinol: state of the science. *In vivo* (Athens, Greece) 2006; 20(2):221–228.

Saller R, Brignoli R, Melzer J, Meier R. An updated systematic review with meta-analysis for the clinical evidence of silymarin. *Forschende Komplementarmedizin* (2006). 2008; 15(1):9–20.

Saller R, Meier R, Brignoli R. The use of silymarin in the treatment of liver diseases. *Drugs* 2001; 61(14):2035–2063.

Sangeetha N, Viswanathan P, Balasubramanian T, Nalini N. Colon cancer chemopreventive efficacy of silibinin through perturbation of xenobiotic metabolizing enzymes in experimental rats. *European Journal of Pharmacology* 2012; 674(2–3):430–438.

Shaarawy SM, Tohamy AA, Elgendy SM, et al. Protective effects of garlic and silymarin on NDEA-induced rats hepatotoxicity. *International Journal of Biological Sciences* 2009; 5(6):549–557.

Smith S, Sepkovic D, Bradlow HL, Auborn KJ. 3,3'-Diindolylmethane and genistein decrease the adverse effects of estrogen in LNCaP and PC-3 prostate cancer cells. *Journal of Nutrition* 2008; 138(12):2379–2385.

Song Z, Deaciuc I, Song M, et al. Silymarin protects against acute ethanol-induced hepatotoxicity in mice. *Alcoholism, Clinical and Experimental Research* 2006; 30(3):407–413.

Szilard S, Szentgyorgyi D, Demeter I. Protective effect of Legalon in workers exposed to organic solvents. *Acta medica Hungarica* 1988; 45(2):249–256.

Taskin E, Dursun N. Recovery of adriamycin induced mitochondrial dysfunction in liver by selenium. *Cytotechnology* 2014.

Thorne Research. Silybum marianum (milk thistle). *Alternative Medicine Review: A Journal of Clinical Therapeutic* 1999; 4(4):272–274.

Uzun MA, Koksal N, Kadioglu H, et al. Effects of N-acetylcysteine on regeneration following partial hepatectomy in rats with nonalcoholic fatty liver disease. *Surgery Today* 2009; 39(7):592–597.

Velussi M, Cernigoi AM, De Monte A, Dapas F, Caffau C, Zilli M. Long-term (12 months) treatment with an anti-oxidant drug (silymarin) is effective on hyperinsulinemia, exogenous insulin need and malondialdehyde levels in cirrhotic diabetic patients. *Journal of Hepatology.* 1997; 26(4):871–879.

Vouldoukis I, Lacan D, Kamate C, et al. Antioxidant and anti-inflammatory properties of a Cucumis melo LC. extract rich in superoxide dismutase activity. *Journal of Ethnopharmacology* 2004; 94(1):67–75.

Wang TT, Schoene NW, Milner JA, Kim YS. Broccoli-derived phytochemicals indole-3-carbinol and 3,3'-diindolylmethane exerts concentration-dependent pleiotropic effects on prostate cancer cells: comparison with other cancer preventive phytochemicals. *Molecular Carcinogenesis* 2012; 51(3):244–256.

Wang Y, Wimmer U, Lichtlen P, et al. Metal-responsive transcription factor-1 (MTF-1) is essential for embryonic liver development and heavy metal detoxification in the adult liver. *FASEB Journal: Official Publication of the Federation of American Societies for Experimental Biology* 2004; 18(10):1071–1079.

Yan F, Zhang QY, Jiao L, et al. Synergistic hepatoprotective effect of Schisandrae lignans with Astragalus polysaccharides on chronic liver injury in rats. *Phytomedicine: International Journal of Phytotherapy and Phytopharmacology* 2009; 16(9):805–813.

Yao J, Zhi M, Minhu C. Effect of silybin on high-fat-induced fatty liver in rats. *Brazilian Journal of Medical and Biological Research [Revista brasileira de pesquisas medicas e biologicas/Sociedade Brasileira de Biofisica . . . [et al.]* 2011; 44(7):652–659.

Yuan L, Kaplowitz N. Glutathione in liver diseases and hepatotoxicity. *Molecular Aspects of Medicine* 2009; 30(1–2):29–41.

Zhang Y, Tang L, Gonzalez V. Selected isothiocyanates rapidly induce growth inhibition of cancer cells. *Molecular Cancer Therapeutics* 2003; 2(10):1045–1052.

Zhou T, Li G, Cao B, et al. Downregulation of Mcl-1 through inhibition of translation contributes to benzyl isothiocyanate-induced cell cycle arrest and apoptosis in human leukemia cells. *Cell Death & Disease* 2013; 4:e515.

Zhu HJ, Brinda BJ, Chavin KD, Bernstein HJ, Patrick KS, Markowitz JS. An assessment of pharmacokinetics and antioxidant activity of free silymarin flavonolignans in healthy volunteers: a dose escalation study. *Drug Metabolism and Disposition: The Biological Fate of Chemicals* 2013; 41(9):1679–1685.

Zhu Y, Zhuang JX, Wang Q, Zhang HY, Yang P. Inhibitory effect of benzyl isothiocyanate on proliferation in vitro of human glioma cells. *Asian Pacific Journal of Cancer Prevention* 2013; 14(4):2607–2610.

BRAIN AND NEUROLOGICAL SUPPORT

Berbert AA, Kondo CR, Almendra CL, Matsuo T, Dichi I. Supplementation of fish oil and olive oil in patients with rheumatoid arthritis. *Nutrition* (Burbank, Calif.) 2005; 21(2):131–136.

Castner SA, Williams GV. Tuning the engine of cognition: a focus on NMDA/D1 receptor interactions in prefrontal cortex. *Brain and Cognition* 2007; 63(2):94–122.

Cosman KM, Boyle LL, Porsteinsson AP. Memantine in the treatment of mild-to-moderate Alzheimer's disease. *Expert Opinion on Pharmacotherapy* 2007; 8(2):203–214.

Covas MI, Konstantinidou V, Fito M. Olive oil and cardiovascular health. *Journal of Cardiovascular Pharmacology* 2009; 54(6):477–482.

Fernandes G, Venkatraman JT. Role of omega-3 fatty acids in health and disease. *Nutrition Research* 1993; 13(Suppl 1):S19 – S45.

Flood JF, Morley JE, Roberts E. Pregnenolone sulfate enhances post-training memory processes when injected in very low doses into limbic system structures: the amygdala is by far the most sensitive. *Proceedings of the National Academy of Sciences of the United States of America* 1995; 92(23):10806–10810.

Hamblin J. *The Atlantic.* The toxins that threaten our brains. March 18, 2014. Available at http://www.theatlantic.com/features/archive/2014/03/the -toxins-that-threaten-our-brains/284466/. Accessed 11/11/2014.

Hige T, Fujiyoshi Y, Takahashi T. Neurosteroid pregnenolone sulfate enhances glutamatergic synaptic transmission by facilitating presynaptic calcium currents at the calyx of Held of immature rats. *European Journal of Neuroscience* 2006; 24(7):1955–1966.

Huang CL, Sumpio BE. Olive oil, the mediterranean diet, and cardiovascular health. *Journal of the American College of Surgeons* 2008; 207(3):407–416.

Kim BW, Koppula S, Kim JW, et al. Modulation of LPS-stimulated neuro-inflammation in BV-2 microglia by Gastrodia elata: 4-hydroxybenzyl alcohol is the bioactive candidate. *Journal of Ethnopharmacology* 2012; 139(2):549–557.

Kim IS, Choi DK, Jung HJ. Neuroprotective effects of vanillyl alcohol in Gastrodia elata Blume through suppression of oxidative stress and anti-apoptotic activity in toxin-induced dopaminergic MN9D cells. *Molecules* 2011; 16(7):5349–5361.

Kumar H, Kim IS, More SV, Kim BW, Bahk YY, Choi DK. Gastrodin protects apoptotic dopaminergic neurons in a toxin-induced Parkinson's disease model. *Evidence-based Complementary and Alternative Medicine: eCAM* 2013; 2013:514095.

Lou-Bonafonte JM, Fito M, Covas MI, Farras M, Osada J. HDL-related mechanisms of olive oil protection in cardiovascular disease. *Current Vascular Pharmacology* 2012; 10(4):392–409.

Manavalan A, Ramachandran U, Sundaramurthi H, et al. Gastrodia elata Blume (tianma) mobilizes neuro-protective capacities. *International Journal of Biochemistry and Molecular Biology* 2012; 3(2):219–241.

Mangone CA, Genovese O, Abel C. [Behavioral-cognitive disorders due to chronic exposure to industrial and environmental toxic substances]. *Vertex* (Buenos Aires, Argentina) 2006; 17(65):16–22.

Maurice T, Gregoire C, Espallergues J. Neuro(active)steroids actions at the neuromodulatory sigma1 (sigma1) receptor: biochemical and physiological evidences, consequences in neuroprotection. *Pharmacology, Biochemistry, and Behavior* 2006; 84(4):581–597.

Mishra M, Huang J, Lee YY, et al. Gastrodia elata modulates amyloid precursor protein cleavage and cognitive functions in mice. *Bioscience Trends* 2011; 5(3):129–138.

Muldoon MF, Ryan CM, Sheu L, Yao JK, Conklin SM, Manuck SB. Serum phospholipid docosahexaenonic acid is associated with cognitive functioning during middle adulthood. *Journal of Nutrition* 2010; 140(4):848–853.

Nikitin VP. A new mechanism of synapse-specific neuronal plasticity. *Neuroscience and Behavioral Physiology* 2007; 37(6):559–570.

Nilius B, Voets T. A TRP channel-steroid marriage. *Nature Cell Biology* 2008; 10(12):1383–1384.

Ramachandran U, Manavalan A, Sundaramurthi H, et al. Tianma

modulates proteins with various neuro-regenerative modalities in differentiated human neuronal SH-SY5Y cells. *Neurochemistry International* 2012; 60(8):827–836.

Reddy BS, Burill C, Rigotty J. Effect of diets high in omega-3 and omega-6 fatty acids on initiation and postinitiation stages of colon carcinogenesis. *Cancer Research* 1991; 51(2):487–491.

Ruiz-Canela M, Martinez-Gonzalez MA. Olive oil in the primary prevention of cardiovascular disease. *Maturitas* 2011; 68(3):245–250.

Sabeti J, Nelson TE, Purdy RH, Gruol DL. Steroid pregnenolone sulfate enhances NMDA-receptor-independent long-term potentiation at hippocampal CA1 synapses: role for L-type calcium channels and sigma-receptors. *Hippocampus* 2007; 17(5):349–369.

Simopoulos AP. Evolutionary aspects of diet, the omega-6/omega-3 ratio and genetic variation: nutritional implications for chronic diseases. *Biomedicine & Pharmacotherapy [Biomedecine & pharmacotherapie]* 2006; 60(9):502–507.

Simopoulos AP. Omega-3 fatty acids in inflammation and autoimmune diseases. *Journal of the American College of Nutrition* 2002; 21(6):495–505.

Sliwinski A, Monnet FP, Schumacher M, Morin-Surun MP. Pregnenolone sulfate enhances long-term potentiation in CA1 in rat hippocampus slices through the modulation of N-methyl-D-aspartate receptors. *Journal of Neuroscience Research* 2004; 78(5):691–701.

Vallee M, Mayo W, Le Moal M. Role of pregnenolone, dehydroepiandrosterone and their sulfate esters on learning and memory in cognitive aging. *Brain Research. Brain Research Reviews* 2001; 37(1–3):301–312.

Vas A, Gulyas B. Eburnamine derivatives and the brain. *Medicinal Research Reviews* 2005; 25(6):737–757.

Vas A, Gulyas B, Szabo Z, et al. Clinical and non-clinical investigations using positron emission tomography, near infrared spectroscopy and transcranial Doppler methods on the neuroprotective drug vinpocetine: a summary of evidences. *Journal of the Neurological Sciences* 2002; 203–204:259–262.

Weinbrenner T, Fito M, de la Torre R, et al. Olive oils high in phenolic compounds modulate oxidative/antioxidative status in men. *Journal of Nutrition* 2004; 134(9):2314–2321.

Wenk GL. Neuropathologic changes in Alzheimer's disease: potential targets for treatment. *Journal of Clinical Psychiatry* 2006; 67 Suppl 3:3–7; quiz 23.

DIGESTIVE AND GASTROINTESTINAL SUPPORT

Anderson JW, Baird P, Davis RH, Jr., et al. Health benefits of dietary fiber. *Nutrition Reviews* 2009; 67(4):188–205.

Clemens R, Kranz S, Mobley AR, et al. Filling America's fiber intake gap: summary of a roundtable to probe realistic solutions with a focus on grain-based foods. *Journal of Nutrition* 2012; 142(7):1390s–1401s.

De-Souza DA, Greene LJ. Intestinal permeability and systemic infections in critically ill patients: Effect of glutamine. *Critical Care Medicine* 2005; 33(5):1125–1135 1110.1097/1101.CCM.0000162680.0000152397.00 00162697.

Frankel WL, Zhang W, Afonso J, et al. Glutamine enhancement of structure and function in transplanted small intestine in the rat. *Journal of Parenteral and Enteral Nutrition* 1993; 17(1):47–55.

Gaby AR. *Nutritional Medicine. Dietary Fiber.* Concord, N.H.: Fritz Perlberg; 2011.

Kuhn KS, Muscaritoli M, Wischmeyer P, Stehle P. Glutamine as indispensable nutrient in oncology: experimental and clinical evidence. *European Journal of Nutrition* 2010; 49(4):197–210.

Lacey JM, Wilmore DW. Is glutamine a conditionally essential amino acid? *Nutrition Reviews* 1990; 48(8):297–309.

Miller AL. Therapeutic considerations of L-glutamine: a review of the literature. *Alternative Medicine Review: A Journal of Clinical Therapeutic* 1999; 4(4):239–248.

Sanders ME. Impact of probiotics on colonizing microbiota of the gut. *Journal of Clinical Gastroenterology* 45 Suppl. (2011): S115–119.

Slavin J. Fiber and prebiotics: mechanisms and health benefits. *Nutrients* 2013; 5(4):1417–1435.

Suarez F, Levitt M.D., Adshead J, Barkin JS. Pancreatic supplements reduce symptomatic response of healthy subjects to a high fat meal. *Digestive Diseases and Sciences* 1999; 44(7):1317–1321.

Vieira AT, Teixeira MM, Martins FS. The role of probiotics and prebiotics in inducing gut immunity. *Frontiers in Immunology* 2013; 4:445.

CARDIOVASCULAR SUPPORT

Aviram M, Rosenblat M, Gaitini D, et al. Pomegranate juice consumption for 3 years by patients with carotid artery stenosis reduces common carotid intima-media thickness, blood pressure and LDL oxidation. *Clinical Nutrition* (Edinburgh, Scotland) 2004; 23(3):423–433.

Canada AT, Calabrese EJ. Superoxide dismutase: its role in xenobiotic detoxification. *Pharmacology & Therapeutics* 1989; 44(2):285–295.

de Nigris F, Williams-Ignarro S, Lerman LO, et al. Beneficial effects of pomegranate juice on oxidation-sensitive genes and endothelial nitric oxide synthase activity at sites of perturbed shear stress. *Proceedings of the National Academy of Sciences of the United States of America* 2005; 102(13):4896–4901.

Dong S, Tong X, Liu H, Gao Q. [Protective effects of pomegranate polyphenols on cardiac function in rats with myocardial ischemia/reperfusion injury]. *Nan fang yi ke da xue xue bao [Journal of Southern Medical University]* 2012; 32(7):924–927.

Eftychiou C, Antoniades L, Makri L, et al. Homocysteine levels and MTHFR polymorphisms in young patients with acute myocardial infarction: a case control study. *Hellenic Journal of Cardiology [Hellenike kardiologike epitheorese]* 2012; 53(3):189–194.

Hassanpour Fard M, Ghule AE, Bodhankar SL, Dikshit M. Cardioprotective effect of whole fruit extract of pomegranate on doxorubicin-induced toxicity in rat. *Pharmaceutical Biology* 2011; 49(4):377–382.

Hao L, Chen L, Sai X, et al. Synergistic effects of elevated homocysteine level and abnormal blood lipids on the onset of stroke. *Neural Regeneration Research* 2013; 8(31):2923–2931.

Hofmann MA, Lalla E, Lu Y, et al. Hyperhomocysteinemia enhances vascular inflammation and accelerates atherosclerosis in a murine model. *Journal of Clinical Investigation* 2001; 107(6):675–683.

Jones ML, Martoni CJ, Parent M, Prakash S. Cholesterol-lowering efficacy of a microencapsulated bile salt hydrolase-active Lactobacillus reuteri NCIMB 30242 yoghurt formulation in hypercholesterolaemic adults. *British Journal of Nutrition* 2012; 107(10):1505–1513.

Jones ML, Martoni CJ, Prakash S. Cholesterol lowering and inhibition of sterol absorption by Lactobacillus reuteri NCIMB 30242: a randomized controlled trial. *European Journal of Clinical Nutrition* 2012; 66(11):1234–1241.

Jurenka JS. Therapeutic applications of pomegranate (Punica granatum L.): a review. *Alternative Medicine Review: A Journal of Clinical Therapeutic* 2008; 13(2):128–144.

Mohan M, Waghulde H, Kasture S. Effect of pomegranate juice on

Angiotensin II-induced hypertension in diabetic Wistar rats. *Phytotherapy Research* 2010; 24 Suppl 2:S196–203.

Osanai T, Fujiwara N, Sasaki S, et al. Novel pro-atherogenic molecule coupling factor 6 is elevated in patients with stroke: a possible linkage to homocysteine. *Annals of Medicine* 2010; 42(1):79–86.

Sica DA, Struthers AD, Cushman WC, Wood M, Banas JS, Epstein M. Medscape. News & Perspectives page. Importance of potassium in cardiovascular disease. Available at http://www.medscape.com/viewarticle/438088_3. Copyright 2002. Accessed 11/12/2014.

Sinatra S. Heart Health, Food and Nutrition, Nutrients and Additives page. Benefits of Magnesium Supplements for Heart Health. Available at http://www.drsinatra.com/benefits-of-magnesium-supplements-for-heart-health. Updated 7/31/2014. Accessed 11/12/2014.

Shaban NZ, El-Kersh MA, El-Rashidy FH, Habashy NH. Protective role of Punica granatum (pomegranate) peel and seed oil extracts on diethylnitrosamine and phenobarbital-induced hepatic injury in male rats. *Food Chemistry* 2013; 141(3):1587–1596.

Zeng X, Dai J, Remick DG, Wang X. Homocysteine mediated expression and secretion of monocyte chemoattractant protein-1 and interleukin-8 in human monocytes. *Circulation Research* 2003; 93(4):311–320.

Zhou S, Palmeira CM, Wallace KB. Doxorubicin-induced persistent oxidative stress to cardiac myocytes. *Toxicology Letters* 2001; 121(3):151–157.

HORMONAL SUPPORT

Berge A, Cladiere M, Gasperi J, Coursimault A, Tassin B, Moilleron R. Meta-analysis of environmental contamination by phthalates. *Environmental Science and Pollution Research International* 2013; 20(11):8057–8076.

Bledzka D, Gromadzinska J, Wasowicz W. Parabens. From environmental studies to human health. *Environment International* 2014; 67:27–42.

Boberg J, Taxvig C, Christiansen S, Hass U. Possible endocrine disrupting effects of parabens and their metabolites. *Reproductive Toxicology* (Elmsford, N.Y.) 2010; 30(2):301–312.

Bolca S, Possemiers S, Maervoet V, et al. Microbial and dietary factors associated with the 8-prenylnaringenin producer phenotype: a dietary intervention trial with fifty healthy post-menopausal Caucasian women. *British Journal of Nutrition* 2007; 98(5):950–959.

Chopin Lucks B. Vitex agnus castus essential oil and menopausal balance: a research update [Complementary Therapies in Nursing and Midwifery 8 (2003) 148–154]. *Complementary Therapies in Nursing & Midwifery* 2003; 9(3):157–160.

Cosentino M, Marino F, Ferrari M, et al. Estrogenic activity of 7-hydroxymatairesinol potassium acetate (HMR/lignan) from Norway spruce (*Picea abies*) knots and of its active metabolite enterolactone in MCF-7 cells. *Pharmacological Research: The Official Journal of the Italian Pharmacological Society* 2007; 56(2):140–147.

Dietz BM, Hagos GK, Eskra JN, et al. Differential regulation of detoxification enzymes in hepatic and mammary tissue by hops (*Humulus lupulus*) in vitro and in vivo. *Molecular Nutrition & Food Research* 2013; 57(6):1055–1066.

Dong Y, Zheng P. Dehydroepiandrosterone sulphate: action and mechanism in the brain. *Journal of Neuroendocrinology* 2012; 24(1):215–224.

Heinonen S, Nurmi T, Liukkonen K, et al. In vitro metabolism of plant lignans: new precursors of mammalian lignans enterolactone and enterodiol. *Journal of Agricultural and Food Chemistry* 2001; 49(7):3178–3186.

Keiler AM, Zierau O, Kretzschmar G. Hop extracts and hop substances in treatment of menopausal complaints. *Planta Medica* 2013; 79(7):576–579.

Kelemen LE, Sellers TA, Vachon CM. Nature Reviews Cancer. Figure 2: Pathways of steroid hormone synthesis, metabolism and sensitivity of tissues. Available at http://www.nature.com/nrc/journal/v8/n10/fig_tab/nrc2466_F2.html. 10/2008. Accessed 11/14/2014.

Labrie F, Labrie C. DHEA and intracrinology at menopause, a positive choice for evolution of the human species. *Climacteric: The Journal of the International Menopause Society* 2013; 16(2):205–213.

Liu J, Burdette JE, Xu H, et al. Evaluation of estrogenic activity of plant extracts for the potential treatment of menopausal symptoms. *Journal of Agricultural and Food Chemistry* 2001; 49(5):2472–2479.

Lucks BC, Sorensen J, Veal L. Vitexagnus-castus essential oil and menopausal balance: a self-care survey. *Complementary Therapies in Nursing & Midwifery* 2002; 8(3):148–154.

Milligan SR, Kalita JC, Heyerick A, Rong H, De Cooman L, De Keukeleire D. Identification of a potent phytoestrogen in hops (*Humulus lupulus L.*) and beer. *Journal of Clinical Endocrinology and Metabolism* 1999; 84(6):2249–2252.

Nagel J, Culley LK, Lu Y, et al. EST analysis of hop glandular trichomes identifies an O-methyltransferase that catalyzes the biosynthesis of xanthohumol. *The Plant Cell* 2008; 20(1):186–200.

Narkwichean A, Maalouf W, Campbell BK, Jayaprakasan K. Efficacy of dehydroepiandrosterone to improve ovarian response in women with diminished ovarian reserve: a meta-analysis. *Reproductive Biology and Endocrinology* 2013; 11:44.

Oberbauer E, Urmann C, Steffenhagen C, et al. Chroman-like cyclic prenylflavonoids promote neuronal differentiation and neurite outgrowth and are neuroprotective. *Journal of Nutritional Biochemistry* 2013; 24(11):1953–1962.

Ohlsson C, Vandenput L, Tivesten A. DHEA and mortality: What is the nature of the association? *Journal of Steroid Biochemistry and Molecular Biology* 2014.

Pluchino N, Drakopoulos P, Bianchi-Demicheli F, Wenger JM, Petignat P, Genazzani AR. Neurobiology of DHEA and effects on sexuality, mood and cognition. *Journal of Steroid Biochemistry and Molecular Biology* 2014.

Possemiers S, Verstraete W. Oestrogenicity of prenylflavonoids from hops: activation of pro-oestrogens by intestinal bacteria. *Environmental Microbiology Reports* 2009; 1(2):100–109.

Rad M, Humpel M, Schaefer O, et al. Pharmacokinetics and systemic endocrine effects of the phyto-oestrogen 8-prenylnaringenin after single oral doses to postmenopausal women. *British Journal of Clinical Pharmacology* 2006; 62(3):288–296.

Rimoldi G, Christoffel J, Wuttke W. Morphologic changes induced by oral long-term treatment with 8-prenylnaringenin in the uterus, vagina, and mammary gland of castrated rats. *Menopause* 2006; 13(4):669–677.

Saarinen NM, Huovinen R, Warri A, et al. Uptake and metabolism of hydroxymatairesinol in relation to its anticarcinogenicity in DMBA-induced rat mammary carcinoma model. *Nutrition and Cancer* 2001; 41(1–2):82–90.

Saarinen NM, Penttinen PE, Smeds AI, Hurmerinta TT, Makela SI. Structural determinants of plant lignans for growth of mammary tumors and hormonal responses in vivo. *Journal of Steroid Biochemistry and Molecular Biology* 2005; 93(2–5):209–219.

Saarinen NM, Warri A, Makela SI, et al. Hydroxymatairesinol, a novel enterolactone precursor with antitumor properties from coniferous tree (*Picea abies*). *Nutrition and Cancer* 2000; 36(2):207–216.

Savineau JP, Marthan R, Dumas de la Roque E. Role of DHEA in cardiovascular diseases. *Biochemical Pharmacology* 2013; 85(6):718–726.

Schmidt J, Peterlin-Masic L. Organic synthetic environmental endocrine disruptors: structural classes and metabolic fate. *Acta chimica Slovenica* 2012; 59(4):722–738.

Soma KK, Rendon NM, Boonstra R, Albers HE, Demas GE. DHEA effects on brain and behavior: Insights from comparative studies of aggression. *Journal of Steroid Biochemistry and Molecular Biology* 2014.

Stevens JF, Page JE. Xanthohumol and related prenylflavonoids from hops and beer: to your good health! *Phytochemistry* 2004; 65(10):1317–1330.

Udani JK, Brown DJ, Tan MO, Hardy M. Pharmacokinetics and bioavailability of plant lignan 7-hydroxymatairesinol and effects on serum enterolactone and clinical symptoms in postmenopausal women: a single-blinded, parallel, dose-comparison study. *Journal of the American College of Nutrition* 2013; 32(6):428–435.

Urbanski HF, Mattison JA, Roth GS, Ingram DK. Dehydroepiandrosterone sulfate (DHEAS) as an endocrine marker of aging in calorie restriction studies. *Experimental Gerontology* 2013; 48(10):1136–1139.

Warner M, Gustafsson JA. DHEA—a precursor of ERbeta ligands. *Journal of Steroid Biochemistry and Molecular Biology* 2014.

Yu D. Agency for Toxic Substance and Disease Registry Case Studies in Environmental Medicine (CSEM). Taking an Exposure History. Available at http://www.atsdr.cdc.gov/csem/exphistory/docs/exposure_history.pdf. 5/12/2008. Accessed 11/14/2014.

MULTIVITAMINS AND VITAMIN D

Annweiler C, Llewellyn DJ, Beauchet O. Low serum vitamin D concentrations in Alzheimer's disease: a systematic review and meta-analysis. *Journal of Alzheimer's Disease* 2013; 33(3):659–674.

Annweiler C, Rolland Y, Schott AM, Blain H, Vellas B, Beauchet O. Serum vitamin D deficiency as a predictor of incident non-Alzheimer dementias: a 7-year longitudinal study. *Dementia and Geriatric Cognitive Disorders* 2011; 32(4):273–278.

Davis DR, Epp MD, Riordan HD. Changes in USDA food composition data for 43 garden crops, 1950 to 1999. *Journal of the American College of Nutrition* 2004; 23(6):669–682.

Grima NA, Pase MP, Macpherson H, Pipingas A. The effects of multi-vitamins on cognitive performance: a systematic review and meta-analysis. *Journal of Alzheimer's Disease* 2012; 29(3):561–569.

Haussler MR, Haussler CA, Bartik L, et al. Vitamin D receptor: molecular signaling and actions of nutritional ligands in disease prevention. *Nutrition Reviews* 66 (10), Suppl. 2 (2008): S98–S112.

Holick M. *Science News* online. Vitamin D is essential to the modern indoor lifestyle. Vol. 178, No. 9. 10/23/2010. Accessed 11/12/2014.

Huang HY, Caballero B, Chang S, et al. Multivitamin/mineral supplements and prevention of chronic disease. *Evidence Report/Technology Assessment* 2006(139):1–117.

Huang Y, Li X, Wang M, et al. Lipoprotein lipase links vitamin D, insulin resistance, and type 2 diabetes: a cross-sectional epidemiological study. *Cardiovascular Diabetology* 2013; 12:17.

Lite J. *Scientific American* online. Vitamin D deficiency soars in the U.S., study says. Available at http://www.scientificamerican.com/article/vitamin-d-deficiency-united-states/. Updated 3/23/2009. Accessed 11/12/2014.

Macpherson H, Pipingas A, Pase MP. Multivitamin-multimineral supplementation and mortality: a meta-analysis of randomized controlled trials. *American Journal of Clinical Nutrition* 2013; 97(2):437–444.

Makishima M, Lu TT, Xie W, et al. Vitamin D receptor as an intestinal bile acid sensor. *Science* 2002; 296(5571):1313–1316.

Matsunawa M, Akagi D, Uno S, et al. Vitamin D receptor activation enhances benzo[a]pyrene metabolism via CYP1A1 expression in macrophages. *Drug Metabolism and Disposition: The Biological Fate of Chemicals* 2012; 40(11):2059–2066.

Mitchell DM, Henao MP, Finkelstein JS, Burnett-Bowie SA. Prevalence and predictors of vitamin D deficiency in healthy adults. *Endocrine Practice: Official Journal of the American College of Endocrinology and the American Association of Clinical Endocrinologists* 2012; 18(6):914–923.

Wacker M, Holick MF. Vitamin D—effects on skeletal and extraskeletal health and the need for supplementation. *Nutrients* 2013; 5(1):111–148.

BIBLIOGRAPHY

Amen, Daniel G., M.D. *Change Your Brain, Change Your Body: Use Your Brain to Get and Keep the Body You Have Always Wanted.* Three Rivers Press, 2010.

Antoniou, Michael, Claire Robinson, and John Fagan. *GMO Myths and Truths.* Earth Open Source, 2012.

Blaylock, Russell L., M.D. *The Blaylock Wellness Report Archive Including Comprehensive Index July 2004–December 2007.* Newsmax Media, 2009.

———. *Natural Strategies for Cancer Patients.* Twin Streams, Kensington Publishing Corp., 2003.

Bollinger, Ty M. *Cancer: Step Outside the Box.* Infinity 510 Squared Partners, 2006.

Bowden, Jonny, Ph.D., and Stephen Sinatra, M.D. *The Great Cholesterol Myth: Why Lowering Your Cholesterol Won't Prevent Heart Disease—and the Statin-Free Plan.* Fair Winds Press, 2012.

Brecher, Harold, and Arline Brecher. *Forty Something Forever: A Consumer's Guide to Chelation Therapy and Other Heart Savers.* Healthsavers Press, 1992.

Campbell-McBride, Natasha, M.D. *Gut and Psychology Syndrome: Natural Treatment for Autism, Dyspraxia, A.D.D., Depression, Schizophrenia.* Amazon.com, 2010.

———. *Put Your Heart in Your Mouth.* Medinform Publishing, 2007.

Clement, Anna Maria, Ph.D., and Brian R. Clement, Ph.D. *Killer Clothes.* Hippocrates Publications, 2011.

Crinnion, Walter, M.D. *Clean, Green & Lean.* John Wiley & Sons, Inc., 2010.

Crook, William G., M.D. *The Yeast Connection: A Medical Breakthrough.* Vintage Books, 1986.

Davis, William, M.D. *Wheat Belly: Lose the Wheat, Lose the Weight and Find Your Path Back to Health.* Rodale, Inc., 2011.

Fahy, Gregory, Michael D. West, L. Stephen Coles, and Steven B. Harris. *The Future of Aging: Pathways to Human Life Extension.* Springer Science + Business Media, 2010.

Fife, Bruce, N.D. *Coconut Cures: Preventing and Treating Common Health Problems with Coconut.* Piccadilly Books, Ltd., 2005.

Hightower, Jane M., M.D. *Diagnosis: Mercury: Money Politics & Poison.* Shearwater Books, 2009.

Junger, Alejandro, M.D., and Amely Greeven. *Clean: The Revolutionary Program to Restore the Body's Natural Ability to Heal Itself.* HarperCollins, 2012.

Kekich, David A. *Life Extension Express: 7 Steps You Can Take Now, to Catch the Emerging Wave of Medical Breakthroughs.* Maximum Life Foundation, 2009.

Kharrazian, Datis, DHSc. *Why Isn't My Brain Working? A Revolutionary Understanding of Brain Decline and Effective Strategies to Recover Your Brain's Health.* Elephant Press, 2013.

Levy, Thomas E., M.D. *Curing the Incurable: Vitamin C, Infectious Diseases and Toxins.* Livon Books, 2002.

Life Extension. *Disease Prevention and Treatment: 130 Evidence-Based Protocols to Combat the Diseases of Aging.* LE Publications, Inc., 2013.

———. *Disease Prevention and Treatment: Scientific Protocols That Integrate Mainstream and Alternative Medicine.* Life Extension Media, 1997.

McHughen, Alan. *Pandora's Picnic Basket: The Potential and Hazards of Genetically Modified Foods.* Oxford University Press, 2000.

McLure, John. *The Cancer Treatment: A Journey on the Transformation Away from Cancer: A Fictionalized Autobiographical Tale.*

Moritz, Andreas. *The Liver and Gallbladder Miracle Cleanse: An All-Natural, At-Home Flush to Purify and Rejuvenate Your Body.* Ulysses Press, 2007.

O'Brien, Robyn, and Rachel Kranz. *The Unhealthy Truth: One Mother's Shocking Investigation into the Dangers of America's Food Supply—and What Every Family Can Do to Protect Itself.* Broadway Books, 2009.

Perlmutter, David, M.D., and Kristin Loberg. *Grain Brain: The Surprising Truth About Wheat, Carbs and Sugar—Your Brain's Silent Killers.* Little, Brown and Company, 2013.

Plourde, Elizabeth, Ph.D. *EMF Freedom: Solutions for the 21st Century Pollution.* New Voice Publications, 2013.

Rogers, Sherry A., M.D. *How to Cure Diabetes.* Prestige Publishing, 2012.

———. *The High Blood Pressure Hoax.* Prestige Publishing, 2008.

————. *Detoxify or Die.* Prestige Publishing, 2002.

————. *Pain Free in 6 Weeks.* Prestige Publishing, 2001.

Shoemaker, Ritchie C., M.D., James Schaller, and Patti Schmidt. *Mold Warriors: Fighting America's Hidden Health Threat.* Gateway Press, Inc, 2005.

Sinatra, Stephen, M.D. *The Healing Kitchen.* Bottom Line, 2013.

————. *The Sinatra Solution.* Basic Health Publications, 2011.

————. *Reverse Heart Disease Now.* Wiley, 2008.

————. *Lower Your Blood Pressure in Eight Weeks.* Ballantine, 2003.

————. *L-Carnitine and the Heart.* McGraw-Hill, 1999.

————. *The Coenzyme Q10 Phenomenon.* McGraw-Hill, 1998.

Somers, Suzanne. *I'm Too Young for This!: The Natural Hormone Solution to Enjoy Perimenopause.* Harmony, 2013.

————. *Bombshell: Explosive Medical Secrets That Will Redefine Aging.* Crown Archetype, 2012.

————. *Sexy Forever: How to Fight Fat After Forty.* Crown Archetype, 2010.

————. *Knockout: Interviews with Doctors Who Are Curing Cancer.* Crown Publishers, 2009.

————. *Breakthrough: Eight Steps to Wellness.* Crown Publishers, 2008.

————. *Ageless: The Naked Truth About Bioidentical Hormones.* Crown Publishers, 2006.

————. *The Sexy Years: Discover the Hormone Connection: The Secret to Fabulous Sex, Great Health and Vitality, for Women and Men.* Crown Publishers, 2004.

Trenev, Natasha. *Probiotics: Nature's Internal Healers.* Penguin Putnam, Inc., 1998.

Turner, Natasha, M.D. *The Carb Sensitivity Program: Discover Which Carbs Will Curb Your Cravings, Control Your Appetite and Banish Belly Fat.* Rodale Books, 2012.

INDEX

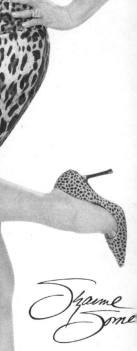

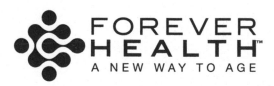